Voice Disorders

Second Edition

Christine Sapienza and Bari Hoffman Ruddy

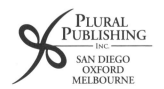

PLURAL
PUBLISHING
INC.
SAN DIEGO
OXFORD
MELBOURNE

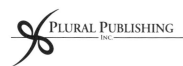

PLURAL PUBLISHING
INC.

5521 Ruffin Road
San Diego, CA 92123

e-mail: info@pluralpublishing.com
Web site: http://www.pluralpublishing.com

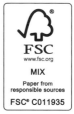

FSC
www.fsc.org
MIX
Paper from
responsible sources
FSC® C011935

Typeset in 11/13 Adobe Garamond by Flanagan's Publishing Services, Inc.
Printed in the United States of America by McNaughton & Gunn
17 16 15   3 4 5

For permission to use material from this text, contact us by
Telephone: (866) 758-7251
Fax: (888) 758-7255
e-mail: permissions@pluralpublishing.com

Every attempt has been made to contact the copyright holders for material originally printed in another source. If any have been inadvertently overlooked, the publishers will gladly make the necessary arrangements at the first opportunity.

Library of Congress Cataloging-in-Publication Data

Sapienza, Christine M.
  Voice disorders / Christine Sapienza and Bari Hoffman Ruddy. — 2nd ed.
     p. ; cm.
  Includes bibliographical references and index.
  ISBN 978-1-59756-493-9 (alk. paper) — ISBN 1-59756-493-1 (alk. paper)
  I. Hoffman Ruddy, Bari. II. Title.
  [DNLM: 1. Voice Disorders. WV 500]

  616.85'56 — dc23
                    2012032271

Contents

Foreword

The study of voice disorders in one sense may be thought to be in its infancy compared to other areas of biobehavioral science. Less than 100 years ago, Grant Fairbanks wrote a textbook entitled *Voice and Articulation Drill-book*, outlining some of the major areas of the study of voice. That was perhaps the first textbook that speech-language pathology students from two or three generations ago used in a course of voice disorders. In that book, only a few short paragraphs were devoted to the respiratory system and its importance in the vibratory control of the vocal folds. It did, however, remain a perennial favorite of many speech-language pathologists, mainly for the exercises related to the treatment of voice disorders. About 20 years later, G. Paul Moore authored a small but rather advanced book entitled *Organic Voice Disorders*, describing the detailed mechanism of phonation using simple line drawings, based on his work with Hans von Leden. The two books by Fairbanks and Moore still remain on many people's shelves as a remembrance of the leaders in previous eras and the contributions they made to the study of the voice and voice disorders. Each of those books contained valuable basic scientific information related to the anatomy and physiology of voice production and practical exercises to treat patients with voice disorders.

It is that unique quality of basic science and treatment strategies that Christine Sapienza and Bari Hoffman Ruddy brought to their first edition of *Voice Disorders* in 2009. That textbook was highly successful due to its detailed descriptions of the anatomy, physi-

ology, and clinical presentations of voice disorders. This second edition of *Voice Disorders* builds on that framework. It is not surprising to see a well-rounded textbook on voice from this duet of scientist and clinician. In fact, to some extent, each of them is both a scientist and a clinician. In their second edition, Sapienza and Hoffman Ruddy have demonstrated that they have kept abreast of the latest developments in the medical, behavioral, and patient-oriented aspects of this rapidly changing discipline. Unlike the early days of Grant Fairbanks, the clinician now needs medical, surgical, and behavioral knowledge of the vocal mechanism and of the structures and systems that contribute to the production of voice. In addition, the authors update the unique role of the speech-language pathologist and his/her relationship with the other members of the voice care team—research scientist, psychologist, surgeon, singing specialist, and vocal coach. Each of those individuals has varying roles in the care of patients with voice disorders.

The authors have chosen to begin their text with a chapter on respiration. That feature makes this book quite different from many other books on voice, which start with the anatomy of the head and neck. Respiratory structures, from the lungs to the subglottis, and their anatomy, physiology, and contribution to phonation are explained with wonderful drawings and graphs. The chapter is written with great detail, yet easy enough to understand thanks to the well-written text to go along with the drawings. The authors make it clear that while the diaphragm is important to phonation, it is the main active muscle of inhalation. Never again will the speech-language pathologist who uses this book tell their patients to "speak from the diaphragm." While the anatomy of the respiratory system is described in many general anatomy books, this book extends the study of respiratory anatomy and physiology specifically as it relates to breathing for phonation. This chapter serves as a basis for the remainder of the book and so it should, as the respiratory system serves as the foundation for the larynx and vocal fold vibration.

There are other fabulous features about this second edition, as well. Sapienza and Hoffman Ruddy update the reader on new medications and their effects on the voice and on the treatment of voice disorders. While medications will change over time, they present medications in terms of classes of drugs so that regardless of which new medication comes out, the clinician will understand the effects of the new drug on the voice once they know the class of the new drug.

Another useful feature of this second edition is the expanded approaches to voice therapy. Again, the authors chose to categorize therapy approaches in terms of type, such as symptomatic, combined modality, and hygienic. For each approach, they describe specific treatment methods and expected outcomes.

It is not surprising that the management of performers and singers gets its own chapter. Both Sapienza and Hoffman Ruddy are well-known to the performing community. In the chapter on vocal performance, they describe the relationship of the speech-language pathol-

ogist to the singer, performer, and other professionals who also take care of singers. This may be the only book used by the voice rehabilitation team in which descriptions of the Alexander Technique and the Feldenkrais Method are found in one place. It is special sections like this that make this book a textbook for today's speech-language pathologist who wants to be up-to-date in treating voice disorders.

The authors have substantially updated the chapter on head and neck cancer, with new statistics on the disease, information on safety for the laryngectomy patient, and more images to guide the reader in understanding the various modes of communication after laryngectomy.

Although not customary in a foreword, I would like to say something about the authors related to this current textbook. I have known Dr. Sapienza since her early postgraduate days and have been impressed with the degree of effort and expertise that she has put in to every project, research proposal, and class syllabus. She reflects the term "teacher-scientist-clinician" perfectly. She understands the needs of students and finds a way to feed those needs in the classroom and in the research lab. It is only recently that I have come to know Dr. Hoffman Ruddy, but it is clear that she was a student of Dr. Sapienza, and she exerts a similar high level of energy into every clinical case and research study that she undertakes. Her attention to detail can be appreciated in her work environment, her writing, and her presentations at national meetings. Both have transformed their keen levels of observation, testing, and analysis into a book that is rich with their experience and knowledge.

Preface

The human ability to produce voice, shape it into meaningful tones and sounds, and use it for so many varied purposes, has allowed for the development of a voice science partnered with a variety of medical disciplines. When disciplines join together in an effort to successfully examine and treat our patients we witness a truly emerging relationship between knowledge and practice.

With enhancements in medical technologies and medical care, treatment plans can be optimized and vocal recovery can be favorable and timely. Continual education is critical to stay contemporary and abreast of new techniques and technologies and respond to the ever changing clinical environment. You will find an increasing responsibility to collaborate and communicate with all members of the patient's health care team and a need to familiarize yourself with the ever-changing medical models. You must continue to educate yourself to keep up with the advances in technology. This need may not be due solely to a rapidity of change in your discipline but also to the rapidity of change in other disciplines (imaging, molecular biology, surgery etc).

The issues surrounding your patients will require more skills and fluid knowledge in human anatomy and physiology, neuroanatomy and physiology, instrumentation, computer applications and multitudes of topics surrounding medical management issues including phonosurgical options and drug treatments Sometimes, the changes to which we, as clinicians, must adapt to are sweeping and sometimes they occur slowly over time.

In writing this textbook we wanted you, the student, to have access to contemporary information that could be easily read. We took pride in developing the anatomical figures for the text so they would portray the structures precisely. Additionally, we wanted to give you the opportunity to have laryngeal examinations of pathology for your reference including opportunity to view phonosurgical procedures and outcomes. In short, we wrote the book in a manner that would enable you and your instructor to have the best resources in one source.

The care of the voice has already evolved from a traditionally behaviorally oriented discipline to one that has responsibilities within the medical domain. For example, the role of the voice pathologist has broadened and includes vocal imaging specialist, researcher, therapist guiding recovery and restoration of healthy voice, trainer guiding effective voice use, counselor and/or more. Our field has developed ad hoc position statements defining the role of the Speech-Language Pathologist and Teacher of Singing in the Remediation of Singers with Voice Disorders (1992). We have guidelines for training in endoscopy and videostroboscopy and guidelines for the Role of the Speech Language Pathologist with respect to the Evaluation and Treatment of Tracheoesophogeal Fistualization/Puncture and Prosthesis. These position statements indicate that a certain level of skill must be obtained prior to administering particular assessment and treatment techniques.

Specific to the assessment and treatment of voice we find ourselves challenged with cases involving syndromic complexities and are asked to delve into histories involving multiple disease processes or polypharmacies. Additionally, the reorganization of the health care industry has created an extensive array of changes in the organization, ownership, and regulation of health care providers and in the delivery of services. Cost concerns, increasing competition, influence of investor priorities, technological advances, changing social attitudes, and an aging and increasingly diverse population, are factors that sustain this dynamic condition.

There is a requirement to objectively document the outcomes of specific treatments in order to provide hard evidence that can be analyzed, data based, studied and modeled. Not all aspects of physiology can be seen. And, while technology is racing forward in the field of laryngeal imaging, subsystem processes that create, for example, the air pressure and airflow for voice are often equally important to examine. At the same time, over collection of data is not a wise way to spend time with a patient. Most of you have probably heard the saying "if it walks like a duck, quacks like a duck — it's a duck. Bottom line, if the collection of more data is not going to alter the treatment plan then does not subject the patient to unnecessary procedures.

Since 1998 there have been significant advances in the following areas of medicine, all of which have impact on the care of the voice:

- pharmacogenomics
- brain damage and spinal cord injury
- cancer therapy and viruses
- antibiotics and resistant infections
- autoimmune disease
- slowing of the aging process

Within our discipline, technological advances include functional magnetic resonance imaging, high-speed video image analysis, computer assisted biofeedback techniques, advanced animal modeling techniques, enhanced surgical procedures, and many others. It wasn't long ago that we witnessed the first laryngeal transplant performed at the Cleveland Clinic in 1999 by Dr. Marshall Strome and his team of physicians.

In order to appreciate such groundbreaking events we need to acknowledge the fact that advances in the core science of our discipline are being made nationally and internationally at facilities dedicated to the advancement of science and medical practice. Recall one area of voice research that began in Groningen at the Institute of Physiology of the Faculty of Medicine by van den Berg in the late 1940's. His fundamental article on the Myoelastic-Aerodynamic Theory of Voice Production in 1958 forever shaped our perceptions on the function of the vocal folds. There are historical lists of contributors to voice, voice care and voice science. Included in that list are the contributors referenced in this book as well as all of our contemporary colleagues dedicated to the study of voice.

We hope this book serves you well in your graduate coursework in voice disorder. We believe it provides the core information needed for your training.

For those practicing in the area of voice and its disorders we currently expect the following academic preparation: understanding of the normal and physiologic process of voice production; understanding of the etiological bases of voice disorders; the ability to examine and interpret laryngeal structure and function; understanding of the instrumentation used to examine laryngeal structure and function; understanding of the principles of diagnosis; understanding of the structural and functional differences across the life span; the ability to assist in differentially diagnosing the disorder and classifying it as structural, functional, idiopathic or neurological; the ability to develop a treatment plan that considers the patient's functional outcome goals; and others.

Additional courses we recommend include issues surrounding continuum of care; interdisciplinary approaches; pharmacology; medical terminology; patient advocacy and accreditations; among others. This is not an inclusive list but one that suggests that our literature, as well as academic course work, must accommodate our needs more fully.

Acknowledgments

To the University of Florida, my colleagues and friends who continually support my research and career in the field of speech-language pathology. To the talented graphic arts of Cindy McMillen and anatomical drawings of Dave Forrestel—true artists. My sincere gratitude to Angie Singh (Plural Publishing) for her support and intelligent decision making on this project. And, to my person(s) that keep my life exceptional, fun and filled with love—Jasmine, Frankie, Kim, Christopher, Jessica, Jake, Ijie, Fahsa, and Zona.

"Do not follow where the path may lead. Go, instead, where there is no path and leave a trail."—Ralph Waldo Emerson

Dr. Christine Sapienza

My sincere appreciation to all physicians at The Ear Nose Throat and Plastic Surgery Associates for providing the ideal collaborative, medical environment. My deepest gratitude to Jeffrey Lehman, MD, for his mentorship, collaboration, and participation in this project. Thank you to my University of Central Florida colleagues for their ongoing support, and to Rebecca Mitchell for her dedicated work. Finally, my eternal gratitude to my husband Michael and daughters Danielle and Alexandra for surrounding me with their love and support.

Dr. Bari Hoffman Ruddy

Dr. Sapienza and Dr. Ruddy wish to sincerely thank:

- The Ear, Nose and Throat Surgical Associates, Orlando, Florida, for providing all endoscopic images and laryngostroboscopic samples;
- Dr. Jeffrey J. Lehman, The Ear, Nose and Throat Surgical Associates, Orlando, Florida, for the surgical videos and images;
- Dr. Bernard Rousseau for his contributions to Chapter 2 on content related to vocal fold biology and histology;
- Dr. Rahul Shrivastav for his contribution on the Acoustic section within Chapter 4;
- Dr. Jeffrey J. Lehman for writing Chapter 8;
- Vicki Lewis, MA, for her contributions to Chapter 9;
- Adam Lloyd, MM, MA, for his contributions to Chapter 10;
- Dr. Kiran Tipernini, Monica Tipernini, and Jeffrey Fichera for contributions for Chapter 11;
- KayPENTAX, InHealth Technologies, and Glottal Enterprises for the provision of images.

To Dr. G. Paul Moore and Dr. Janina Casper, who in their greatness paved the pathway that we traveled on in our professional endeavors, shadowing us with guidance and mentorship.

To Dr. Dave Ingram for creating opportunity through his continuous mentorship and excellence in teaching students about voice and patient care. Your integrity and excitement for student learning is unmatched.

Chapter 1

Respiratory
Anatomy and Physiology

This chapter describes the anatomy of the respiratory system and explains how it functions to produce voice. Anatomy is the study of structure(s) and physiology is the study of how structures function to produce a particular action. In the case of voice production, respiratory structures play a very important role by providing the necessary driving force to initiate and sustain vocal fold vibration.

Breathing appears to be a relatively simple process—seemingly automatic, and unconscious. Yet, it is highly controlled and complex. And, breathing for voice production is a unique process, different from the act of ventilation or circulation for the life purpose of exchanging O_2 and CO_2. Anatomically, the most basic elements of the respiratory system are the lungs, rib cage, and diaphragm/abdominal unit.

After reading this chapter, you will:

- Understand the basic components of respiratory anatomy
- Understand the passive and active forces involved in breathing
- Understand the role of the respiratory system for producing voice
- Understand how disordered respiratory function may affect voice production

> Ventilation means bringing oxygen into the lungs. Circulation is the transporting of oxygen all over the body, to where it is needed.

The Lungs

The lungs are elastic tissue that inflate and deflate and, as a result of the inflation and deflation, move air. Anatomically, there are three lobes on the right lung and two lobes on the left lung. The right lung is larger than the left lung to make room for the heart (Figure 1–1).

Inspiration is the act of taking air into the lungs and expiration is the act of expelling air out of the lungs. By bringing air into the lungs during inspiration, oxygen can be circulated into the bloodstream to the cells in the body. Expiration allows for the release of carbon dioxide (CO_2).

The Trachea

The trachea is a cartilaginous structure that allows air to pass from the nose and mouth into the lungs. It is made up of 16 cartilaginous

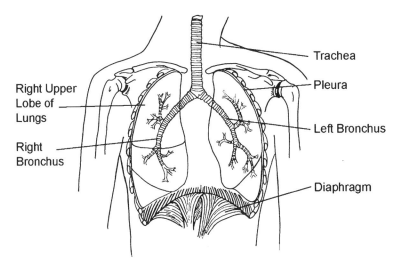

Figure 1–1. Lower airway and right and left lungs.

rings. The larynx sits on top of the upper most tracheal ring. The trachea, if damaged is potentially life threatening. In the event the trachea is damaged, a tube is placed into the airway to allow air to flow into the lungs. This is called intubation.

The Bronchi

There are two main bronchi that branch off of the trachea, one going to each lung. Smaller branches from the bronchi continue to divide, known as secondary bronchi. There are three secondary bronchi supplying the right lung and two secondary bronchi supplying the left lung. Bronchioloes are the smallest branches stemming from the secondary bronchi and lead to the alveoli where gas exchange occurs allowing air to enter into the blood. The cartilage and mucous membrane of the primary bronchi are similar to that in the trachea. The amount of hyaline cartilage in the bronchial walls decreases, as the branching continues throughout the bronchial tree. Hyaline cartilage is absent in the smallest bronchioles (Figure 1–2).

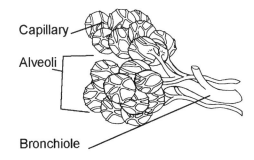

Figure 1–2. Final branches of the respiratory tree where primary gas exchange occurs.

Hyaline cartilage forms most of the fetal skeleton and is found in the trachea, larynx (see Chapter 2), and joint surfaces of the adult.

The Thorax

The thorax is the chest cavity that surrounds and protects the lungs as well as the heart and other respiratory structures like the bronchial tree. Made up of the ribs and muscles, the most inferior aspect of the thorax is the diaphragm.

The Ribs

There are 12 pairs of ribs. Ribs 1 to 7 are called the true ribs and ribs 8 to 10 are called the false ribs. Ribs 11 and 12 are called floating ribs because they do not attach to the sternum like ribs 1 to 10.

The Diaphragm

The diaphragm anatomically separates the chest from the abdomen. It is the major muscle of inspiration (Figures 1–3 and 1–4). At rest, the diaphragm sits in a dome-shaped position and when it contracts during inspiration it moves downward and flattens, enlarging the chest cavity. As the diaphragm moves downward the force is transferred to the lower ribs moving them outward. This happens because, as the diaphragm contracts, it is opposed by the passive properties of the abdominal wall, the tone of its muscles, and the inertia of the abdominal contents. When this occurs, the intra-abdominal pressure rises and the lower rib cage expands (Goldman, Rose, Morgan, & Denison, 1986). This, in turn, enlarges the thoracic dimension, creating an inspiratory maneuver.

> When the diaphragm contracts, during normal breathing, it moves down about 1 to 2 cm and interestingly can move as much as 10 cm during deep inspiration.

The Abdominal Wall

The abdominal wall is a layered structure with external, internal and innermost regions. Made up of central and lateral muscles that arise from the ribs and the pelvic girdle, the

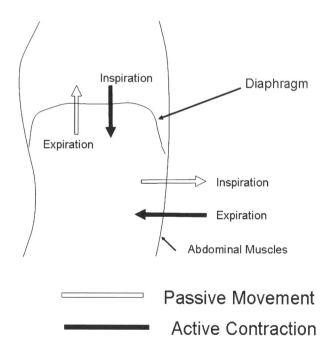

Figure 1–3. Direction of thoracic cavity movement with inspiration and expiration.

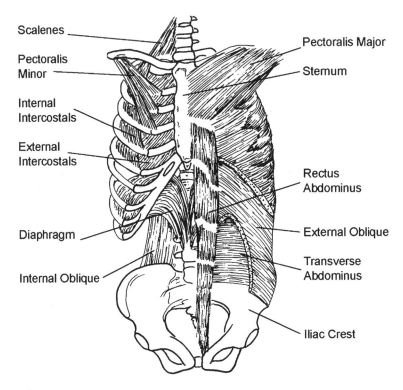

Figure 1–4. The abdominal musculature and supporting structures.

abdominal wall has passive and active properties that are described in more detail below. During passive expiration, the abdominal wall draws in, and during effortful tasks like coughing, sneezing, and certain voicing tasks the abdominal muscles contract to compress the abdominal contents. This in turn, increases the intra-abdominal pressures. This compression is also important for other functions like defecation and childbirth. The next section describes other important anatomical structures to the respiratory system.

Sternum

The sternum has three processes that serve as attachments for respiratory muscles like the diaphragm and intercostal muscles. The three processes include the manubrium, body, and xiphoid process.

The first seven ribs are attached to the sternum. The manubrium appears as a handle and serves as an attachment for ribs 1 and 2, the corpus is the body of the sternum and serves as the attachment for ribs 2 to 7, and the xiphoid process is the smallest of the three parts and serves as a partial attachment for many muscles including some of the abdominal wall muscles.

When giving CPR, pressure on the xiphoid process should be avoided as it can cause a piece of the xiphoid process to break off causing potential damage to the heart lining and muscle and/or result in punctures or lacerations of the diaphragm.

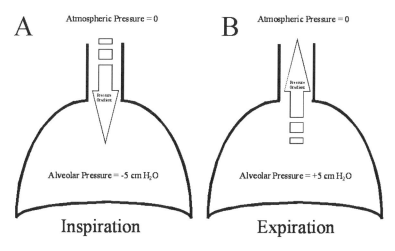

Figure 1–5. Schematic depicting pressure relationships for inspiration and expiration. The arrow indicates the direction of the driving force.

Clavicle

The clavicle is known as the collar bone and the two bones of the clavicle extend from the manubrium. The clavicle serves for attachment of certain respiratory muscles like the trapezius, pectoralis major, and sternocleidomastoid.

Driving Forces of the Respiratory System

The process of moving air requires a driving force. The force comes from a pressure gradient or difference between the alveolar pressure and the atmospheric pressure (Figures 1–5 and 1–6). Alveolar pressure is the pressure within the alveoli.

> Alveolar pressure is the smallest gas exchange unit of the lung and is about 105 mm Hg or 142.8 cm H_2O.

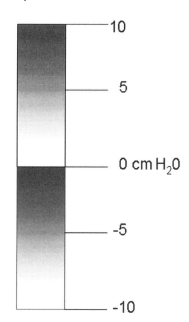

Figure 1–6. Schematic depicting positive pressure and negative pressure generation relative to atmospheric pressure (0 cm H_2O).

Alveolar pressure is typically referenced with respect to atmospheric pressure, which is always set to zero. When alveolar pressure is above atmospheric pressure, it is positive; when alveolar pressure is below atmospheric pressure it is negative.

For the lungs to inflate, the inward driving force must be an alveolar pressure less than atmospheric pressure. This creates a pressure gradient that causes air to flow into the lung (inspiration). On the other hand, for air to flow out of the lung (expiration), the driving force must be an alveolar pressure greater than atmospheric pressure. The pressure of a gas equals the perpendicular force exerted by the gas divided by the surface area on which the force is exerted.

In order to produce voice, air moves from the alveolar spaces through the conducting airways, including the trachea, through the glottis or the space between the vocal folds, vibrating the medial edges of the vocal folds. Sound from the vocal folds is then transferred to the pharynx and oral cavity, where it is shaped by the articulators into speech sounds. Discussion of vocal fold vibration is continued in Chapter 2.

How Does the Human Body Generate These Respiratory Forces?

The alveolar pressure is changed by two forces. The first, a passive force, is due to the elastic properties of the respiratory system. The second force, an active force, is developed by the contraction of the respiratory muscles. One example that is often used to illustrate and explain the passive and active forces of the respiratory system is a balloon as it helps explain the concepts of respiratory forces (Figure 1–7). Inflation of a balloon requires an active stretching of the balloon. This illustration shows how inspiratory muscles contract to expand the chest wall. It takes active muscle force to overcome the balloon stiffness and force air into the balloon. This increases the balloon's volume, just as the lungs increase in volume, creating a pressure gradient that allows air to flow into the balloon/lungs. With the balloon inflated and the opening to the balloon closed, the balloon retracts toward its rest position and produces a pressure inside the balloon causing the air inside the balloon to compress. This is an elastic force, which is an inherent property of the balloon just like the lungs (see Figure 1–7). The strength of the elastic force is a *passive* property of the balloon/lungs and is directly proportional to the stretch of the balloon/lungs. The greater the balloon/lung volume, (i.e., the greater stretch of the balloon/lung wall) the greater the elastic recoil of the balloon/lung and the greater the pressure inside the balloon/lung. The pressure inside the balloon/lung can be further increased if the outside of the balloon/lung is squeezed (see Figure 1–7). This "squeeze" is the result of the *active* contraction of expiratory muscles and is referred to as an active pressure. The total pressure within the balloon/lung is then the sum of the passive elastic pressure and the active "squeeze" pressure.

When the respiratory system is at rest, the lung is partially inflated to approximately 40% of the total lung capacity (TLC). This is important to remember because the lungs are actually not deflated at "rest" but rather are partially inflated. This rest position is called the Functional Residual Capacity or FRC (Figure 1–8). At FRC, neither the lung nor the thorax is really at its respective rest position.

The lungs are apposed (or connected) to the thorax by pleural linkage. In fact, three-quarters of the lung's surface contacts the thoracic wall by pleural linkage. With a pneumothorax, the lung immediately collapses *but* the thorax expands. A pneumothorax occurs when the pleural space is disrupted.

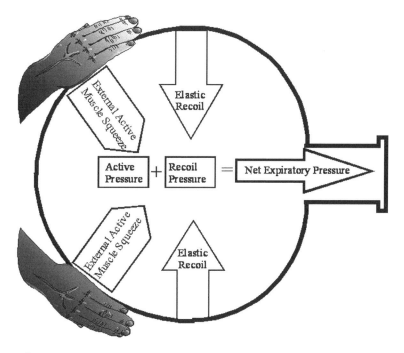

Figure 1–7. Schematic of a balloon depicting active and passive mechanisms during expiration. The hands squeezing the balloon illustrate the addition of an active expiratory force.

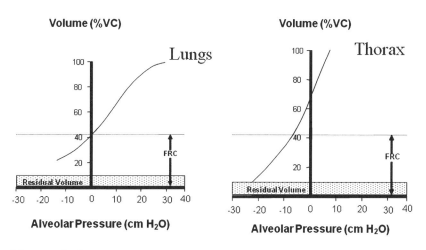

Figure 1–8. Pressure-volume curves for lungs and thorax.

A pneuomothorax can happen with a blast injury, as a result of a fractured rib, and sometimes with diseases like cystic fibrosis and chronic obstructive pulmonary disease.

When a pneumothorax occurs the lungs and thorax achieve a natural position, which they would prefer if they were anatomically independent from one another. The lungs natural position then is a volume much smaller than FRC. That is why the lung(s) has a natural tendency to collapse. The thorax's natural position is a volume much greater that FRC, approximately 70% of TLC, which means the thorax, has a natural tendency to expand at FRC (see Figure 1–8).

When the lung is placed in the thorax, the outer surface of the lung is apposed to the inner surface of the thorax by the pleural linkage mentioned above. The pleural linkage is actually a hydrostatic force. A membrane called the visceral pleura covers the lung. A similar membrane called the parietal pleura covers the thorax. A small amount of fluid, the pleural fluid, separates these membranes. If you were to place two smooth surfaces against each other with fluid between them, like two microscope slides with water between them, you would see how easily they move back and forth but how very hard they are to pull apart. This is the hydrostatic force "holding" the two smooth surfaces together yet allowing free movement between the surfaces. In the respiratory system, the pleural fluid between the visceral and parietal pleurae holds the lung against the thoracic wall while allowing the lung to slide freely during volume changes. However, mechanically linking the lung and thorax means that the combined systems' elastic behavior is a result of the interaction of the lung and thoracic elastic forces. As stated above, this causes the lung to be at a volume that is above its elastic natural position, yielding a collapsing force. The thorax is at a volume smaller than its elastic natural position yielding an expanding force. At FRC, the expanding elastic force of the thorax balances the collapsing elastic force of the lung.

Passive and Active Forces of the Respiratory System

Active inspiration is a muscle action that increases the dimensions of the chest wall. A por-

tion of the inspiratory muscle energy used to expand the thorax is recaptured by the passive collapsing force of the elastic recoil pressure that is volume dependent. This is the passive property of expiration. *Remember*, the act of inspiration is *always* active. This means that in order for inspiration to occur, muscle contraction must happen. Mentioned briefly above, the diaphragm is the main muscle of inspiration. It is actually a large sheet of muscle and tendons. It attaches to the lumbar vertebrae of the spinal column, the lower ribs (ribs 7–12) and the xiphoid process of the sternum. The cervical nerves of the spinal cord called C3, C4, and C5, also known as the phrenic nerves, supply innervation to the diaphragm.

> A saying goes "C3, C4, C5, keeps you alive" . . . but there is now evidence that bilateral loss of the phrenic nerve might not necessarily result in death.

> Did you know that a hiccup is caused by a spasmodic, involuntary contraction of the diaphragm?

The external intercostal muscles are the other primary muscles of inspiration and are found between the ribs. The external intercostal muscles slant downward and outward and their diagonal position allows them to do more work upon their contraction. Because they are hinged at the spine and sternum, when they contract they lift the ribs up and outward (Figure 1–9). Other secondary inspiratory muscles are listed in Table 1–1. Accessory muscles of inspiration are only most active with high ventilatory tasks (e.g., deep inspiration) and are not used during quiet inspiration.

Active expiratory pressure can be added to the passive elastic expiratory driving force by generating muscle contraction that decreases the chest wall dimension. The decrease in

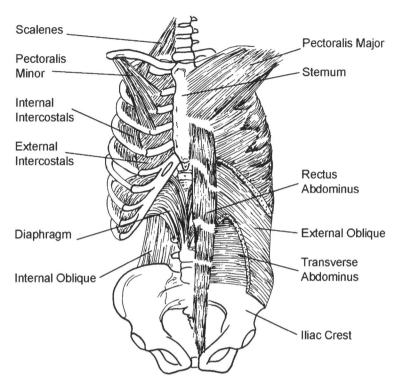

Scalenes

Pectoralis Minor

Internal Intercostals

External Intercostals

Diaphragm

Internal Oblique

Pectoralis Major

Sternum

Rectus Abdominus

External Oblique

Transverse Abdominus

Iliac Crest

Figure 1–9. External and internal intercostal muscles, and abdominal wall muscles.

chest wall dimension can happen by pulling the ribs downward. The ribs are attached at the costochondral joint of the thoracic vertebrae and the sternum or costal arch. The arch of the ribs is oriented downward. Pulling the ribs up produces a "bucket handle" effect (Figure 1–10) and increases the diameter of the upper chamber. Pulling the ribs down similarly decreases the diameter of the upper chamber. Any muscle that acts to pull the ribs *down* will assist in producing an active *expiratory* driving force. Keep in mind, the active expiratory driving force is like squeezing the balloon from the outside and the force of the squeeze generates a pressure that adds to the passive, elastic recoil pressure.

The muscles that produce this squeezing pressure are usually identified as the internal intercostal muscles and abdominal muscles.

The internal intercostal muscles attach to the inner, lower margin of the cranial rib and the inner, upper margin of the adjacent caudal rib.

> *Cranial* means toward the head of the body. *Caudal* means toward the posterior end of the body.

The fibers are oriented ventrodorsally. When "turned on" during active breathing efforts, the internal intercostal muscles contract in synchrony with expiratory airflow. Contraction of these muscles decreases the intercostal space and pulls the ribs down.

The abdominal muscles include the rectus abdominis, external abdominal oblique, internal abdominal oblique, and transversus abdominis (see Figure 1–9). The rectus abdominis is

Table 1–1. Accessory Inspiratory Muscles and Their Origins and Insertions and Major Expiratory Muscles and Their Origins and Insertions

Muscle	Function	Origin	Insertion
Levatores costartum	Accessory Inspiratory	Transverse processes of C7 to T12 vertebrae	Superior surfaces of the ribs immediately inferior to the preceding vertebrae
Serratus posterior superior	Accessory Inspiratory	The spinous processes of C7 through T3	The upper borders of the 2nd through 5th ribs
Sternocleido-mastoid	Accessory Inspiratory	Manubrium and medial portion of the clavicle	Mastoid process of the temporal bone
Scalenus	Accessory Inspiratory	C2–C7 vertebrae	The first and second ribs
Trapezius	Accessory Inspiratory	The spinous processes of the vertebrae C7–T12	At the shoulders, into the *lateral* third of the clavicle, and into the spine of the scapula
Pectoralis major	Accessory Inspiratory	The anterior surface of the clavicle; the anterior surface of the sternum, as low down as the attachment of the cartilage of the 6th or 7th rib	The crest of the greater tubercle of the humerus
Pectoralis minor	Accessory Inspiratory	3rd to 5th ribs, near their costal cartilages	The medial border and upper surface of the scapula
Serratus anterior	Accessory Inspiratory	The surface of the upper eight ribs	The entire anterior length of the medial border of the scapula
Subclavius	Accessory Inspiratory	Arises by a short, thick tendon from the first rib and its cartilage at their junction, in front of the costoclavicular ligament	The groove on the under surface of the clavicle
Levator scapulae	Accessory Inspiratory	Arises by tendinous slips from the transverse processes of the atlas and axis and from the posterior tubercles of the transverse processes of the 3rd and 4th cervical vertebrae.	The vertebral border of the scapula

Table 1-1. *continued*

Muscle	Function	Origin	Insertion
Rhomboideus major	Accessory Inspiratory	The spinous processes of T2 to T5	The medial border of the scapula
Rhomboideus minor	Accessory Inspiratory	The spinous processes of C7 and T1	The vertebral border near the point that it meets the spine of the scapula
Transversus thoracis	Accessory Inspiratory	The posterior surface of the body of the sternum, from the posterior surface of the xiphoid process, and from the sternal ends of the costal cartilages of the lower 3 or 4 true ribs	The lower borders and inner surfaces of the costal cartilages of ribs 2-6
Quadratus lumborum	Accessory Inspiratory	Arises by aponeurotic fibers from the iliolumbar ligament and the adjacent portion of the iliac crest	The lower border of the last rib for about half its length, and the apices of the transverse processes of the upper 4 lumbar vertebrae
Subcostal	Accessory Inspiratory	The inner surface of one rib	The inner surface of the 2nd or 3rd rib above, near its angle
Serratus posterior	Accessory Inspiratory	The spinous processes of T11 and T12 and L1-L3	The inferior borders of the lower 4 ribs, a little beyond their angles
Latissimus dorsi	Accessory Inspiratory	The spinous processes of T6-T12, iliac crest and inferior 3 or 4 ribs	The humerus
Internal oblique abdominis	Expiratory	Inguinal ligament, Iliac crest and the lumbodorsal fascia	Linea alba, xiphoid process, and the inferior ribs.
External oblique abdominis	Expiratory	Lower 8 ribs	Crista iliaca, ligamentum inguinale
Rectus abdominis	Expiratory	Pubis	Costal cartilage of ribs 5-7, xiphoid process of sternum

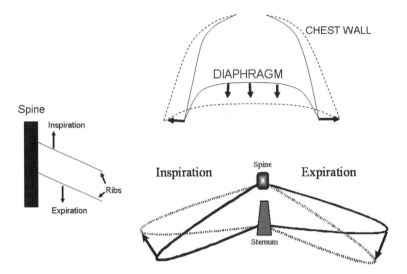

Figure 1–10. Schematic representation of the motion of the diaphragm and ribs during respiratory muscle contraction. The diaphragm contracts and flattens producing an upward pulling force on the ribs and an outward distending force on the abdomen. The intercostal muscles assist the upward pulling force on the ribs during inspiration and downward pulling force on the ribs during expiration. The bucket-handle nature of the parasternal ribs is illustrated with the ends attached to a vertebra and the sternum. Inspiratory muscles pull the rib up and increase the thoracic diameter. Expiratory muscles pull the rib down and decrease the thoracic diameter.

attached to the lower margin of the sternum and the lower edge of the lower parasternal ribs a few centimeters lateral to the sternum. The caudal attachment is ventral (pertaining to the front) to the pelvic girdle. The internal and external abdominal oblique muscles attach cranially to the caudal edge of the costal ribs. The caudal attachment is the rectus abdominis and the pelvic girdle. The external abdominal oblique fibers are oriented from a cranial to caudal direction, dorsventral angle. The internal abdominal oblique fibers are oriented cranial to caudal in a ventrodorsal angle.

The transversus abdominis fibers are oriented circumferentially (forming a circumference) between the rectus abdominis and the spine. The action of the rectus abdominis is to stabilize the ventral midline and stiffen the ventral abdominal midline. The external abdominal oblique, internal abdominal oblique, and transversus abdominis act to decrease the diameter of the abdomen and pull the costal ribs down. This increases the abdominal pressure and forces the abdominal contents upward providing the force that drives the piston action of the diaphragm up into the thorax.

Any muscle group that attaches to the rib cage with a fiber orientation acts to pull the ribs downward or to compress the abdomen in an expiratory direction. The longissimus dorsi, iliocostalis dorsi, iliocostalis lumborum, and serratus posterior inferior muscles in the dorsal side of the back attach to the lower margin of the ribs with the pelvic girdle spine. Portions of the quadratus lumborum on the ventral side of the spine attach the caudal border of the last rib with the pelvic girdle. These muscles are found on the dorsal and ventral sides of the spine. Their orientation provides a downward pull of the ribs, decreasing the diameter of the thorax. The dorsal muscles are also in a position to stabilize the spine during strong ventral contraction of the ventral abdominal muscles, preventing a forward bending action from rectus abdominis contraction. Thus, an erect posture is important in the action of these muscles, assisting in the generation of an active compression of the thorax producing the active expiratory pressure.

In summary, the act of breathing on the generation of alveolar pressure is an inspiratory action caused by the contraction of the diaphragm and external intercostal muscles to increase the lung volume. The active expiratory pressure driving force is the coordinated action of a variety of muscles that decrease the diameter of the thorax and compress the abdomen. Compressing the abdomen increases abdominal pressure, thus providing the driving force for the piston action, which then stretches the relaxed diaphragm.

The Respiratory System and Voice Production

Adequate control of lung volume and respiratory muscle activity during expiration is crucial for the regulation of subglottal pressure (Hixon, Goldman, & Mead, 1973). It is the subglottal pressure that controls a variety of parameters related to voice production such as airflow, glottal area, fundamental frequency (the pitch of the sound), and sound pressure level (the loudness of the sound). Subglottal pressure is the driving force for the initiation of vocal fold vibration. As stated above, both active and passive forces regulate the main alveolar pressure and in turn a certain percent-

age of the generated alveolar pressure is used for voice production.

> Alveolar pressure is the pressure within the alveoli of the lungs. Subglottal pressure is the pressure directly below the vocal folds that is used to dynamically move the vocal folds by airflow.

Relaxation Pressure Curve

The clinician can use an image of the relaxation pressure curve to educate a patient about the respiratory mechanisms used to produce voice/ speech and to explain what parts of voice/speech are active and passive during its production. Of course, the concepts of passive and active properties of the respiratory system described above must be simplified for the patient. Having a clear understanding of the respiratory mechanisms that are used to develop pressure for voice production can help the clinician determine if a particular breathing technique used with a patient should or should not be applied in voice therapy. Figure 1–8 depicts a relaxation pressure curve produced along the lung volume continuum of 0% lung volume to total lung capacity (TLC; 100%). The relaxation pressure curve is presented here again in order to explain the types of forces generated by the respiratory system.

At each percentage of lung volume there is a pressure generated by the inherent recoil forces of the lung, thorax, and abdominal-diaphragm unit. Figure 1–8 illustrates that pressures produced at lung volumes between 45 to 60% VC produce pressures on the order of 5 to 10 cm H_2O. It is at these lung volumes where inspiratory or expiratory work to produce voice is minimal. Work, for the purpose of this description, is the recruitment of muscular forces used to depart from the relaxation pressure. By recruiting muscular effort, higher pressures can be generated and this may be necessary in order to meet the demands of certain voicing or speech tasks.

When a higher lung volume is approached, as indicated by Figure 1–8, at about 80% VC, an active inspiratory muscle force must be generated to combat the high recoil forces generated by the lung-thorax unit. At volumes as high as 80%, the tendency to recoil to those resting volumes is very high. In order to resist the high recoil force, inspiratory muscles must be recruited in a "checking" like fashion (Hixon, 1987). At very low lung volumes, on the order of 20% VC, it is apparent from Figure 1–8 that there is not enough pressure to meet the demands required for comfortable effort voice/speech production.

The pressure needed to produce comfortable effort level voice production is on the order of 4 to 5 cm H_2O and, as the patient's vocal loudness increases, the subglottal pressure increases. At 20% TLC, on Figure 1–8, the relaxation pressure is negative. In order to create a positive pressure for voice, recruitment of abdominal musculature is necessary to decrease the volume within the chestwall. A "piston-like" force is generated, increasing the pressure needed to meet the demands of the voice/speech task. The fact that abdominal muscles must be "turned on" for voice/speech to occur at very low lung volumes means the mechanism of action is active (i.e., muscle contraction). This active mechanism from the clinician/patient perspective is "work."

A clinician's ability to interpret the relaxation pressure diagram helps in providing appropriate recommendations to the voice patient. For example, having your patient "take big breaths" before they start to voice does not make good physiologic sense as they would have to recruit inspiratory muscles to resist high recoil forces. Rather, counsel the patient to take a small breath in before starting to voice, and finally, seek to determine if there are any lower or upper airway limitations that may be preventing them from utilizing the lung volumes they have generated effectively.

Therapeutic Considerations

There are many clinical instances where alveolar pressure cannot be generated effectively. Chronic obstructive pulmonary disease (COPD) is one such condition. With COPD, narrowing of the upper airway occurs, as a compensatory mechanism, in an attempt to regulate airflow and maintain lung volume during voice production. Symptoms self-reported by patients with COPD suggest both respiratory and laryngeal involvement and include dyspnea (sensation of breathlessness), reduced vocal loudness, and hoarseness. Lee, Friesen, Lambert, and Loudon, (1998), developed a dyspnea questionnaire because questionnaires that are sensitive to those with lung disease are not plentiful in the voice literature. Lee et al.'s (1998) results showed that dyspnea is a relevant factor when assessing speech and voice abilities in those with lung disease from both personal and vocational standpoints and advocated the need for scales that are sensitive to the variable of dyspnea. The scale developed by Lee et al., although not used specifically with patients with voice disorders, could be used as a supplement to acquire information not available from other voice handicap indexes.

Cases involving spinal cord injury and neuromuscular degenerative diseases such as multiple sclerosis may lack muscular integrity, resulting in a disability to generate high enough muscular forces to deviate from the relaxation pressure. Developing adequate subglottal pressure is critical for generating vocal loudness, varying the frequency of the voice, and sustaining the sound duration. And although the demands of speech will vary, pressure will be required to be constant regardless of the lung volume and task duration.

Some patients with voice disorders have a laryngeal condition creating high laryngeal airway resistance. Cases such as adductor spasmodic dysphonia, muscle tension dysphonia or other dynamic laryngeal dysfunction conditions that result in increased glottal closed time cause high laryngeal airway resistance, restricting airflow (see Chapter 6). Static laryngeal conditions on the other hand like laryngeal webbing, subglottal stenosis, bilateral abductor vocal fold paralysis, arytenoid joint dislocation, and others can also result in high laryngeal airway resistance (see Chapter 5). There are other patients who present with low laryngeal airway resistance. These are cases of hypofunctional voice disorders, and may include adductor vocal fold paralysis or any other condition that limits vocal fold mobility (Saarinen, Rihkanen, Malmberg, Pekkanen, & Sovijarvi 2001). With these conditions it is difficult to control expiratory airflow because of inadequate vocal fold movement. These patients may also complain of breathing symptoms.

Laryngeal compensation, documented by visual examination of the larynx, and verified with laryngeal airway resistance measures has been found in those with vocal nodules (Sapienza & Stathopoulos, 1994), and adductor spasmodic dysphonia (Finnegan, Luschei, Barkmeier, & Hoffman, 1996; Plant & Hillel, 1998; Witsell, Weissler, Donovan, Howard, & Martinkosky, 1994). Initial research on breathing patterns in those with voice disorders comes from the work of Hixon (1987), Sapienza and Stathopoulos (1994), Sapienza, Stathopoulos, and Brown (1997), Hillman et al. (1998) and others. These studies indicate an interactive role between the shape of the glottal space and breathing behavior. Specifically, when high glottal airflows are produced during voice production, larger lung volumes are used during voicing, the voice task is ended at lower lung volumes, particularly below FRC, and there is deviant phrasing.

Dyspnea, mentioned previously, is the conscious awareness of labored breathing or air hunger and occurs most commonly with heavy exercise but can occur with certain laryngeal conditions (Brunner et al., 2011; West & Popkess-Vawter, 1994).

> Dyspnea is a critical symptom to try to understand because it is common to many pulmonary and laryngeal function disorders. However, its definition is complex and as such requires both psychological assessment and physiologic assessment of both the upper and lower airways.

Those with voice disorders often complain of dyspnea when they are walking or having to walk and talk simultaneously. Physiologically, the origin of dyspnea can be multifaceted and understanding the cause of dyspnea requires assessment of both lower and upper airway function. Clinically, your responsibilities when presented with patients complaining of dyspnea, is twofold. Your first responsibility is to make your patient aware of the importance of understanding the relationship between glottal configuration, upper airway resistance, and respiration. Your second responsibility, prior to treating any breathing symptoms, and in conjunction with other medical professionals, is to rule out that the dyspnea is not related to heart disease, lung disease, or the psychological state (i.e., anxiety) of the patient.

Pulmonary Function Testing: Important to Make the Right Referral

Referral of your patient to a pulmonologist is recommended to help discern the cause of dyspnea. The standard pulmonary function tests that are used to help determine the origin of the dyspnea and or any other lower airway condition, are the forced vital capacity (FVC) maneuver, the forced expiratory volume in one second (FEV1) maneuver or maximum voluntary ventilation (MVV) maneuver, and the maximum inspiratory and expiratory flow-volume loop. These tests are done with spirometry. In particular, the flow-volume relationships diagnose the presence and assess the effect of large (central) airway obstruction. Characteristic patterns of the flow-volume loop also distinguish fixed from variable obstruction and extra- from intrathoracic location. The speed of air movement in and out of the lungs is assessed by the flow rate, and the volume that is measured indicates the amount of air moved.

Interpreting the Results of the Flow-Volume Loop

There will be a time when flow-volume loop data is sent to you as a record of a patient's pulmonary condition. Therefore, your familiarity with the major landmarks of a flow-volume loop is important for the clinical interpretation of the patient's condition.

The major landmarks of a flow-volume loop are shown in Figure 1–11. Peak Expiratory Flow Rate (PEFR) is the first peak of air exhaled from the patient. The measure of peak flow rate can be used to help judge if the patient is giving maximal effort, tests overall strength of expiratory muscles, and

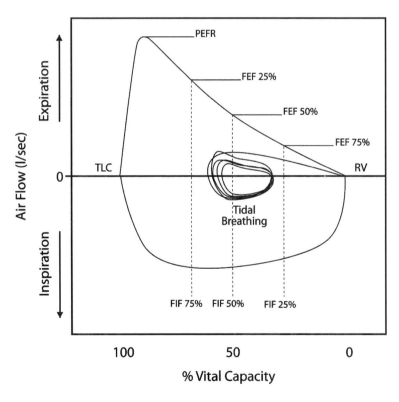

Figure 1–11. Flow-volume loop indicating major flow and volumetric landmarks during expiratory and inspiratory cycle. PEFR = peak expiratory flow rate; FEF = forced expiratory flow; RV = residual volume; FIF = forced inspiratory flow.

the general condition of the large airways, such as the trachea and main bronchi. Forced Expiratory Flow at 25% of FVC (FEF25%) is the flow rate at the 25% point of the total volume (FVC) exhaled. Assuming maximal effort from the patient during the generation of the flow-volume loop, this flow rate indicates the condition of the large to medium size bronchi. Forced Expiratory Flow at 50% of FVC (FEF50%) is the flow rate at the 50% point of the total volume (FVC) exhaled. This landmark is at the midpoint of the FVC and indicates the status of the medium to small airways. Forced Expiratory Flow at 75% of FVC (FEF75%) is the flow rate at the 75% point of the total volume (FVC) exhaled. This landmark indicates the status of the small airways.

Forced Inspiratory Flow at 25% of FVC (FIF25%) is the flow rate at the 25% point of the total volume inhaled. Abnormalities here are indicators of upper airway obstructions. Areas of the mouth, upper and lower pharynx (back of the throat), and glottis impact the inspiratory flow rates. Peak Inspiratory Flow Rate is the fastest flow rate achieved during inspiration. Forced Inspiratory Flow at 50% of FVC (FIF50%) is the flow rate at the 50% point of the total volume inhaled. Forced Inspiratory Flow at 75% of FVC is the flow rate at the 75% point of the total volume inhaled.

When a clinical report is received from a pulmonary clinic or pulmonologist, the spirometry values are typically presented in absolute numbers as well as percent predicted based on normative values. The normative values are race, sex, and age dependent and the standards may vary across clinical laboratories. If the spirometric data rule out lower airway disease, and the flow-volume loop data indicate upper airway obstruction, then appropriate care can focus on the remediation of the laryngeal condition and with intervention the sensation of dyspnea should diminish.

Using the Right Terminology

It is important to use the right terminology in clinical report writing. In the speech pathologist's assessment and treatment of voice disorders, many terms related to breathing have prevailed in the literature. These terms include "support," "diaphragmatic breathing," "clavicular breathing," "circular breathing," "breathing exercises," and others. Use of the term "support" can be vague, and often when used in clinical report writing does not tell much about the physiologic status of the respiratory system. When the term "support" is used, it likely relates to the physiologic driving force (i.e., pressure) for voicing. As such, using the term pressure is definitive and physiologically more correct then the term "support" or "breath support."

Likewise, the term "diaphragmatic breathing," particularly when referring to voice production, is a bit of a misnomer, given that the diaphragm is a muscle of inspiration. Consequently, it doesn't make much physiologic sense to use this term when directing instruction of expiration to the patient. If the term is used to indicate the piston-like mechanism of the abdominal wall then the term should be changed to abdominal force thus making more physiologic sense with regard to the discussion of mechanics of breathing. Similarly, the term clavicular breathing should only be used when a patient breathes by raising the pectoral area of the chest wall and shoulders. The term clavicular breathing has now become overused to identify patients with presumed poor "breath support." And, in fact, many times it is used to classify the way women breathe. But, typically the term clavicular breathing is inaccurately used since those who have healthy respiratory structure and function of the chest wall do not use a less efficient system of breathing, like clavicular breathing, voluntarily or reflexively.

For those with solely laryngeal conditions, and intact respiratory muscle tone, clavicular breathing is unlikely. In fact, the human body likes to work less, not more, per any given task. So unless completely exhausted, patients that have voice disorders, and who have no neurologic impairment or lower airway disease, are unlikely to be clavicular breathers. Use of the term clavicular breathing should be cautiously employed to describe only those to whom it really applies. Finally, there is a breathing type called circular breathing and it is associated with musicians (i.e., saxophonists). Difficult to achieve, the process starts with a half-full lung. The mouth is then supposedly filled with an air pocket, while still breathing out from the lungs. The person then switches from lung to mouth air with no interruption and forces air out from the mouth with the cheeks. The person then switches back to the now full lungs and repeats the process.

In the behavioral treatment of voice disorders we often come across the term "breathing exercises." This is again a broad categorical phrase covering a spectrum of exercises from relaxation to yoga methods. Many of these exercises have merit, particularly those that are focused on teaching coordination of inspiration and expiration, postural alignment, and use of the abdomen to help produce pressure for speech. However, there are some exercises that do not offer specific physiologic guidelines. For example, within some promoted exercise programs there have been regimens that place people on their back to facilitate better breathing or relaxation. Hoit (1995) examined how breathing differs in the upright and supine positions, and discussed in detail the clinical implications with the different postures when treating patients with voice disorders. It is our responsibility to realize which factors are being manipulated during these breathing exercises and which are valid to use with patients that have voice disorders.

Biofeedback Techniques

Finally, biofeedback techniques may help the patient monitor and control the inspiratory and expiratory cycles of breathing during voice production. Biofeedback is the feedback of biological information to gain control of bodily processes that normally cannot be controlled voluntarily. Electromyography (EMG) is one way to measure muscle activity through the use of strategically placed electrodes. Most commonly, because it is a noninvasive procedure, surface electrodes are placed on the general area of muscle that is being tested for its activity.

Theoretically, in the treatment of those with voice disorders, the clinician should have the patient monitor both perceptual and physiological processes associated with the voice disorder while implementing a particular treatment regimen that attempts to reduce hyperfunctional behaviors. Murdoch, Pitt, Theodoro, and Ward (1999) used biofeedback with the inductance plethysmography (or Respitrace) to provide real-time, continuous visual biofeedback of rib cage circumference during breathing in a child with traumatic brain injury. Results showed very good success with the biofeedback technique when compared to traditional instructions for proper speech breathing. Murdoch and colleagues believed that the visual biofeedback techniques brought about far superior outcome when compared to traditional methods. The use of biofeedback with patients appears effective and is easily incorporated into treatment program with a variety of patient types.

Summary

The respiratory system is considered the power source for voice production and deterioration of its function can significantly impact a patient's ability to generate adequate ventilation for life purposes and subglottal air pressure for voice production. As such the respiratory system is one of the most important subsystems requiring evaluative and treatment attention in the care of the voice. The next chapter describes the sound source for voice production by description of laryngeal anatomy and physiology.

References

Brunner, E., Friedrich, G., Kiesler, K., Chibidziura-Priesching, J., & Gugatschka, M. (2011). Subjective breathing impairment in unilateral vocal fold paralysis. *Folia Phoniatric Logopedica*, *63*(3), 142–146.

Finnegan, E. M., Luschei, E. S., Barkmeier, J. M., & Hoffman, H. T. (1996). Sources of error in estimation of laryngeal airway resistance in persons with spasmodic dysphonia. *Journal of Speech and Hearing Research*, *39*(1), 105–113.

Goldman, J. M., Rose, L. S., Morgan, M. D., & Denison, D. M. (1986). Measurement of abdominal wall compliance in normal subjects and tetraplegic patients. *Thorax*, *41*(7), 513–518.

Hillman, R. E., Holmberg, E. B., Perkell, J. S., Walsh, M., & Vaughan, C. (1998). Objective assessment of vocal hyperfunction: An experimental framework and initial results. *Journal of Speech and Hearing Research*, *32*(2), 373–392.

Hixon, T. J. (1987). *Respiratory function in speech and song*. Boston, MA: College-Hill Press/Little Brown and Company.

Hixon, T. J., Goldman, M. D., & Mead, J. (1973). Kinematics of the chest wall during speech production: Volume displacement for the rib cage, abdomen and lung. *Journal of Speech and Hearing Research*, *19*, 297–356.

Hoit, J. D. (1995). Influence of body position on breathing and its implications for the evaluation and treatment of speech and voice disorders. *Journal of Voice*, *9*(4), 341–347.

Lee, L., Friesen, M., Lambert, I. R., & Loudon, R. G. (1998). Evaluation of dyspnea during physical and speech activities in patients with pulmonary diseases. *Chest*, *113*(3), 625–632.

Murdoch, B. E., Pitt G., Theodoros D. G., & Ward E. C. (1999). Real-time continuous visual biofeedback in the treatment of speech breathing disorders following childhood traumatic brain injury: Report of one case. *Pediatric Rehabilitation*, *3*(1), 5–20.

Plant, R. L., & Hillel, A. D. (1998). Direct measurement of subglottic pressure and laryngeal resistance in normal subjects and in spasmodic dysphonia. *Journal of Voice*, *12*(3), 300–314.

Saarinen, A., Rihkanen, H., Malmberg, L. P., Pekkanen, L., & Sovijarvi, A. R. (2001). Disturbances in airflow dynamics and tracheal sounds during forced and quiet breathing in subjects with unilateral vocal fold paralysis. *Clinical Physiology*, *21*(6), 712–717.

Sapienza, C. M., & Stathopoulos, E. T. (1994). Respiratory and laryngeal measures of children during vocal intensity variation. *Journal of the Acoustical Society of America*, *94*(5), 2531–2543.

Sapienza, C. M., Stathopoulos, E. T., & Brown, W. S. (1997). Speech breathing during reading in women with vocal nodules. *Journal of Voice*, *11*(2), 195–201.

West, N., & Popkess-Vawter, S. (1994). The subjective and psychosocial nature of breathlessness. *Journal of Advanced Nursing*, *20*(4), 622–626.

Witsell, D. L., Weissler, M. C., Donovan, M. K., Howard, J. F., & Martinkosky, S. J. (1994). Measurement of laryngeal resistance in the evaluation of botulinum toxin injection for treatment of focal laryngeal dystonia. *Laryngoscope*, *104*(1), 8–11.

Chapter 2

Laryngeal Anatomy and Physiology

*J*ust like the information provided in Chapter 1, for respiratory anatomy and physiology, this chapter describes laryngeal anatomy and physiology and includes a general explanation of the theories of sound production, effects of development and aging on the larynx, and variations of physiology that accompany sound production. As you read this chapter think about what the anatomical structures can accomplish based on their morphology (form and shape) and how they function via the structures they are attached to. Use the anatomic diagrams to help visualize the movements of the laryngeal structures and how these movements occur during voice production (phonation). Then, as you watch the examples of both normal and disordered voice production that are included with this textbook, use the anatomic drawings to help guide the identification of these structures on the laryngeal videoendoscopic examinations.

After reading this chapter, you will:

- Understand the basic components of laryngeal anatomy
- Understand the basic developmental process of the larynx

- Understand laryngeal structural differences between males and females and between the young and the old
- Understand how the larynx functions to produce sound and its variations

Laryngeal Anatomy

Basic Structure and Function

As a multistructured organ within the vocal tract, the larynx serves as a passageway between the upper and lower airway (Figure 2–1). It is composed of one bone, multiple cartilages, numerous muscles, membranous and connective tissue, and movable joints, much like other structures in our body. The larynx acts as a sphincter, closing to protect the lower airways from foreign material, opening to aid breathing, and serving as the sound source for voice production as pressure from the respiratory system is transferred from the subglottal space through the glottal space into the supraglottal cavity (Figure 2–2).

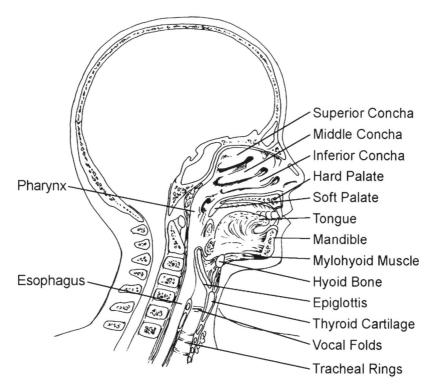

Pharynx

Esophagus

Superior Concha
Middle Concha
Inferior Concha
Hard Palate
Soft Palate
Tongue
Mandible
Mylohyoid Muscle
Hyoid Bone
Epiglottis
Thyroid Cartilage
Vocal Folds
Tracheal Rings

Figure 2–1. Lateral view of head and neck structures.

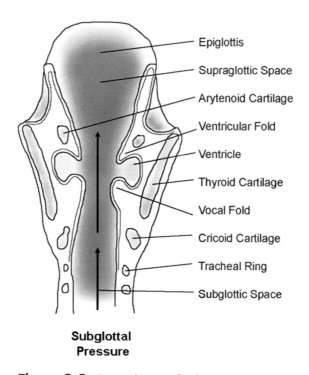

Epiglottis
Supraglottic Space
Arytenoid Cartilage
Ventricular Fold
Ventricle
Thyroid Cartilage
Vocal Fold
Cricoid Cartilage
Tracheal Ring
Subglottic Space

**Subglottal
Pressure**

Figure 2–2. Coronal view of sub and supraglottic space.

With their protective and pivotal role, the vocal folds within the larynx act like a valve to open and close the airway. The open airway allows the passage of air into and out of the lungs. Closure of the vocal folds acts in a protective function. The protective function of the larynx is completely reflexive (this means automatic) and involuntary (not under control) as occurs during a reflexive cough. The phonatory functions, on the other hand are initiated voluntarily, but regulated involuntarily.

The glottis is simply the space between the vocal folds and its size and shape changes as a function of the vibratory behavior of the vocal folds. When the vocal folds are open, the glottis widens and this is called abduction (Figure 2–3). When the vocal folds are closed no air can flow through the glottis; this is called adduction (Figure 2–4). There

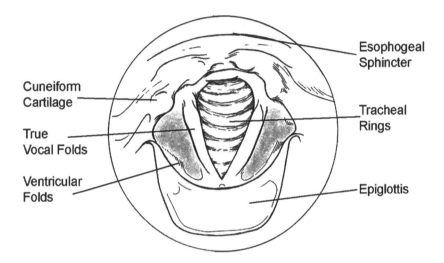

Figure 2–3. Superior view of laryngeal structures (vocal fold opening).

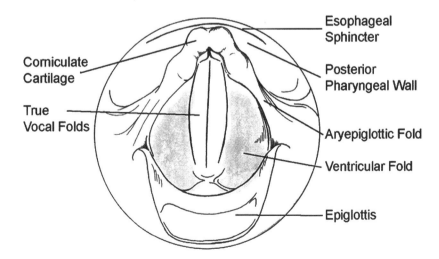

Figure 2–4. Superior view of laryngeal structures (vocal fold closure).

are varying states of abduction and adduction as seen in Figure 2–5. For example, during a maximum inspiration, when the goal is to achieve maximum inspiratory flow into the lungs, the vocal folds are maximally abducted, representing the functional synergy between vocal fold function and respiratory function. For the initiation of phonation, the vocal folds are positioned near the midline.

As indicated earlier, the larynx is part of the critical pathway for sustaining the life function of breathing. The function of the intrinsic laryngeal muscles for abducting and adducting the vocal folds serves to widen and narrow the glottal space. Without the movement of the primary laryngeal cartilages by the intrinsic laryngeal muscles for abduction, air could not flow into the lungs and be controlled as it passes out of the lungs. Therefore, in order for normal breathing to occur, the larynx must be healthy. That is, the muscles of the larynx must receive the appropriate neurologic signal from the brain and the peripheral nerve endings must be anatomically intact to control the function of the laryngeal muscles.

Paralysis of the vocal folds (altered neurologic signaling to the vocal fold muscle) can result in a reduction of the glottal space thereby jeopardizing a patient's ability to ventilate adequately. If the glottal space is too narrow, then airway resistance is increased, altering normal inspiration and expiration.

The muscles, in turn, must be able to produce the appropriate forces to move the laryngeal cartilages and then the laryngeal cartilages themselves must be flexible. The muscles of the larynx are skeletal, meaning they are under voluntary control for voice production, controlled by the central nervous system. Not every part of the larynx has a critical role in voice production yet every laryngeal structure has a *supporting* role in voice production, whether it is anatomic or functional. If the larynx is unhealthy, then there could be serious repercussions for regulating airflow as discussed in Chapter 1.

Biological Functions of the Larynx

In addition to its sphincteric function during breathing, the larynx plays another important biological role and that is during the act of swallowing. During swallowing the vocal folds adduct tightly to prevent food or liquid from entering into the glottal space and subsequently into the trachea or lower airway. This action helps in avoiding the possibility of getting a bacterial infection in the tracheobronchial tree, commonly known as aspiration pneumonia. The larynx, with its extrinsic muscle connections to the hyoid bone, elevates (both anteriorly and superiorly) during swallowing, closing off the laryngeal space and stopping breathing (Davenport, Bolser, Morris, 2011; McCulloch, Van Dael, & Ciucci, 2011). This stoppage of breathing is called apnea. The movements of the larynx

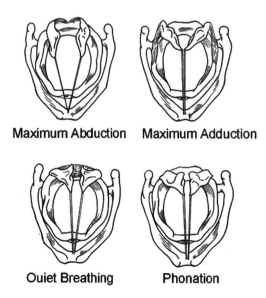

Maximum Abduction   Maximum Adduction

Quiet Breathing   Phonation

Figure 2–5. Depiction of glottal configurations during maximum abduction and adduction, quiet breathing, and phonation.

during swallow are vital and cofunction with the movements of the hyoid bone due to their anatomic connections.

The larynx also serves another biological function such as thoracic fixation, which occurs when lifting heavy weights or performing activities like bearing a child. Thoracic fixation requires tight vocal fold adduction in order to build high intra-thoracic pressure. After the high effort task is completed, the vocal folds abduct, and air is rapidly released through the glottal space. Inability to close off the glottis can result in a disability in completing high effort fixative functions. Other functions that require vocal fold adduction are cough and bowel movements.

Nonbiological Functions of the Larynx

Although the functions of breathing, swallowing, and thoracic fixation are considered to be primary biological functions of the larynx, the act of phonation is considered a nonbiological function. It is classified as a nonbiological function because our vitality is not reliant on the ability to produce voice. In fact, being able to produce voice in the way we do; talking, laughing, screaming, and singing are unique human characteristics.

> Excised larynges from animals (dog, cat, pig, rabbit) are often used to develop models of laryngeal function or test the outcome of new treatments prior to human use, such as the use of injectable substances for aiding vocal fold mobility problems or to study the process of vocal fold healing. By studying animal models, scientists learn about the intricacies of the larynx and transfer their knowledge to the care of the human larynx.

The sophistication of our voice production as well as the complexity of our laryngeal anatomy and oral structures provides us with distinction from other lower animals.

> Although the dog larynx is often used in laryngeal research, cross-species comparisons have revealed that the layered structure of the pig vocal fold shares more similarities with the human vocal fold (Hahn, Kobler, Starcher, Zeitels, & Langer, 2006; Hahn, Kobler, Zeitels, & Langer, 2006; Hunter & Titze, 2004).

Laryngeal Structure: Pieces and Parts

The main part of the laryngeal framework is made up of cartilage and there are two types of cartilage that require description before describing the individual structures of the larynx. The first is hyaline cartilage, which is flexible and elastic, made up of collagen (basic building block of cartilage) and other proteins. Hyaline cartilage forms the thyroid, cricoid, and arytenoids cartilages within the larynx and ossifies with age. The next is elastic cartilage. Elastic cartilage is similar to hyaline cartilage, but in addition to the collagenous fibers, the matrix of the elastic cartilage also contains a network of branched yellow elastic fibers, and these *do not* ossify. The epiglottis is elastic cartilage.

Ossification is a process whereby cartilage is replaced by bone. Although it is often taught that cartilage with age, "turns into bone," as we age cartilage is actually *replaced* by bone. Cartilage that does not go through the process of ossification is referred to as permanent cartilage, like that found in the tip of the nose, the external ear, the walls of the trachea, and the epiglottis among others. In the larynx the thyroid cartilage ossifies more frequently than the cricoid but each starts to ossify about the third decade of life (Mupparapu & Vuppalapati, 2004).

The Hyoid Bone

A U-shaped bone consisting of several parts, the hyoid bone, is suspended just above the thyroid cartilage, and is an important site for the muscular attachments of the larynx via the suprahyoid and infrahyoid muscles that are discussed further below. The hyoid bone is considered by some as an anatomic structure separate from the laryngeal framework, acting as a supporting structure to the laryngeal framework by providing muscular attachments linking tongue and laryngeal positions. The hyoid bone is attached to the tongue via a ligament called the glossoepiglottic ligament and its unique position with the tongue is only present in humans. For our purposes, we consider the hyoid bone part of the laryngeal framework.

The hyoid includes two greater cornu (protrusions) and two lesser cornu. The greater cornu are posteriorly directed limbs of the U-shaped bone and articulate with the lesser cornua anteriorly (Figures 2–6 and 2–7). The lesser cornu provide a place for stylohyoid ligaments to attach. Connection of the hyoid bone to the thyroid cartilage occurs by the thyrohyoid ligament and the thyrohyoid membrane.

Thyroid Cartilage

The thyroid cartilage is the largest unpaired cartilage in the laryngeal framework and is the most visible when looking at the front of the neck and the most palpable (to touch). The thyroid cartilage has several parts: two lami-

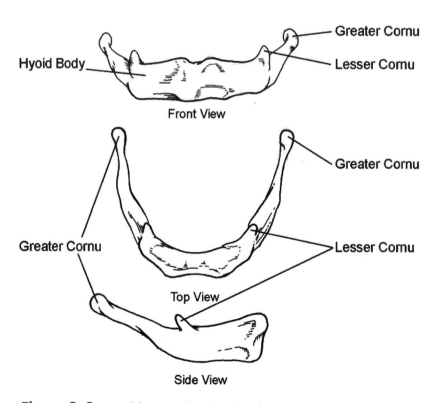

Figure 2–6. Hyoid bone and its landmarks.

nae, two superior cornu, 2 inferior cornu, an oblique line, and a superior thyroid notch. The thyroid cartilage is most often recognized for its anterior angle which results in a prominence of the cartilage, commonly known as "the Adam's apple." This angle is wider in females (120 degrees in females) and more acute in males (approximately 90 degrees), resulting in a more prominent Adam's apple in men. The thyroid cartilage also connects to the cricoid cartilage as described below.

Thyroid Laminae

The thyroid laminae are broad flat plates of cartilages. The laryngeal prominence is a line of fusion of the two laminae. Each lamina is connected above to the hyoid bone by the thyrohyoid membrane. There exists an oblique line on each thyroid lamina that descends diagonally from superior to inferior on the lateral surface of the thyroid lamina. It is the place for other muscular attachments to the thyroid cartilage.

Superior and Inferior Thyroid Cornu

Again, cornua are simply projections of the cartilage and serve as points of attachments for ligaments or muscles. The superior horn of the thyroid cartilage attaches to the hyoid bone via ligaments. Ligaments in the human body attach either bone to bone or cartilage to cartilage. In the larynx the superior horn of the thyroid cartilage attaches to the hyoid bone by the lateral thyrohyoid ligament. The inferior

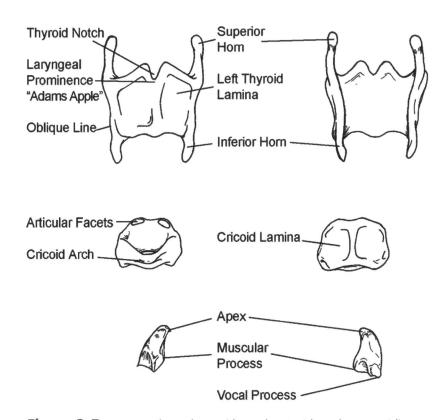

Figure 2–7. Laryngeal cartilages (thyroid, cricoid, and arytenoid).

horn of the thyroid cartilage helps connect the thyroid to the cricoid cartilage, discussed next. Rather than a ligament attaching the thyroid to the cricoid, the inferior horn of the thyroid cartilage forms a joint with the cricoid cartilage, called the cricothyroid joint. This joint is referred to as a synovial joint (freely movable and the most common joint in the body). The cricothyroid joint specifically allows the thyroid to rotate anteriorly or posteriorly on the cricoid cartilage. When the thyroid is rotated anteriorly, the distance between the front arch of the cricoid to the lower border of the thyroid cartilage is decreased. This lengthens the vocal folds, assuming the arytenoids are fixed in position, thus increasing the tension of the vocal ligaments. Both of the cricothyroid joints operate symmetrically during this movement.

Interestingly, the articulation between the cricoid and thyroid cartilages forms a narrower angle in men than women. This is important to know because it might explain the greater difficulty in exposing the cartilages during laryngeal framework surgery for men, which is discussed in more detail in Chapter 8.

> A prominent Adam's apple can be reduced for those seeking reduction as an elective procedure for gender transition. This procedure is called a thyroid chondroplasty.

Cricoid Cartilage

The cricoid cartilage is a single cartilage made up of hyaline tissue and forms the base or inferior aspect of the laryngeal framework. With a shape often compared to a signet ring, the cricoid cartilage has a broad posterior aspect and thinner arch anteriorly. It is connected to the thyroid cartilage, via the inferior horn, as explained previously, and superiorly by the cricothyroid membrane. The cricoid also attaches to the first tracheal ring by the cricotracheal ligament or membrane.

Arytenoid Cartilage

The arytenoid cartilages are paired and situated on the superior margin of the cricoid lamina and consist of hyaline and elastic tissue. Usually described as pyramidal shaped, the arytenoids are connected to the epiglottis by a muscle called the aryepiglottic muscle or fold and to the thyroid cartilage anteriorly by the vocal ligament. Arytenoid movement allows for vocal fold abduction and adduction and these movements occur because of the cricoarytenoid joint. The arytenoid cartilages sit on top of the cricoid cartilage and the cricoarytenoid joint allows the arytenoid joints to slide medially and rock at these joints (Selbie, Zhang, Levine, & Ludlow, 1998). These joints are also synovial joints and allow for downward and inward and upward and outward movement. When the vocal process of the arytenoid moves medially the vocal folds adduct. When there is lateral movement the vocal folds abduct. Sliding of the arytenoid cartilages toward each other causes adduction and sliding away from each other causes abduction.

There are two main processes on the arytenoids cartilage; one is called the vocal process and the other muscular process. The vocal process is the anterior and medial extension of the arytenoid cartilages where the posterior vocal fold ligament attaches via a tendinous-like structure called the macula flava. Ultrastucture examination by Sato, Hirano, and Nakashima (2000) showed the vocal processes are very firm in forming the glottis with greatest pliability at the tip of the vocal process. The muscular processes of the arytenoids on the other hand are the extensions where the posterior and lateral cricoarytenoid muscles attach, hence the name "muscular process."

A laryngeal injury such as a laryngeal fracture due to a motor vehicle accident, sporting activity, or fight can possibly disrupt or dislocate the cricothyroid and cricoarytenoid joints, creating possible airway limitation and subsequent need for a tracheostomy.

Vocal process granulomas are benign lesions of the posterior glottis that are commonly centered over the tips of the cartilaginous vocal processes of the arytenoids.

The arytenoid cartilages also serve as the posterior attachment for the false vocal folds.

Corniculate Cartilage

As paired elastic cartilages, the corniculate cartilages appear mounted on top of the arytenoid cartilages. Although considered one of the primary cartilages of the laryngeal framework, functionally, the corniculate cartilages serve no role in voice production.

Cuneiform Cartilages

The cuneiform cartilages are paired and small, rod-shaped elastic cartilages embedded in the aryepiglottic muscle/fold. Biologically, they serve the supportive framework of the larynx but have no apparent role in voice production.

Epiglottis

The epiglottis is considered the superior part of the larynx, located posterior to the hyoid bone and base of the tongue. A direct view to the back of a child's oropharynx may allow a glimpse of the superior border of the epiglottis. A single cartilage, covered by a mucous membrane, the epiglottis is leaf shaped, broad at its top and narrow at its base; this narrowing is referred to as the petiolus. The epiglottis is composed of elastic cartilage. It attaches to the angle of the thyroid cartilage by a ligament called the thyroepiglottic ligament and to the tongue by several ligaments called glossoepiglottic ligaments. The movement of the epiglottis is an important reflex mechanism during swallowing, helping to close the laryngeal space or vestibule. Closure at the arytenoid to epiglottic base is done by active anterior tilting of the arytenoid cartilage and posterior projection of the epiglottic base as the larynx elevates during swallow. Epiglottic downward movement to closure is the biomechanical effect of hyolaryngeal movement, downward bolus movement, and tongue base retraction (Logemann et al., 1992) (Figure 2–8).

Epiglottitis is an inflammation of the epiglottis. As a result, the epiglottis becomes infected and swollen, and it can obstruct the airway, which may be fatal unless promptly treated.

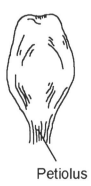

Petiolus

Figure 2–8. Epiglottis and its petiolus.

Laryngeal Muscles

There are two groups of laryngeal muscles. The first group contains the intrinsic laryngeal muscles, which are responsible for the movements of the laryngeal cartilages and finer control of the laryngeal structures. The second group contains the extrinsic laryngeal muscles and they are responsible for larger laryngeal movements, like elevation and depression of the larynx. We first discuss the intrinsic laryngeal muscles.

Intrinsic Laryngeal Muscles

The intrinsic laryngeal muscles are found within the larynx and include a total of five, all of which are paired. These muscles work to regulate the tension in the vocal ligament and the size and shape of the glottal space.

Thyroarytenoid

The thyroarytenoid muscle (TA) shortens the vocal folds when it contracts. It originates on the inner surface of the thyroid cartilage and inserts into the muscular process of the arytenoid cartilage. Upon contraction, it shortens the vocal fold by decreasing the distance between the vocal process and the thyroid angle. The TA muscle is also referred to as the deepest layer of the vocal fold structure. There are two sections to the TA, the more medial section is the thyrovocalis and the more lateral section is the thyromuscularis.

The thyrovocalis section of the TA tenses the vocal fold when it contracts. The thyromuscularis section of the thyroarytenoid relaxes the vocal fold when it contracts (Figures 2–9 and 2–10).

Posterior Cricoarytenoid

The posterior cricoarytenoid muscle (PCA) originates on the posterior surface of the cri-

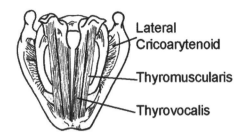

Figure 2–9. Thyroarytenoid muscle and its two sections, thryrovocalis and thyromuscularis.

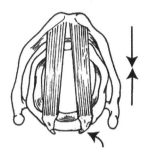

Figure 2–10. Depiction of thyroarytenoid muscle contraction and subsequent vocal fold shortening.

coid lamina and courses up and forward to insert in the muscular process of the arytenoids. Upon contraction it abducts the vocal fold by moving the muscular process medially and rotating the vocal process laterally. Of interest is the synergistic relationship that exists between the PCA and the diaphragm. Recall, the diaphragm is the major muscle of inspiration. Given the primary abductory role of the PCA, it should not be surprising that PCA muscle activity is exhibited with diaphragmatic activity during the inspiratory cycle of breathing. In fact, PCA activity starts just before the activity of the diaphragm starts and when loss of PCA activity occurs, in spite of diaphragmatic activity, obstruction of the airway can occur (Sherrey & Megirian, 1980; Waldbaum, Hadziefendic, Erokwu, Zaidi, & Haxhiu, 2001) (Figures 2–11 and 2–12).

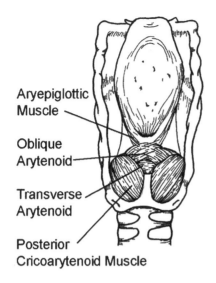

Aryepiglottic Muscle

Oblique Arytenoid

Transverse Arytenoid

Posterior Cricoarytenoid Muscle

Figure 2–11. Posterior cricoarytenoid muscle.

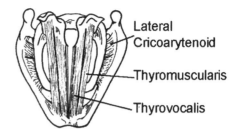

Lateral Cricoarytenoid

Thyromuscularis

Thyrovocalis

Figure 2–13. Lateral cricoarytenoid muscle.

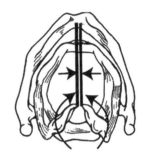

Figure 2–14. Vocal fold movement associated with lateral cricoarytenoid contraction.

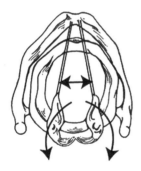

Figure 2–12. Vocal fold movement associated with posterior cricoarytenoid contraction.

Lateral Cricoarytenoid

Shaped like a fan, the lateral cricoarytenoid muscle (LCA) has its origin on the upper border of the anterolateral arch of the cricoid cartilage. It courses upward and backward to insert into the muscular process of arytenoid cartilage. Upon contraction it adducts the vocal fold by moving the muscular process posterolaterally and the vocal process medially (Figures 2–13 and 2–14).

The Cricothyroid Muscle.

The cricothyroid muscle (CT) has its origin in the anterolateral arch of the cricoid cartilage and its fibers course vertically upward to insert into the lower margin of the thyroid lamina. There are two sections of the cricothyroid muscle belly, called the pars recta and pars oblique. Hong, Kim, and Kim (2001), from electromyographic study of the cricothyroid muscles, found that during speech the combined activities of the pars recta and pars oblique are central in the adjustment of the vocal fold length by pulling downward and forward on the thyroid cartilage (Figures 2–15 and 2–16).

Arytenoid Muscles/Arytenoideus/ Interarytenoids

There are two sets of interarytenoid muscles, the oblique fibers and the transverse fibers.

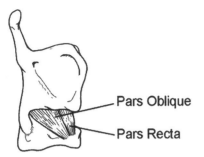

Pars Oblique

Pars Recta

Figure 2–15. Cricothyroid muscle, showing two bellies of the pars recta and par oblique.

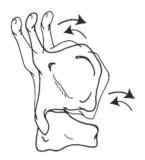

Figure 2–16. Vocal fold movement associated with cricothyroid contraction.

The oblique fibers have their origin on the posterolateral surface of the arytenoid cartilage and they course diagonally to insert near the tip of the opposite arytenoid cartilage. The transverse fibers have their origin on the lateral and posterior surface of the arytenoid cartilages and course horizonatally to insert into the lateral and posterior surface of the opposite arytenoid cartilage. When contracted, the oblique and transverse fibers adduct the vocal folds (Figure 2–17, Table 2–1).

Ventricular Vocal Folds

The ventricular (vestibular) folds or false vocal folds anatomically sit superior and lateral to the true vocal folds. They stretch from the

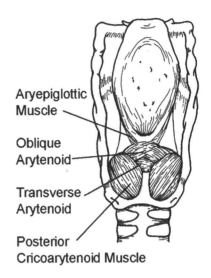

Aryepiglottic Muscle

Oblique Arytenoid

Transverse Arytenoid

Posterior Cricoarytenoid Muscle

Figure 2–17. Interarytenoid muscles (oblique and transverse).

angle of the thyroid cartilage, just below the attachment of the epiglottis to the arytenoid cartilages, attaching onto the anterolateral surface, a short distance above the vocal process.

The ventricular folds are composed of seromucous glands and a truly complex layer of fibroelastic and adipose tissue and predominantly fast-twitch oxidative glycolytic muscle fibers, meaning that they are resistant to fatigue and use an aerobic metabolism. The ventricular folds play a major role in preventing invasion of pathogenic agents onto the true vocal folds and serve as an important level of airway protection during swallowing (Kutta, Steven, Kohla, Tillman, & Paulsen, 2002; Kutta, Steven, Veroga, & Paulsen, 2004). Ultrastructural analysis of the epithelial layer shows ciliated cells and gland duct openings on the surface. Between the ventricular vocal folds and true vocal folds is a recess or space called the ventricle. The ventricle leads upward to an appendage or sac called the saccule and there exist secretory cells that provide secretion to moisten the vocal folds. Cysts can form in the saccule (Figure 2–18).

Table 2–1. Summary of the Intrinsic Laryngeal Muscles' Function

Muscle	*Abduction*	*Adduction*	*Length*	*Tension*	*Relaxation*
Cricothryoid			Increase	X	
Lateral cricoarytenoid		X	Decrease		
Oblique arytenoid		X			
Posterior cricoarytenoid	X				
Thyromuscularis			Decrease		X
Thyrovocalis		X	Decrease	X when acting in tandem as an antagonist to cricothyroid	
Transverse arytenoid		X			

Abduction: opening of the vocal folds.
Adduction: closing of the vocal folds.
Tension: increasing vocal fold length and stiffness.
Relaxation: decreasing vocal fold stiffness.

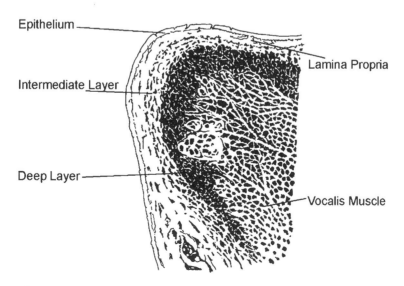

Figure 2–18. Histologic layers, as seen from a cross-section of the vocal fold mid-portion.

33

Did you know that the ventricular vocal folds can regenerate completely if surgically removed?

What Are the Vocal Folds Made of, Exactly?

The true vocal folds are made up of a unique combination of connective tissue, epithelium and muscle with each layer providing an essential biomechanical property to allow for optimal vocal fold vibration. Dr. Minoru Hirano, described the unique anatomic multilayered characteristics of the vocal folds (Hirano, 1966). Appreciation of the layered structure is critical for understanding the effects of vocal fold lesions on tissue viscoelascity, healing of the vocal fold mucosa after phonomicrosurgery, and, finally, appreciation of the complex dynamics of vocal fold vibration.

The five layers originally proposed by Hirano include the following.

Epithelium

The epithelium, which may be found in other parts of the body, is a thin covering (100–180 μm) of the vocal folds, protecting them from their intrinsic and extrinsic environment. As such, the vocal fold epithelium provides an important barrier function. The epithelium is composed of stratified squamous cells which are flat or plate-like in shape. At the outermost edge of the cell membrane are microvilli and microridges of various patterns, which contribute to the distribution and retention of mucus on the vocal fold. These microridges may also increase the absorbance of oxygen and nutrients and facilitate the movement of water and molecules across the cell surface. Individual epithelial cells are joined together

at the junctional complex. These junctional complexes are made up of proteins refereed to as "tight junction proteins" and are responsible for creating and maintaining the integrity of the physical barrier. Tight junction proteins may also have an important role in protecting the underlying mucosa from the mechanical stresses that occur during vocal fold vibration (Rousseau, Suehiro, Echemendia, & Sivasankar, 2011). Considering the repeated trauma that the vocal folds are exposed to during human voice production, disruption of the epithelium and epithelial barrier integrity may play a significant role in the development of vocal fold pathology.

Superficial Layer of the Lamina Propria

The superficial layer of the lamina propria, also referred to as Reinke's space, is made up of a loose network of connective tissue. The superficial layer contains very few fibrous proteins and interstitial elements (Butler, Hammond, & Gray, 2001; Ward, Thibeault, & Gray, 2002). This unique composition allows the superficial layer to move freely over the denser underlying connective tissue layers during vocal fold vibration. The collagens and elastic fibers contribute to tissue strength and flexibility. These fibrous proteins provide the lamina propria with structural support. Hammond et al. (1997) found that the superficial layer of the lamina propria contained very few of the large elastic fibers compared to the deeper layers of the lamina propria. Elastic fibers are easily stretched and deformed but when moved away from their resting position can easily recover their original size and shape. The interstitial elements of the lamina propria are comprised of proteoglycans and glycoproteins. These tissue components are primarily responsible for regulating tissue and cellular functions. For example, hyaluronic acid (HA), or hyaluronan, is a ubiquitous glycosamino-glycan found throughout the lamina propria. Hyaluronic acid serves an important space filling function in the lamina propria, occupying the spaces between fibrous tissue elements and providing "shock absorption." (Butler, Hammond, & Gray, 2001; Ward, Thibeault, & Gray, 2002). Hyaluronic acid also contributes significantly to the superficial layer's biomechanical properties (Chan, Gray, & Titze, 2001). The superficial layer of the lamina propria and epithelium are commonly referred to as the "cover" (Hirano, 1981). Together, these tissues are most markedly involved during vocal fold vibration (Finck, 2005).

Intermediate Layer of the Lamina Propria

The intermediate layer of the lamina propria is composed mostly of elastic fibers and hyaluronic acid. The elastic fibers run parallel to the vibrating free edge of the vocal fold. The intermediate layer is chiefly made up of mature elastic fibers (Hahn, Kobler, Starcher, Zeitels, & Langer, 2006). The distinction between the intermediate layer and superficial layer is that unlike the superficial layer which contains sparse elastin and hyaluronic acid, the intermediate layer of the human vocal fold stains richly for elastin and hyaluronic acid (Hahn, Kobler, Starcher, Zeitels, & Langer, 2006).

Deep Layer of the Lamina Propria

The deep layer of the lamina propria is abundant in collagenous fibers. The collagen fibers are arranged in a "wicker basket" like pattern and run parallel to the vibrating free edge of the vocal fold (Madruga de Melo, Lemos, Filho, et al., 2003). Interestingly, collagen constitutes approximately 43% of total protein in the human vocal fold, which is much lower than human dermis, where collagen constitutes nearly 70% of total protein. (Goldsmith, 1991; Hahn, Kobler, Zeitels, & Langer, 2006). Studies have demonstrated age and gender related differences in the deposition of vocal fold collagen. Adult and geriatric vocal folds have a higher average concentration of collagen compared to infant vocal folds; adult males have a higher average concentration of vocal fold collagen compared to adult women; adult women have a higher average concentration of vocal fold collagen compared to geriatric women; and geriatric men have a higher average concentration of vocal fold collagen compared to geriatric women (Hammond, Gray, & Butler, 2000). Albeit present in the deep layer of the human vocal fold, average concentrations of elastin and hyaluronic acid are less dense relative to concentrations of these same substances in the intermediate layer (Hahn, Kobler, Starcher, Zeitels, & Langer, 2006).

Thyrovocalis Muscle

The thyrovocalis muscle, which is the most medial portion of the thyroarytenoid muscle, makes up the bulk of the vocal fold structure.

Vocal Fold Ligament

The intermediate and deep layers of the lamina propria form the vocal ligament. The vocal ligament is rich in fibrous tissue components. The dense distribution of elastic fibers and collagen subtypes I and III distinguish the vocal ligament from the overlying vocal fold cover (superficial layer of the lamina propria and epithelium). This unique arrangement of fibrous tissue proteins comprising the stiffer vocal fold ligament provides a truly unique structure. This highly specialized tissue unlike any other in the body allows for vibration capable of generating sound and musically useful pitches from roughly 80 to 1100 Hz.

Vocal Fold Architecture

More detail about the architecture of the vocal fold has been gained over the last 20 years or so by the profound work of Dr. Steven Gray and colleagues. Dr. Gray revealed the presence of the basement membrane zone between the epithelium and the superficial layer of the lamina propria, which appears to anchor or secure basal cells to the superficial layer of the lamina propria (see also Thibeault & Gray [2004]). The basement membrane zone or BMZ is considered the junction between the epithelial layer and lamina propria. As Thibeault and Gray (2004) explained, the BMZ is a complex layer of proteins. The BMZ does not have capillaries or blood vessels. Therefore, if bleeding occurs in the vocal fold layer, it implies injury to the superficial layer of the lamina propria.

There are several collagen subtypes in the human vocal folds and by analyzing the different features of these subtypes from human cadaveric specimens it was found that types I, III, IV, and V, as well as elastin exists. Type III is distributed throughout the whole lamina propria, helping to maintain its structure. Type I is found just below the basal membrane of the epithelium, the deep layer of the lamina propria, and in the anterior and posterior maculae flava, providing increased tensile strength to help withstand the vibratory forces during voice production.

> Maculae flavae are dense tissues at the anterior and posterior ends of the membranous vocal fold. The maculae flavae are rich in cells and extracellular matrix components.

Collagen subtypes IV and V are found in the epithelium. In the BMZ there are several proteins that facilitate attachment of the epithelium to the underlying lamina propria. This includes Collagen Type IV which is a tough layer of collagen and makes up the anchoring filaments. Type VIII makes up the anchoring fibers which loop into the superficial layer of the lamina propria and attach to the lamina densa.

The epithelium, BMZ, and lamina propria all have specific roles in oscillating tissue. The vocal folds are comprised of three predominant cell types: fibroblasts, myofibroblasts, and macrophages. These cells are present in varying concentrations throughout the human vocal fold and play an important role in maintenance of the vocal fold layers and protection of the vocal fold from injury (Catten, Gray, Hammond, Zhou, & Hammond, 1998). A thorough understanding of the composition of the vocal fold ECM and tissue layered structure is important for selection of the best available options for surgical reconstruction and the most suitable therapeutic candidates for replacement and repair of vocal fold defects.

> Interstitial proteins are important in wound repair, The interstitial proteins include proteoglycans, glycosaminoglycans and structural glycoproteins.

The Extracellular Matrix (ECM)

The vocal fold ECM is made up of a number of important molecules that contribute to tissue characteristics during oscillation. The superficial, intermediate and deep layers of the vocal fold lamina propria are comprised of various ECM components including elastin, decorin, fibronectin, hyaluronic acid, laminin, and the collagen types referred to above, types I, III, and IV. Fibronectin is an interstitial glycoprotein found in abundance in the vocal fold lamina propria. Fibronectin plays an important role in cell adhesion, angiogenesis, and cell migration, thus it is particularly dense in embryonic, healing and regenerating tissues (Hirschi, Gray, & Thibeault, 2002). Healing of the damaged vocal fold ECM involves a complex interplay of cells, extracellular matrix substances, and soluble growth factors (Branski, Rosen, Verdolini, & Hebda, 2005; Ling, Yamashita, Waselchuk, Raasch, Bless, & Welham, 2009; Rousseau, Ge, Ohno, French, & Thibeault, 2008; Thibeault, Rousseau, Welham, Hirano, & Bless, 2004).

The healing of post-natal wounds is most commonly characterized by a dense and poorly reconstructed ECM (Martin, 1997). The end product of vocal fold wound healing is often scar formation, which can result in poor viscoelastic tissue properties and functional voice outcomes (Rousseau, Sohn, Montequin, Tateya, & Bless, 2004; Thibeault, Gray, Bless, Chan, & Ford, 2002). This has led to the application of tissue engineering techniques, such as the use of decellularized ECM scaffolds to repair laryngeal tissue defects (Ringel, Kahane, Hillsamer, Lee, & Badylak, 2006). These techniques have shown great promise. Manipulation of the vocal fold using ECM derived hydrogels and other candidate agents has also been shown to be useful in the treatment of vocal fold injuries and glottal insufficiency (Jia et al., 2006; Lim, Kim, Kim, Kim, & Choi, 2008; Perazzo, Duprat Ade, Lacelotti, & Donati, 2007).

Hyaluronic Acid (HA)

HA is a ubiquitous glycoaminoglycan found throughout connective, epithelial and neural tissues. Interestingly, HA is the most promi-nent ECM substance found in regenerating fetal wounds, which heal scarlessly. HA is particularly abundant in the intermediate layer of the human vocal fold lamina propria. Selective removal of HA from the human vocal fold cover impairs tissue biomechanical properties, leading to a significant decrease in tissue elasticity or stiffness, and a significant increase in tissue viscosity (Chan, Gray, & Titze, 2001). HA levels are significantly decreased during acute vocal fold injury (Rousseau, Sohn, Montequin, Tateya, & Bless, 2004; Thibeault, Rousseau, Welham, Hirano, & Bless, 2004) Reduced HA levels are associated with increased phonation threshold pressure (i.e., the minimum pressure needed to sustain vocal fold oscillation) and decreased vocal economy (Rousseau, Sohn, Montequin, Tateya, & Bless, 2004). These findings provide support for the theory that reduced vocal fold HA may lead to less than optimal biomechanical properties for phonation. These data also appear to provide a rationale for maintaining HA levels in the vocal fold during acute wound healing to lessen the impact of scar formation on clinically relevant measures of phonation (Rousseau, Sohn, Montequin, Tateya, & Bless, 2004).

Several studies have reported gender differences in the concentration of HA in the human vocal fold. Hammond et al. (1997) reported a threefold increase in the amount of HA in male vocal folds compared to female vocal folds (Hammond, Zhou, Hammond, Pawlak, & Gray, 1997). Butler et al (2001) corroborated these findings, demonstrating a nearly twofold difference in ECM HA in the superficial layer of the female vocal fold compared to the male vocal fold. Specifically, ECM HA in the superficial layer of the male vocal fold was higher than HA in the female vocal fold (Butler, Hammond, & Gray, 2001). In contrast, Lebl et al. (2007) found that the average concentration of HA in the female vocal fold was twice as high as HA in the male vocal fold. Although conflicting, the results of these studies suggest that there are likely gender related differences in the concentration of HA in the human vocal fold. These differences may help to explain clinically observed disparities in the incidence of vocal pathology between men and women.

> An age-dependent slowing down of extracellular matrix turnover appears to be a hallmark feature associated with aging of the vocal fold lamina propria (Ding & Gray, 2001a, 2001b; Ohno, Hirano, & Rousseau, 2009).

Extrinsic Laryngeal Muscles

Table 2–2 summarizes the origins, insertions, and innervation of the extrinsic laryngeal muscles, which include the suprahyoid and infrahyoid muscles. When a muscle contracts, it shortens and the structure where the muscle inserts into moves closer to the structure of the muscle's origin; thus, there are two primary functions of the extrinsic muscles. The first function of the extrinsic laryngeal muscles is to elevate the larynx within the vocal tract. This is done by the action of the suprahyoid extrinsic muscles.

The suprahyoid muscles elevate the hyoid bone and larynx primarily with their other functions serving jaw movement. Laryngeal elevation occurs during swallowing and some singing tasks, helping to manipulate vocal pitch along with cricothyroid activity (Roubeau, Chevrie-Muller, & Lacau Saint Guily, 1997). The second function of the extrinsic laryngeal muscles is to accomplish laryngeal depression. The infrahyoid extrinsic muscles accomplish this task. Laryngeal depression occurs during some singing tasks and inspiration. Finally, the extrinsic laryngeal muscles support the position of the larynx in the neck

so that the intrinsic laryngeal muscles can apply their forces on the laryngeal cartilages (Figures 2–19 and 2–20).

Suprahyoid Muscles

Digrastric Muscle

The digastric has two muscular bellies (anterior and posterior), which are joined by an intermediate tendon. Acting like one muscle, the paired digastric muscles either elevate the hyoid bone or depress the mandible. In elevating the hyoid bone, the anterior belly pulls the hyoid forward and upward and the posterior belly pulls the hyoid back and upward.

Mylohyoid

A flat, triangular muscle located on the underside of the chin, the mylohyoid helps form the muscular floor of the mouth. When the mylohyoid muscle contracts it elevates the floor of the mouth and tongue and depresses the jaw as long as the hyoid is stabilized.

Geniohyoid

The geniohyoid muscle is a narrow muscle arising from the inferior mental spine of the mandible to the front surface of the hyoid bone. When contracted, the geniohyoid elevates the hyoid bone, raises the floor of the mouth for swallowing and depresses the mandible when the hyoid is stabilized.

Stylohyoid

The stylohyoid originates from the styloid process of the temporal bone and inserts into the body of the hyoid bone. When contracted, the stylohyoid muscle pulls the hyoid upward and back and during swallowing fixes the hyoid bone for infrahyoid action.

Table 2–2. Origins, Insertion, and Innervation for the Supra and Infrahyoid Muscles of the Larynx

	Origin	*Insertion*	*Innervation*
SUPRAHYOID			
Anterior Belly of Digrastric	Lower border of the mandible	Intermediate tendon	CN V: Trigeminal nerve
Geniohyoid	Mandibular symphysis of mandible	Anterior surface of the hyoid body	A branch of cervical nerve 1 (ansa cervicalis) through hypoglossal
Mylohyoid	Inner surface of the mandible	Fibers cross to the midline raphe which extends to the hyoid body	CN V: Trigeminal nerve
Posterior Belly of Digrastric	Mastoid process	Intermediate tendon connecting to the hyoid bone	CN VII: Facial nerve
Stylohyoid	Styloid process of the temporal bone	Body of the hyoid	CN VII: Facial nerve
INFRAHYOID			
Omohyoid	Inferior belly: surface of the scapula	Inferior belly: intermediate tendon extending to the hyoid bone	CN C1–C3: through ansa cervicalis
	Superior belly: intermediate tendon extending to the hyoid bone	Superior belly: greater horn of the hyoid	CN C1–C3: through ansa cervicalis
Sternohyoid	Manubrium and end of the clavicle	Hyoid body	CN C1–C3: through ansa cervicalis
Sternothyroid	Manubrium and costal cartilage of the first rib	Oblique line of the thyroid cartilage	CN C1–C3: through ansa cervicalis
Thyrohyoid	Oblique line of the thyroid lamina	Greater horn of the hyoid bone	CN C1: through Hypoglossal

C1–C3 = Cervical vertebrae

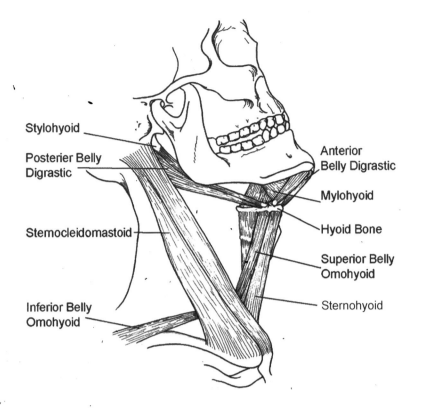

Figure 2–19. Lateral view of extrinsic muscle complex showing individual extrinsic laryngeal muscles.

Stylohyoid

Posterier Belly Digrastic

Stemocleidomastoid

Inferior Belly Omohyoid

Anterior Belly Digrastic

Mylohyoid

Hyoid Bone

Superior Belly Omohyoid

Sternohyoid

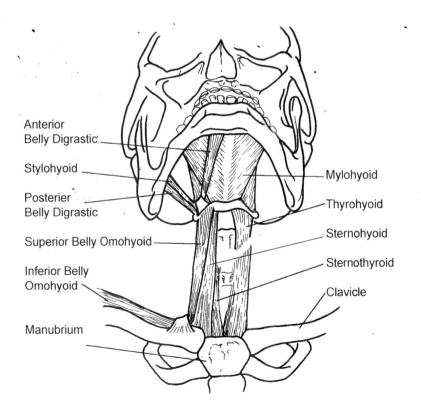

Figure 2–20. Anterior view of suprahyoid and infrahyoid muscle complex.

Anterior Belly Digrastic

Stylohyoid

Posterier Belly Digrastic

Superior Belly Omohyoid

Inferior Belly Omohyoid

Manubrium

Mylohyoid

Thyrohyoid

Sternohyoid

Sternothyroid

Clavicle

> The suprahyoid muscle complex is often implicated in extrinsic laryngeal muscular tension in patients with voice disorders (Aronson, 2004).

Infrahyoid Muscles

The infrahyoid muscles primarily depress the hyoid and larynx with its other functions serving jaw movement. These muscles include the following.

Sternohyoid

The sternohyoid attaches the hyoid bone to the sternum. When the sternohyoid muscle contracts it depresses the hyoid bone and therefore the larynx.

Sternothyroid

The sternothyroid muscle is beneath the sternohyoid, originates from the manubrium of the sternum and inserts into the oblique line of the thyroid cartilage. When the sternothyroid muscle contracts it depresses the larynx.

Omohyoid

The omohyoid muscle is at the front of the neck and consists of two bellies separated by an intermediate tendon. When the omohyoid muscle contracts, its action depresses the hyoid bone and as a result, it depresses the larynx.

Thyrohyoid

This muscle is actually a continuation of the sternothyroid muscle. It originates from the oblique line on the thyroid lamina and inserts into the greater cornu of the hyoid bone. When the thyrohyoid muscle contracts it moves the hyoid bone closer to the larynx.

Laryngeal Ligaments and Membranes

Other aspects of the laryngeal structure are the membranes and ligaments which hold the laryngeal cartilages together, forming slings for movement in both the superior and inferior direction. The ligaments and membranes are divided into extrinsic and intrinsic categories. As stated earlier, ligaments serve to attach bone to bone or cartilage to bone, in this case. Ligaments also help with range of joint motion (Figure 2–21).

Mucous Membrane

The mucous membrane of the larynx is a continuation of the mucous membrane from the trachea inferiorly and the membrane of the mouth superiorly. It is made up of two types of epithelium, columnar and squamous. It is the squamous type that covers the true and false vocal folds and appears to be the most common location for the origin of laryngeal cancer (see Chapters 5 and 11).

Extrinsic Membranes

The extrinsic laryngeal membranes connect the laryngeal cartilages to structures outside of the larynx providing anatomic support of the larynx.

Thyrohyoid Membrane

The thyrohyoid membrane is a broad, unpaired, fibroelastic membrane that extends from the superior border of the thyroid cartilage lamina, extending to front of its superior cornu, to the superior margin of the body and

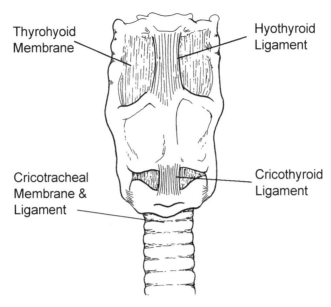

Figure 2–21. Anterior view of laryngeal framework showing primary ligamentous and membranous structures.

greater cornu of the hyoid bone. The thicker part is referred to as the median thyrohyoid ligament. The posterior borders of the thyrohyoid membrane are called the lateral thyrohyoid ligaments and extend from the tips of the superior thyroid cornu to the posterior ends of the greater hyoid cornu. There is an opening in the lateral aspect of the membrane to allow passage of the internal laryngeal nerve and artery.

The thyroepiglottic membrane appears to fill in the space between the hyoid bone and the thyroid cartilage. The cricotracheal membrane extends from the inferior border of the cricoid cartilage to the first tracheal ring.

The cricotracheal membrane is the site perforated for entrance for tracheostomy as there are no major blood vessels in this membrane and less chance for the development of edema or stenosis (narrowing of space).

Intrinsic Membranes

The intrinsic laryngeal membranes connect laryngeal cartilages and help to control cartilaginous movement.

Quadrangular Membrane

The quadrangular membrane is paired and lies just above the laryngeal ventricle (recall the ventricle is the space between the true vocal folds and the ventricular folds). The membrane thickens along its inferior edge forming ligaments known as the vestibular ligaments. The front portion of the ligament attaches to the epiglottis and the back portion of the ligament attaches to the lateral margin of the arytenoid and corniculate cartilages. The free upper portion of the ligament is underneath the mucosa of the aryepiglottic fold and helps form the aryepiglottic fold structure. The free inferior borders of the quadrangular membrane forms the structure of the ventricular vocal folds as the ventricular ligament.

Conus Elasticus

The conus elasticus is a submucous elastic membrane attached to the upper margin of the cricoid cartilage and connects the cricoid cartilage with the thyroid and arytenoid cartilages. Described as having two parts, the medial cricothryoid ligament connects the anterior part of the cricoid arch with the inferior border of the thyroid membrane. The lateral cricothyroid membrane comes from the superior surface of the cricoid arch and connects with the vocal process of the arytenoid cartilage. Its thickened upper margin forms the vocal ligament.

Ligaments

The vocal ligament is an elastic band of connective tissue located in the vocal fold. It attaches to the inner surface of the thyroid cartilage at the level of the thyroid angle, and to the vocal process of the arytenoid cartilage.

- The thyroepiglottic ligament attaches the epiglottis to the thyroid cartilage at the level of the thyroid angle.
- The hyoepiglottic ligament attaches the lower part of the anterior surface of the epiglottis to the body of the hyoid bone.
- The ventricular ligament is above and parallel to the vocal ligament and is part of the ventricular fold.

The cricothyroid ligament has two sections, a lateral and medial section. The median cricothyroid ligament joins the cricoid and thyroid ligaments together and the lateral section is known as the cricothyroid membrane (also known as the conus elasticus). Important to note is that the edge of the cricothryoid ligament is the vocal ligament. The anterior part or middle cricothyroid ligament is thick and strong. It connects together the front parts of the adjoining margins of the thyroid and cricoid cartilages. The lateral portions are thin and lie close under the mucous membrane of the larynx; they extend from the superior border of the cricoid cartilage to the inferior margin of the vocal ligaments, with which they are continuous.

Aryepiglottic Folds

The aryepiglottic folds extend bilaterally between the arytenoid cartilages and the lateral margin of the epiglottis and serve as a lateral anatomic border of the laryngeal space. The aryepiglottic folds consist of the corniculate and cuneiform cartilages, as well as numerous groups of mucous glands (Reidenbach, 1997). The aryepiglottic folds are pliable enough to allow their movement inward during swallow but yet stiff enough to withstand collapse during inspiration.

Cavities

The cavity of the larynx has as its boundaries the epiglottis, the aryepiglottic folds and the apexes of the arytenoids cartilages posteriorly. The most glottal opening, as previously defined, is the space between the vocal folds. The anterior glottal space is the anterior commissure. The space between the arytenoid cartilages is the posterior commissure. The supraglottal space within the laryngeal cavity is the ventricle. The space below the glottis is referred to as the subglottis.

Arterial Supply of the Larynx

The arterial supply to the larynx comes from a variety of local vessels. Extending from the external carotid artery is the superior thyroid artery that supplies the pharynx, larynx, and upper esophagus. The superior thyroid artery also supplies the thyroid gland. The ascending pharyngeal artery also arises from the external carotid artery to supply the lower pharynx and larynx (Figure 2–22).

> The thyroid gland should not be confused with the thyroid cartilage. The thyroid gland functions as one of the endocrine glands, which makes the thyroid hormone to regulate physiologic functions in your body. It is located in the middle of the lower neck, below the larynx (see Figure 2–22).

The inferior thyroid artery arises from the thyrocervical trunk (a branch of the subclavian artery), passes posterior to the carotid sheath, and supplies the inferior portion of the corresponding lobe of the thyroid gland; its branches can course anterior or posterior to or between branches of the recurrent laryngeal nerve.

> Often intra-arterial chemotherapy for laryngeal cancer is accomplished via the superior thyroid artery.

Laryngeal Nerve Supply

The function of the intrinsic laryngeal muscles is accomplished by bilateral innervation from peripheral nerves that extend from cranial nerve 10, the vagus. The vagus is the longest of the 12 cranial nerves that originate from

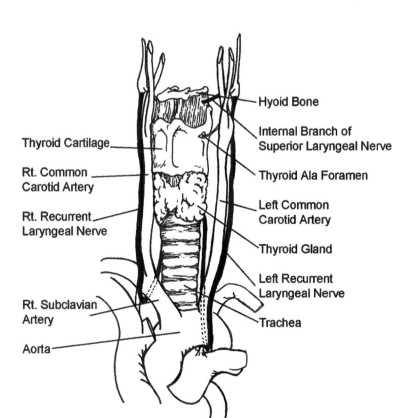

Thyroid Cartilage

Rt. Common Carotid Artery

Rt. Recurrent Laryngeal Nerve

Rt. Subclavian Artery

Aorta

Hyoid Bone

Internal Branch of Superior Laryngeal Nerve

Thyroid Ala Foramen

Left Common Carotid Artery

Thyroid Gland

Left Recurrent Laryngeal Nerve

Trachea

Figure 2–22. Depiction of laryngeal blood supply, laryngeal nerve supply, and location of thyroid gland.

the brainstem. Although the vagus nerve carries sensory information from various organs and structures, it is the motor component that moves the laryngeal muscles. The motor component of the vagus nerve originates in the medulla of the brainstem in the nucleus ambiguus. The nucleus ambiguus gives rise to three branches, the pharyngeal branch, the recurrent laryngeal branch, and the superior laryngeal branch. Two small branches from the superior laryngeal nerve that exists; the internal and external branches. All muscles of the larynx are controlled by right and left-sided branches of each of the nerves described below. For example there is a right recurrent laryngeal nerve and a left recurrent laryngeal nerve, and so forth (see Figure 2–22).

The Recurrent Laryngeal Nerve

The recurrent laryngeal nerves supply the motor control or function to all of the intrinsic laryngeal muscles except the cricothyroid muscle. The recurrent laryngeal nerve is often referred to as the RLN. The RLN divides into anterior and posterior branches. The right sided recurrent branch leaves the vagus nerve just in front of the subclavian artery. It wraps back around the artery and travels up posteriorly into a groove between the trachea and esophagus. The left recurrent branch leaves the vagus nerve on the aortic arch and loops posteriorly crossing the arch to travel up through the superior mediastinum. The anterior branch supplies the lateral cricothyroid muscles and thyroarytenoid muscles, as well as the interarytenoids, aryepiglottic, and thryoepiglottic muscles. The posterior branch supplies the posterior cricoarytenoid.

The left recurrent branch ascends along a groove between the esophagus and trachea entering into the larynx behind the thyroid and cricoid cartilages. Both recurrent branches enter the larynx just below the inferior constrictor muscles.

> The left recurrent laryngeal nerve has a long course, making it vulnerable to injury at various sites. Injury can occur during thyroidectomy surgery or after anterior entrance for cervical disk surgery or open heart surgery.

The Superior Laryngeal Nerve

The superior laryngeal nerve branches are distal to the pharyngeal branch and descend lateral to the pharynx. The superior laryngeal nerve is often referred to as the SLN. It divides into an internal and external branch. The internal branch is sensory and autonomic. It pierces the thyrohyoid membrane along with the superior laryngeal artery and supplies sensory fibers of the laryngeal mucosa, middle of the laryngeal cavity, and superior surface of the vocal folds. The external branch is motor and it travels and supplies the cricothyroid muscle.

Sensation from the Larynx

The laryngeal mucosa contains some of the densest concentrations of sensory receptors in the human body (Sanders & Mu, 1998). Laryngeal sensation (afferent) from the supraglottic areas travels via the intrinsic branch of the SLN. The intrinsic branch of the SLN has three divisions, the superior, middle, and inferior divisions. The superior division senses information from the mucosa of the epiglottis, the middle division senses information from the mucosa of the true and ventricular vocal folds, and the aryepiglottic folds and the inferior division senses information from the mucosa of the arytenoids, subglottis, anterior wall of the hypopharynx, and the upper esophageal sphincter. Research shows that the most sensitive areas of the larynx include the epiglottis, the true and false vocal folds, and the arytenoid region (Sanders & Mu,

1998). Rather than being classified based on their location within the larynx, the receptors are classified based on their function. There are receptors that respond to airflow, pressure, and motion. Laryngeal sensation is important for the reflexive functions of swallow and cough and its testing can help with understanding the degeneration of laryngeal function associated with certain diseases, like Parkinson's disease, amyotrophic lateral sclerosis, and stroke (Amin et al., 2006; Aviv et al., 1997) and for testing response in patients with unilateral vocal fold immobility (Tabaee, Murry, Zschommler, & Desloge, 2005). Testing laryngeal sensation in patient groups is relatively easy with available equipment. One way in which laryngeal sensation is tested is by using calibrated air puffs applied to the region of the aryepiglottic folds near the muscular attachment on the arytenoid cartilage (Aviv et al., 1998).

The recurrent laryngeal nerve is responsible for sensation from the subglottic region which is a region below the vocal fold level. Mostly known for its motor function, the RLN's role in sensation should not go overlooked, particularly for its role in sensory innervation from the subglottal region.

The next section describes the main anatomic differences between pediatrics and adults and males and females that contribute to the functional voice differences between the groups.

Laryngeal Development (Infancy to Adulthood)

Around the fourth or fifth week of fetal development the laryngotracheal sulcus appears and there are thearytenoids of the larynx become definite. In the third month of fetal development the thyroid lamina fuse and the laryngeal ventricle appears between the true and false vocal folds. By the 24th week, the maculae flavae are identified as are the fetal vocal folds. Interestingly, by the second trimester diaphragmatic and laryngeal movements can be identified and the coordination between the respiratory and laryngeal systems is apparent.

It is obvious that the size of the laryngeal anatomy is smaller in a newborn child versus an adult (adult being defined as postpubescent).

> The vocal folds are complete, and the baby can and does sometimes cry silently by the 12th week of fetal development.

The anteroposterior dimensions as well as the transverse dimensions of the larynx are similar across the developmental span until about 13 years of age (Litman, Weissend, Shibata, & Westesson, 2003). In newborns, the length of the vocal fold is 2.5 to 3.0 mm with continual linear growth as a function of age. The membranous portion of the vocal fold comprises less of the total vocal fold length in comparison to the adult. Furthermore, the cartilaginous glottis accounts for 60 to 75% of the vocal folds' length in children below two years of age. The reason for the larger posterior glottis in infants and young children is that it aids the feeding and breathing process. Histologic differences also exist in the vocal fold with a thinner vocal fold mucosa in newborns and young children, with the ratio of the mucosa to the length of the membranous portion of the vocal fold greater as compared to the adult structure. Furthermore, the layered structure of the vocal folds is not differentiated in newborns and young children; the lamina propria is very uniform in structure. In adults, there is clear differentiation between the superficial, intermediate, and deep layers of the lamina propria as described earlier. There is no ligamentous structure in newborns, with an immature vocal ligament emerging between the age of 1 and 4 years (Hirano, Kurita, & Nakashima, 1981). The vocal ligament continues in its immaturity until after puberty, which can range from age 10 until 16 years of age depending on the child's sex. Additional histological distinctions include a greater percentage of collagen in the pediatric vocal fold muscle and less dense anterior and posterior macula flava fibers, which implies less anchoring strength of the laryngeal structures (Hirano et al., 1981). Moreover, the subglottal space in pediatric patients is the narrowest part and least pliable of the airway in comparison to the adult airway, with the full-term infant diameter of the subglottal space cited as 4 mm.

There is no appearance of sex differences in vocal fold length until sometime between 9 and 15 years of age. As mentioned earlier, the adult vocal fold length is approximately 17 to 21 mm in adult males and 11 to 15 mm in adult females (Hirano et al., 1981). Both sexes reach full maturity of their vocal fold size by puberty but the male vocal folds increase by over two times that of the female during this important growth and development period (Kahane, 1978).

The change in the larynx with puberty in males is quite dramatic. Puberty starts in males because of an increase in the hormone testosterone resulting in a greater overall skeletal growth in boys in comparison to females. In addition to the many other physical changes that occur to males during puberty, the increased testosterone results in thickening of the laryngeal cartilages and vocal fold growth. This is why the voice begins to lower and crack in boys as it transitions through this growth period.

Further distinctions are that the pediatric larynx maintains a higher laryngeal position between the first and third cervical level in comparison to an adult's laryngeal position, which continues to lower with advancing age, with the lower border of the cricoid cartilage hovering between the sixth and seventh cervical vertebrae (Hudgins, Siegel, Jacobs, & Abramowski, 1997). Also, in the pediatric larynx, the laryngeal framework descends into the neck with growth and elongates the oropharynx and hypopharynx, taking it from a conical shape to a more cylindrical contour. With development, laryngeal-pharyngeal widening occurs along with an increased diameter of the cricoid cartilage and expansion of the alar wings of the thyroid cartilage.

The epiglottis is omega-shaped in approximately 50% of the pediatric population and it is soft and pliable. It is often in direct contact with the soft palate and tongue base, particularly in infants.

Furthermore, the cricoid ring is the only portion of the airway that is surrounded completely by cartilage. It is this area that is most susceptible to the development of laryngeal trauma and laryngeal stenosis (Wiatrak, 2000). Finally, there is little calcification to the pediatric laryngeal cartilages. The whole laryngeal framework in children is much softer than in adults, which makes it less susceptible to blunt trauma but developed during breathing. The pliability of the young larynx, along with edema (swelling) can create substantial airway limitation. For example, 1 mm of edema can limit the subglottic space by more than 60%.

In the immature larynx, there is no vertical prominence in the thyroid cartilage. The presence of the thyroid prominence does not occur until substantial changes happen in vocal fold length (approximately between the ages of 10 and 14 years). The thyroid cartilage does not assume its adult configuration until adolescence. The cricothyroid membrane is a slit rather than a palpable space. Figure 2–23 shows a posterior view of the larynx depicting the cartilaginous framework of an immature versus mature structure. Note that the hyoid cartilage assumes a much lower anatomic position and actually overlaps the thyroid cartilage. The arytenoids are proportionally larger as compared to the other laryngeal structures.

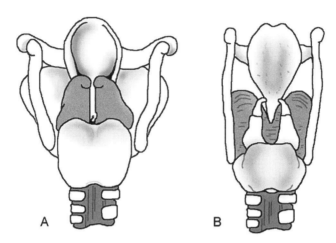

Figure 2–23. Posterior view of immature laryngeal structure (**A**) and mature laryngeal structure (**B**).

The posterior glottis plays important respiratory and protective functions during this age as described above (Hirano et al., 1981). Because of these anatomic distinctions, the internal examination of the larynx is unlike an adult's. As well, the external examination of the larynx and anatomical landmarks are distinctly unique in children.

Figure 2–23 also depicts the furled epiglottis and proportionately larger arytenoids in the pediatric larynx. The large arytenoids, the shape of the epiglottis, as well as large aryepiglottis folds may obscure the view of the true vocal folds and glottis during laryngoscopic examination. Furthermore, the pediatric vocal folds also have a downward slant from posterior to anterior, which is a characteristic not found in the adult.

Adult Male and Female Differences in Laryngeal Anatomy

Human laryngeal anatomy differs between the sexes on a variety of different levels, which include distinctions in cartilaginous size and vocal fold dimensions. And, as discussed previously, these differences are due to the increased testosterone that occurs during puberty in males. A recap of the most apparent differences between men and women is that men have:

- a larger thyroid lamina
- a more acute thyroid angle, giving prominence to the thyroid notch or larger "Adam's apple"
- thicker vocal folds
- larger glottal space

The larger and more massive vocal folds in men are responsible for the lower pitch production as compared to women. Women tend to have a larger posterior cartilaginous space then men which seems to be related to distinctions in anatomy rather than function but might, in fact, be contributed to in part by the way women use their voices culturally, with a softer more feminine presentation of voice, creating a larger glottal space and breathier voice quality. The open phase within a vibratory cycle is typically longer in women. If the glottis is open longer than typical, air is allowed to pass into the vocal tract, producing a breathy quality. One interesting study found that women had more difficulties with increasing vocal loudness when having to speak against background noise. Men were able to phonate louder than the women suggesting that women may be more susceptible to harming their voices when confronted with the need to talk loud (Sodersten, Ternstrom, & Bohman, 2005).

Age Effects on Laryngeal Anatomy

Aging causes general changes to the entire body including the skeletal and muscular systems. These changes affect the normal function of the respiratory, laryngeal, and supralaryngeal structures resulting in deterioration and alteration to voice production. Preventive measures can be taken to help slow the aging process and there is evidence, in particular, that exercise aids in reducing the changes that occur in the muscular system of the body by helping to prevent muscle wasting known as sarcopenia (Suetta, Magnusson, Beyer, & Kjaer, 2007). With age, the muscle systems can experience structural change and fatigue that reduce the muscle contractile force capability.

More evidence suggests marked vocal fold atrophy, vocal fold edema (Kendall, 2007) and reduced number of myelinated fibers in the recurrent and superior laryngeal nerves (Tiago, Pontes, & do Brasil, 2007). Other results from rat animal models indicate reduced blood flow to the larynx with age, reductions in the amount of hyaluronic acid and increased collagen content (Abdelkafy et al., 2007; Ohno, Hirano, & Rousseau, 2009). The vocal folds, upon laryngoscopic examination may appear thin with vocal fold closure incomplete because of muscle mass loss. Muscular changes along with reduced flexibil-

ity in the laryngeal joints can result in significant changes to voice production and create alterations in the vibratory pattern of the vocal folds resulting in aperiodicity. The aperiodic nature of the vocal fold vibration results in perceived voice qualities ranging from breathiness, hoarseness to roughness. Pontes, Yamasaki, and Behlau (2006) found the following parameters common for the older larynx including vocal fold bowing, prominence of the vocal process, glottic proportion, phase and amplitude symmetry of the mucosal wave, and tremor of the laryngeal structures. Presbylaryngis is the term used to refer to the changes associated with the aging larynx (see Chapter 5).

> A retrospective study by Cannito, Kahane, & Choma (2008) on vocal aging and adductor spasmodic dysphonia showed a markedly reduced positive response to botulinum toxin treatment in the older patients.

Phonation

Phonation is the production of sound. In order to produce sound the vocal folds vibrate at hundreds of times per second or at a frequency, which on average ranges from about 100 to 250 Hz for adults. During phonation, the vocal fold movement varies from a state of nearly adducted to a state of partial abduction. Each cycle per second finds the vocal folds moving through a series of events (Figure 2–24). Other functions like breathing and cough represent the opposite ends of the movement continuum with maximum inhalation requiring maximum vocal fold abduction and cough requiring complete vocal fold adduction, necessary to build high amounts of intrathoracic pressure for expulsion of foreign material.

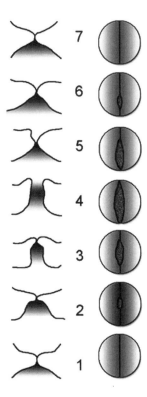

Figure 2–24. Illustration of coronal view depicting phases of one cycle of vocal fold vibration.

A hertz (Hz) is the number of vibrations which occur per second. One Hz is equal to one cycle per second. The average number of cycles produced by the adult male vocal folds is about 100 Hz, the average number for the adult female is about 200 Hz and for the young child 300 Hz.

Myoelastic Theory of Voice Production

First introduced by Muller in 1843 (van den Berg, 1958), the myoelastic aerodynamic theory of voice production described how vocal fold movement occurred. It replaced the neurochronaxic theory put forth by Husson in the 1950s which held that each cycle of vocal fold vibration occurred by a nervous impulse to the vocal fold muscle causing an impulse to create vocal fold vibration (Rubin, 1960). Given the neurophysiologic constraints of neural input (i.e., impulse rate, refractory rates, differing lengths of the right versus left recurrent laryngeal nerve, etc.), the neurochronaxic theory was deemed invalid.

The myoelastic aerodynamic theory holds that continued air pressure is developed and built up underneath the vocal folds, at an amount great enough to displace the inertial property of the vocal fold tissue and sustain the vibration of the vocal folds over time. The pressure moves the nearly adducted vocal folds laterally and because of their elastic properties, the vocal folds return to their original closed position, again offering resistance to the flow of air, creating again a high enough pressure to once more displace the vocal folds laterally. This repetitive cycle of movement is continuous. As long as the pressure is sustained and the vocal folds are healthy, vocal fold movement occurs hundreds of times per second. The aerodynamic component defined within the theory is the force of pressure and the resulting flow as the air moves through the glottal space. The Bernoulli effect is also a feature of the aerodynamic component of vocal fold movement within this theory and occurs due to the constriction in the airways as the vocal folds are returning to the adducted state via tissue elasticity. As the airway narrows, the air velocity increases, increasing the kinetic energy. In order for the Bernoulli effect to occur, potential energy must decrease if kinetic energy is increased. What happens is that the pressure exerted on the walls of the airway decreases and the vocal folds are pulled toward each other. As the glottal space narrows, the air velocity increases even more. This results in an even greater pulling force on the vocal folds with the eventual effect being vocal fold adduction as the vocal folds are sucked together. The vocal folds again move apart as the subglottal pressure is now higher underneath the vocal folds then above.

Myo—muscle contraction of the lateral cricoarytenoid and thryroarytenoid muscle which postures the vocal folds in a nearly adducted position.

Elastic—elastic properties of the vocal folds which are capable of being stretched, compressed and deformed and returning to their original shape or state.

Aerodynamic—branch of fluid dynamics concerned with the properties of airflow such as airflow velocity, air pressure, density, and so forth.

When the bottom part of the vocal folds is farther apart than the upper part of the folds it is referred to as a convergent shape because the airflow is converging. Air pressure within the glottis is high with a convergent glottal shape.

One full cycle of vocal fold vibration and the steps to this action are as follows (see Figure 2–24):

1. The initial production of sound requires activation of the intrinsic laryngeal muscles, specifically the lateral cricoarytenoid and thyroarytenoid muscles to posture the vocal folds in a position of near closure (often called vocal fold approximation).

2. In this position, the vocal folds offer enough resistance to the flow of air coming from the lower airway until the subglottal pressure in the lower airway builds to a great enough amount to displace the "adducted" vocal folds.

3. The lower border of the vocal folds separates first, followed by the upper border.

The minimum pressure amount needed to sustain vocal fold vibration is called the phonation threshold pressure (PTP) (Titze, Schmidt, & Titze, 1995). Many factors can alter PTP including hydration level, vocal skill, vocal fatigue, and sound intensity and vocal pitch as they relate to glottal diameter (Plant, 2005; Titze et al., 1995).

4. The lateral movement of the vocal folds continues and the glottal space reaches a position of maximum abduction.

5. A pressure differential occurs with the subglottal pressure below the vocal folds greater than the pressure above the vocal folds. Subsequently, the positive pressure provides enough force to separate the medial edges of the vocal folds and airflow moves upward through the glottal space.

6. The natural elasticity of the tissue causes the lower border of the vocal folds to start to return to their rest position and the vocal folds move back to their original, closed position.

7. The repositioning of the vocal folds creates a Bernoulli effect whereby a negative pressure between the vocal folds is developed. The glottal shape is divergent; the airway resistance is low with a narrower opening at the glottal entrance as compared to the glottal exit.

8. The negative air pressure causes an inward pull on the vocal folds, closing them.

9. The cycle is repeated, starting again with step 2. Only after phonation is stopped would the cycle be repeated starting with step 1.

More discussion has evolved since the introduction of the myoelastic aerodynamic theory of voice production. Complex modeling using in vivo models, ex vivo models, and computer simulations has led to a better understanding of the biomechanical intricacies of the human vocal folds, the complex interaction between subglottal and supraglottal loading and energy transfer (e.g., Hunter & Titze, 2000; Jiang & Tao, 2007; Titze & Laukkanen, 2007; Zanartu, Mongeau, & Wodicka, 2007). The complexity of laryngeal movement is better understood from the development of new biomechanical models and these new models will ultimately help shape the practice guidelines for both behavioral and phonosurgical interventions.

Mechanisms for Changing Pitch

There are several mechanisms for changing the pitch and loudness of the voice. The mechanism for changing the pitch of the voice primarily is related to changes in vocal fold length which affects vocal fold tension and stiffness, primarily the stiffness in the epithelial layer of the vocal fold. By lengthening the vocal folds the relative mass decreases, the cross-sectional area and thickness of the vocal folds decrease, all of which create a faster vibratory rate.

Increasing vocal fold length and tension can vary the pitch of the voice up to two or three octaves. When the vocal folds vibrate at a faster rate per unit time the frequency is higher and the perception of a higher pitch voice results. This phenomenon was observed by Moore when using high-speed motion film (1937) and others who measured change in vocal fold length from film and photographs (Brackett, 1947; Hollien, 1960) (Figure 2–25).

The primary intrinsic muscle that controls vocal fold length is the cricothyroid muscle. But also, when the thyroartyenoid muscle contracts it can make the vocal fold more rigid and this can create a faster rate of vocal fold vibration, particularly at large vibratory amplitudes (Scherer, 1991). This interaction between thyroarytenoid and the cricothyroid muscle activity is complex for changing fundamental frequency. It is not as straightforward as might be expected. Rather, the direction and extent of the change in fundamental frequency with either thyroarytenoid or cricothyroid muscle activity is dependent on the starting fundamental frequency (i.e., whether

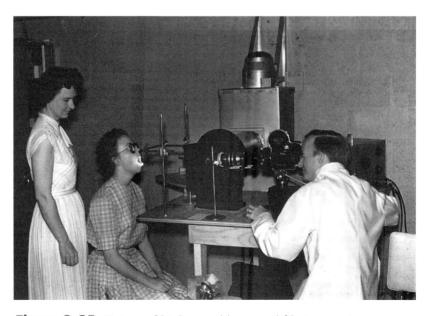

Figure 2–25. Picture of high-speed laryngeal filming equipment.

it is high or low) and also the degree of vibratory amplitude associated with the voicing task (i.e., how loud the voice is being produced (see Scherer, 1991).

Next, fundamental frequency can be increased by elevations in subglottal pressure. Subglottal pressure increases the vibratory amplitude of the vocal folds, resulting in a greater lateral excursion of the vocal folds and an increased vocal fold stretching and tension. An elevation in subglottal pressure at a low fundamental frequency starting point will have a greater effect on increasing the vibrating frequency than it will at a higher fundamental frequency.

What Is a Vocal Register?

A great number of definitions have existed for vocal register. That is why determining a set number of existing vocal registers is a difficult task. In fact well over 100 terms have been used to identify one register or another. A definition is given here but realize that vocal registration is a complex voice phenomenon that differs depending on speaking versus singing. García in 1840 stated that registers are a series of succeeding sounds of equal quality, a scale from low to high produced by the application of the same mechanical principle, the nature of which differs basically from another series of sounds of equal quality produced by another mechanical principle. So, some are low, some are high. Each is produced with a different biomechanical action, and this action results in a distinct perception. Hollien (1974) defined a register as a series or range of consecutive phonated frequencies which can be produced with nearly identical voice quality, and the mechanism is laryngeal in action.

Three registers have been described by Hollien that relate to the speaking voice and these are the pulse, modal, and falsetto (Hollien, Moore, Wendahl, & Michel, 1966). They are distinct in their fundamental frequency range.

Pulse register is a fundamental frequency range at the low end of the frequency scale (approximately 35 to 50 Hz) (McGlone & Shipp, 1971). The vocal folds are closed for a longer proportion of time within the vibratory cycle followed by short pulses of opening and closing within one vibratory cycle (Childers & Lee, 1991). A low subglottal air pressure, on the order of 2 cm H_2O can sustain the vibration associated with pulse register. Visual features noted during pulse register are thick and short vocal folds. Pulse register is perceived as a low pitch and is commonly identified at the termination of statements during speech production, and is considered a normal phenomenon. However, when pulse register is used markedly, it can be classified as a voice disorder.

Modal register is the range of fundamental frequency most commonly used by a speaker. Perceived as the "normal mode" of vocal fold vibration, the subglottal pressure for sustaining this vibratory frequency is about 4 to 5 cm H_2O, the vocal fold appearance is neither lax nor stretched and the airflow values are higher during modal than during pulse register (Blomgren, Chen, Ng, & Gilbert, 1998).

Falsetto or loft register is a fundamental frequency range at the upper end of the vocal folds vibrating capacity. The vocal folds are highly elongated with only the edges of the vocal fold participating in phonation. Vibratory amplitude is small compared to the vocal fold vibratory amplitude during low-frequency phonation. Vocal fold opening predominates within the vibratory cycle. The sound pressure level of the voice is low when compared to the modal register. Subglottal pressures need to be higher to sustain the vibrating frequency associated with the falsetto register compared to pulse and modal registers (McGlone & Shipp, 1971).

Mechanism for Changing Loudness

As was the case for changing pitch, there are several mechanisms for changing the loudness of the voice. Increasing subglottal pressure is the primary mechanism for increasing the loudness variation. A doubling of lung pressure can increase the sound source output by 9.5 dB. The increased lung pressure causes an increase in peak flow rate and greater vibratory amplitude of the vocal folds (Scherer, 1991). In Chapter 4, the measure of maximum flow declination rate, which is the negative peak amplitude of a differentiated glottal airflow signal is defined (Figure 2–26). As the negative peak amplitude of the differentiated flow signal increases, the loudness of the voice increases due to the increase in peak flow during the vibratory cycle and greater vibratory amplitude of the vocal folds. Sundberg and Gauffin detailed this relationship (1979). Increased mouth opening accounts for an increase in loudness as does an increase in the fundamental frequency of the voice. Scherer (1991) further discusses other mechanisms, like a reduction in the cross-sectional area of the epilaryngeal region and alterations in the phase lag between the lower and upper margins of the vocal folds.

These mechanisms basically alter the shape of the glottal airflow waveform, resulting in improved regulation of the glottal sound source for increasing vocal loudness.

> The excised human larynx is being used to help understand the chaos associated with register jumps and may alter the conventional thinking on the laryngeal mechanisms controlling shifts in registers (Tokuda, Haracke, Svec, & Herzel, 2008).

Summary

The laryngeal system is considered the source for voice production. Degradation of its function affects the ability to adequately produce pitch, loudness, and quality that are considered perceptual normal for a person's age and sex. Like the respiratory system, the laryngeal system is one of the most important subsys-

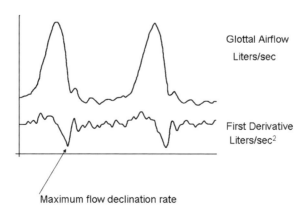

Figure 2–26. Glottal airflow waveform and its first derivative depicting the measure of maximum flow declination rate.

tems requiring evaluative and treatment attention in the care of the voice. The next chapter describes the impact of poor vocal health on laryngeal structure and function.

References

Abdelkafy, W. M., Smith, J. Q., Henriquez, O. A., Golub, J. S., Xu, J., Rojas, M., . . . Johns, M. M. (2007). Age-related changes in the murine larynx: Initial validation of a mouse model. *Annals of Otology, Rhinology, and Laryngology, 116*(8), 618–622.

Amin, M. R., Harris, D., Cassel, S. G., Grimes, E., & Heiman-Patterson, T. (2006). Sensory testing in the assessment of laryngeal sensation in patients with amyotrophic lateral sclerosis. *Annals of Otology, Rhinology, and Laryngology, 115*(7), 528–534.

Aronson, A. E. (2004). Extrinsic muscular tension in patients with voice disorders. *Journal of Voice, 18*(2), 275.

Aviv, J. E., Kim, T., Thomson, J. E., Sunshine, S., Kaplan, S., & Close, L. G. (1998). Fiberoptic endoscopic evaluation of swallowing with sensory testing (FEESST) in healthy controls. *Dysphagia, 13*(2), 87–92.

Aviv, J. E., Sacco, R. L., Thomson, J., Tandon, R., Diamond, B., Martin, J. H., et al. (1997). Silent laryngopharyngeal sensory deficits after stroke. *Annals of Otology Rhinology and Laryngology, 106*(2), 87–93.

Blomgren, M., Chen, Y., Ng, M. L., & Gilbert, H. R. (1998). Acoustic, aerodynamic, physiologic, and perceptual properties of modal and vocal fry registers. *Journal of the Acoustical Society of America, 103*(5), 2649–2658.

Brackett, I. (1947). *An analysis of the vibratory action of the vocal fold during the production of tones at selected frequencies.* Ph.D. dissertation, Northwestern University, Chicago, IL.

Branski, R. C., Rosen, C. A., Verdolini, K., & Hebda, P. A. (2005). Acute vocal fold wound healing in a rabbit model. *Annals of Otology, Rhinology, and Laryngology, 114*(1), 19–24.

Butler, J. E., Hammond, T. H., & Gray, S. D. (2001). Gender related differences of hyal-uronic acid distribution in the human vocal fold. *Laryngoscope, 111*, 907–911.

Catten, M., Gray, S. D., Hammond, T. H., Zhou, R., & Hammond, E. (1998). Analysis of cellular location and concentration in vocal fold lamina propria. *Otolaryngology-Head and Neck Surgery, 118*(5), 663–667.

Chan, R. W., Gray, S. D., & Titze, I. R. (2001). The importance of hyaluronic acid in vocal fold biomechanics. *Otolaryngology-Head and Neck Surgery, 124*(6), 607–614.

Childers, D. G., & Lee, C. K. Vocal quality factors: Analysis, synthesis, and perception. *Journal of the Acoustical Society of America, 90*(5), 2394–2410.

Davenport, P. W., Bolser, D. C., & Morris, K. F. (2011), Swallow remodeling of respiratory neural networks. *Head and Neck, 33*, S8–S13. doi: 10.1002/hed.21845

Ding, H., & Gray, S. D. (2001a). Senescent expression of genes coding collagens, collagen degrading metalloproteinases, and tissue inhibitors of metalloproteinases in rat vocal folds: comparison with skin and lungs. *Journals of Gerontology Series A: Biological Sciences and Medical Sciences, 56*, B145–B152.

Ding, H., & Gray, S.. D. (2001b). Senescent expression of genes coding tropoelastin, elastase, lysyl oxidase, and tissue inhibitors of metalloproteinases in rat vocal folds: comparison with skin and lungs. *Journal of Speech, Language, and Hearing Research, 44*(2), 317–326.

Finck, C. (2005). Vocal fold structure and speech pathologies. *Review of Laryngology Otology and Rhinology (Bord), 126*(5), 295–300.

García, M. (1840). *The art of singing.* Philadephia, PA: Oliver Ditson.

Goldsmith, L. A. (1991). *Physiology, biochemistry, and molecular biology of the skin.* New York, NY: Oxford University Press.

Gray, S. D. (2000). Cellular physiology of the vocal folds. *Otolaryngology Clinics of North America, 33*(4), 679–698.

Hahn, M S., Kobler, J. B., Starcher, B. C., Zeitels, S. M., & Langer, R. (2006). Quantitative and comparative studies of the vocal fold extracellular matrix I: Elastic fibers and hyaluronic acid. *Annals of Otology, Rhinology, and Laryngology, 115*(2), 156–164.

Hahn, M. S., Kobler, J. B., Zeitels, S. M., & Langer, R. (2006). Quantitative and comparative studies of the vocal fold extracellular matrix II: Collagen. *Annals of Otology, Rhinology, and Laryngology, 115*(3), 225–232.

Hammond, T. H., Gray, S. D., & Butler, J. E. (2000). Age and gender related collagen distribution in human vocal folds. *Annals of Otology, Rhinology, and Laryngology, 109*(10), 913–920.

Hammond, T. H., Zhou, R., Hammond, E. H., Pawlak, A., & Gray, S. D. (1997). The intermediate layer: A morphologic study of the elastin and hyaluronic acid constituents of normal human vocal folds. *Journal of Voice, 11*(1), 59–66.

Hirano, M. (1966). Structure and behavior of the vibratory vocal folds. In T. Sawashima & D. Cooper (Eds.), *Dynamic aspects of speech production*. Tokyo, Japan: University of Tokyo Press.

Hirano, M. (1981). *Clinical examination of voice*. Wien; New York, NY: Springer-Verlag.

Hirano, M., Kurita, S., & Nakashima, T. (1981). The structure of the vocal folds. In K. N. Stevens & M. Hirano (Eds.), *Vocal fold physiology* (pp. 22–43). Tokyo, Japan: University of Tokyo Press.

Hirschi, S. D., Gray, S. D., & Thibeault, S. L. (2002). Fibronectin: An interesting vocal fold protein. *Journal of Voice, 16*(3), 310–316.

Hollien, H. (1960). Some laryngeal correlates of vocal pitch. *Journal of Speech and Hearing Research, 3*, 52–58.

Hollien, H. (1974). On vocal registers. *Journal of Phonetics, 2*, 125–143.

Hollien, H., Moore, P., Wendahl, R.W., & Michel, J.F. (1966). On the nature of vocal fry. *Journal of Speech and Hearing Research, 9*(2), 245–247.

Hong, K. H., Kim, H. K., & Kim, Y. H. (2001). The role of the pars recta and pars oblique of cricothyroid muscle in speech production. *Journal of Voice, 15*(4), 512–518.

Hudgins, P. A., Siegel, J., Jacobs, I., & Abramowsky, C. R. (1997). The normal pediatric larynx on CT and MR. *AJNR American Journal of Neuroradiology, 18*(2), 239–245.

Hunter, E. J., & Titze, I. R. (2000). Review of range of arytenoid cartilage motion. *Acoustics Research Letters Online, 6*(3), 112–117.

Jia, X., Yeo, Y., Clifton, R. J., Jiao, T., Kohane, D. S., Kobler, J. B., et al. (2006). Hyaluronic acid-based microgels and microgel networks for vocal fold regeneration. *Biomacromolecules, 7*(12), 3336–3344.

Jiang, J. J., & Tao, C. (2007). The minimum glottal airflow to initiate vocal fold oscillation. *Journal of the Acoustical Society of America, 121*(5 Pt. 1), 2873–2881.

Kahane, J. C. (1978). A morphological study of the human prepubertal and pubertal larynx. *American Journal of Anatomy, 151*(1), 11–19.

Kendall, K. (2007). Presbyphonia: A review. *Current Opinions in Otolaryngology-Head and Neck Surgery, 15*(3), 137–140.

Kim, M. J., Hunter, E. J., & Titze, I. R. (2004). Comparison of human, canine, and ovine laryngeal dimensions. *Annals of Otology, Rhinology, and Laryngology, 113*(1), 60–68.

Kutta, H., Steven, P., Kohla, G., Tillmann, B., & Paulsen, F. (2002). The human false vocal folds—an analysis of antimicrobial defense mechanisms. *Anatomy and Embryology (Berl.). 205*(4), 315–323.

Kutta, H., Steven, P., Varoga, D., & Paulsen, F. P. (2004). Tff peptides in the human false vocal folds of the larynx. *Peptides, 25*(5), 811–818.

Lebl, M. D., Martins, J. R., Nader, H. B., Simoes Mde, J., & De Biase, N. (2007). Concentration and distribution of hyaluronic acid in human vocal folds. *Laryngoscope, 117*(4), 595–599.

Lim, J. Y., Kim, H. S., Kim, Y. H., Kim, K. M., & Choi, H. S. (2008). PMMA (polymethylmetacrylate) microspheres and stabilized hyaluronic acid as an injection laryngoplasty material for the treatment of glottal insufficiency: In vivo canine study. *European Archives of Otorhinolaryngology, 265*(3), 321–326.

Ling, C., Yamashita, M., Waselchuk, E. A., Raasch, J. L., Bless, D. M., & Welham, N. V. (2009). Alteration in cellular morphology, density, and distribution in rat vocal fold mucosa following injury. *Wound Repair and Regeneration, 18*, 89–97.

Litman, R. S., Weissend, E. E., Shibata, D., & Westesson, P. L. (2003). Developmental changes of laryngeal dimensions in unparalyzed, sedated children. *Anesthesiology, 98*(1), 41–45.

Logemann, J. A., Kahrilas, P. J., Cheng, J., Pauloski, B. R., Gibbons, P. J., Rademaker, A. W.,

& Lin, S. 1992). Closure mechanisms of laryngeal vestibule during swallow. *American Journal of Physiology, 262*(2 Pt. 1), G338–G344.

Madruga de Melo, E. C., Lemos, M., Filho, J. A. X., Sennes, L. U., Saldiva, P. H. N., & Tsuji, D. H. (2003). Distribution of collagen in the lamina propria of the human vocal fold. *Laryngoscope, 113*, 2187–2191.

Martin, P. (1997). Wound healing—aiming for perfect skin regeneration. *Science, 276*, 75–81.

McCulloch, T. M., Van Daele, D., & Ciucci, M. R. (2011), Otolaryngology-head and neck surgery: An integrative view of the larynx. *Head and Neck, 33*, S46–S53. doi:10.1002/hed.21901

McGlone, R., & Shipp, T. (1971). Some physiologic correlates of vocal fry phonation. *Journal of Speech and Hearing Research, 7*, 17–29.

Moore, P. (1937). Vocal fold movement during vocalization. *Speech Monographs, 4*, 44–55.

Mupparapu, M., & Vuppalapati, A. (2004). Ossification of laryngeal cartilages on lateral cephalometric radiographs. *Angle Orthodontis, 75*(2), 196–201.

Ohno, T., Hirano, S., & Rousseau, B. (2009). Age associated changes in the expression and deposition of vocal fold collagen and hyaluronan. *Annals of Otology, Rhinology, and Laryngology, 118*(10), 735–741.

Perazzo, P. S., Duprat Ade, C., Lancelotti, C., & Donati, F. (2007). A study of the histological behavior of a rabbit vocal fold after a hyaluronic acid injection. *Review of Brasilian Otorrinolaringology (Engl. ed.), 73*(2), 171–178.

Plant, R. L. (2005). Aerodynamics of the human larynx during vocal fold vibration. *Laryngoscope, 115*(12), 2087–2100.

Pontes, P., Yamasaki, R., & Behlau, M. (2006). Morphological and functional aspects of the senile larynx. *Folia Phoniatrica et Logopaedia, 58*(3), 151–158.

Reidenbach, M. M. (1997). Aryepiglottic fold: Normal topography and clinical implications. *Clinical Anatomy, 11*(4), 223–235.

Ringel, R. L., Kahane, J. C., Hillsamer, P. J., Lee, A. S., & Badylak, S. F. (2006). The application of tissue engineering procedures to repair the larynx. *Journal of Speech, Language and Hearing Research, 49*(1), 194–208.

Roubeau, B., Chevrie,-Muller, C., & Lacau Saint Guily, J. (1997). Electromyographic activity of strap and cricothyroid muscles in pitch change. *Acta Otolaryngology, 117*(30), 459–464.

Rousseau, B., Ge, P. J., Ohno, T., French, L. C., & Thibeault, S. L. (2008). Extracellular matrix gene expression after vocal fold injury in a rabbit model. *Annals of Otology, Rhinology, and Laryngology, 117*(8), 598–603.

Rousseau, B., Sohn, J., Montequin, D. W., Tateya, I., & Bless, D. M. (2004). Functional Outcomes of reduced hyaluronan in acute vocal fold scar. *Annals of Otology, Rhinology, and Laryngology, 113*, 767–776.

Rousseau, B., Suehiro, A., Echemendia, N., & Sivasankar, M. (2011). Raised intensity phonation compromises vocal fold epithelial barrier integrity. *Laryngoscope, 121*, 346–351.

Rubin, H. J. (1960). The neurochronaxi theory of voice production—a refutation. *American Medical Association Archives of Otolaryngolgy, 71*, 913–920.

Sanders, I., & Mu, L. (1998). Anatomy of the human internal superior laryngeal nerve. *Anatomical Record, 252*(4), 646–656.

Sato, K., Hirano, M., & Nakashima, T. (2000). Ultrastructure of the vocal process of the arytenoid cartilage. *Annals of Otology, Rhinology and Laryngology, 109*(7), 650–653.

Scherer, R. (1991). Physiology of phonation: A review of basic mechanics. In C. N. Ford & D. M. Bless (Eds.), *Phonosurgery: Assessment and management of voice disorders.* New York, NY: Raven Press.

Selbie, W. S., Zhang, L., Levine, W. S., & Ludlow, C. L. (1998). Using joint geometry to determine the motion of the cricoarytenoid joint. *Journal of the Acoustical Society of America, 103*(2), 1115–1127.

Sherrey, J. H., & Megirian, D. (1980). Respiratory EMG activity of the posterior cricoarytenoid, cricothyroid, and diaphragm muscles during sleep. *Respiratory Physiology, 39*(3), 355–365.

Sodersten, M., Ternstrom, S., & Bohman, M. (2005). Loud speech in realistic environmental noise: Phonetogram data, perceptual voice quality, subjective ratings, and gender differences in healthy speakers. *Journal of Voice, 19*(1), 29–46.

Suetta, C., Magnusson, S. P., Beyer, N., & Kjaer, M. (2007). Effect of strength training on muscle function in elderly hospitalized patients.

Scandinavian Journal of Medicine and Science in Sports, 17(5), 464–472.

Sundberg, J., & Gauffin, J. (1979). Waveform and spectrum of the glottal voice source. In B. Lindblom & S. Ohman (Eds.), *Frontiers of speech communication research* (pp. 301–320). New York, NY: Academic Press.

Tabaee, A., Murry, T., Zschommler, A., & Desloge, R. B. (2005). Flexible endoscopic evaluation of swallowing with sensory testing in patients with unilateral vocal fold immobility: Incidence and pathophysiology of aspiration. *Laryngoscope, 115*(4), 565–569.

Thibeault, S. L., & Gray, S. (2004). Response of the vocal mechanism to trauma. In J. Casper & C. M. Sapienza (Eds.), *Vocal rehabilitation for medical speech-language pathology, For clinicians by clinicians* (pp. 11–28). Austin, TX: Pro-Ed.

Thibeault, S. L., Gray, S. D., Bless, D. M., Chan, R. W., & Ford, C. N. (2002). Histologic and rheologic characterization of vocal fold scarring. *Journal of Voice, 16*(1), 96–104.

Thibeault, S. L., Rousseau, B., Welham, N. V., Hirano, S., & Bless, D. M. (2004). Hyaluronan levels in acute vocal fold scar. *Laryngoscope, 114*(4), 760–764.

Tiago, R., Pontes, P., & do Brasil, O. C. (2007). Age-related changes in human laryngeal nerves. *Otolaryngology-Head and Neck Surgery, 136*(5), 747–751.

Titze, I. R., & Laukkanen, A. M. (2007). Can vocal economy in phonation be increased with an artificially lengthened vocal tract? A computer modeling study. *Logopedics, Phoniatrics and Vocology, 32*(4), 147–156.

Titze, I. R., Schmidt, S. S., & Titze, M. R. (1995). Phonation threshold pressure in a physical model of the vocal fold mucosa. *Journal of the Acoustical Society of America, 97*(5 Pt. 1), 3080–3084.

Tokuda, I. T., Horacek, J., Svec, J. G., & Herzel, H. (2008). Bifurcations and chaos in register transitions of excised larynx experiments. *Chaos, 18*(1), 013102.

van den Berg, J. (1958). Myoelastic-aerodynamic theory of voice production. *Journal of Speech and Hearing Research, 1*(3), 227–244.

Waldbaum, S., Hadziefendic, S., Erokwu, B., Zaidi, S. I. A., & Haxhium, M. A. (2001). CNS innervation of posterior cricoarytenoid muscles: A transneuronal labeling study. *Respiration Physiology, 126*(2), 113–125.

Ward, P. D., Thibeault, S. L., & Gray, S. D. (2002). Hyaluronic acid: Its role in voice. *Journal of Voice, 16*(3), 303–309.

Wiatrak, B. J. (2000). Congenital anomalies of the larynx and trachea. *Otolaryngological Clinics of North America, 33*(1), 91–110.

Zanartu, M., Mongeau, L., & Wodicka, G. R. (2007). Influence of acoustic loading on an effective single mass model of the vocal folds. *Journal of the Acoustical Society of America, 121*(2), 1119–1129.

Chapter 3

Vocal Health

There are many unique and challenging issues involved when working with patients with disordered voice. Contributing factors that are involved with the onset, maintenance, and rehabilitation of voice disorders include the patient's personality, their family dynamics, medical history, the daily environmental influences to which they are exposed, their occupational demands, as well as their intrinsic expectations about the perceived voice quality. A patient's perceived vocal impairment will certainly relate to the amount of daily activities involving voice use; greater voice use will subsequently increase the perceived functional impact the voice disorder has on the patient's quality of life. Likewise, each voice has its physiologic limits and the sooner patients with voice disorders acknowledge these limits, the sooner they can take full responsibility for their voice and its overall care and maintenance.

After reading this chapter, you will:

- Understand what phonotraumatic factors contribute to vocal pathology
- Understand why phonotraumatic factors contribute to vocal pathology
- Understand how to help your patient minimize poor health habits that are adverse to healthy voice production

Phonotrauma

Phonotrauma is defined as the behavior(s) that contribute to laryngeal/vocal fold tissue injury, inflammation, or other forms of damage. In the past, terms like vocal abuse and misuse were used to describe the behaviors that contributed to laryngeal injury. These terms have been substituted with the term phonotrauma for several reasons. First, the terms abuse and misuse have a negative connotation associated with their meaning. Sometimes a patient engaging in a phonotraumatic behavior is simply not aware that the behavior is damaging to the laryngeal structure. *Abuse* implies a purposeful action and when used by a clinician may be perceived by the patient as an insulting term. The same reasons hold true for the term misuse (e.g., Aronson, 1990; Boone, McFarlane, & Von Berg, 2004; Colton & Casper, 1996; Sataloff, 1991; Stemple, Glaze, & Klaben, 2000). As such, the term phonotrauma has a more neutral connotation and the contributions of phonotraumatic behaviors can be professionally addressed with the patient without risk of causing personal insult (Behrman, Rutledge, Hembree & Sheridan, 2008). Avoiding the use of terms such as "abuse" and "misuse" may further enhance patient willingness to participate in voice therapy," as the focus is instead on the environmental and mechanical factors contributing to the voice disorder (Verdolini, Hess, Titze, Bierhals, & Gross, 1999).

A crucial role for the clinician is to identify potentially phonotraumatic behaviors contributing to a patient's vocal symptoms of interest. Recognition and review of these factors is one of the first steps in a patient's rehabilitation program. Elimination of identified phonotraumatic behaviors will help lay the groundwork for effective voice use.

The following information reviews the concepts of vocal health and provides a general, practical, and informative guide for the clinician in order to help prepare for the assessment of vocal health and hygiene. This informative section explains the effects of poor vocal health habits on both the structure and functioning of the vocal folds and, where appropriate, provides evidence for a cause and effect relationship between specific phonotraumatic behaviors and voice disorder(s). In cases where only anecdotal evidence exists to support the elimination of a phonotraumatic behavior, the best rationale for minimizing a phonotraumatic activity is provided.

Basic Issues Related to Vocal Health

The core issues surrounding basic vocal health (adequate hydration, nutrition, no smoking, limited alcohol intake, allergies, stress, etc.) are addressed in this section. Continual reinforcement of these concepts throughout the course of voice therapy is necessary until the patient has accepted responsibility for maintaining a vocally healthy lifestyle. There are numerous facets of vocal health and as many of these important issues as possible are covered in this chapter.

The last decade has brought an intense focus to the idea of maintaining a healthy lifestyle. Increasing awareness of the importance of general body exercise, including strength training and stretching, permeates our national news media. Fad diets, organic diets, and diets put forth by nutritionists and medical staff can be found on the Internet, and in books and magazines. These diets focus on altering eating habits and promoting the use of proper nutrition in disease prevention. Natural health food stores, homeopathic remedies, and the use of vitamins and supplements is an ever increasing area of popular interest and use. Because exercise and general body health are known to increase vitality and positively affect the ongoing process of aging (Blacklock, Rhodes, & Brown, 2007; Kramer & Erickson, 2007), programs that inspire mental and physical health in elderly individuals are being encouraged as the medicine of the new *millennium.*

Exercise increases circulation, potentially contributing to greater mental strength and increased physiologic power. The effect of exercise is systemic or holistic, affecting all bodily physiologic systems, including those involved in sound production. As the outcome of general body exercise is holistic, overall body health is a critical factor for creating optimum sound production. For children, the latest focus has been on dealing with the national problem of obesity and developing recommendations for creating a healthier nutritional environment while assisting children and adolescents in balancing their busy lives.

The concept of vocal health has a different focus from that endorsed through the concepts of general body exercise. If the key word "vocal health" is entered into an Internet search, many Web sites will emerge providing general information regarding factors that can potentially be damaging to the vocal fold structure. These factors can be further subdivided into those that are considered intrinsic (factors that the patient has less control over), and those that are extrinsic (factors to which the patient may be exposed). An example of an intrinsic factor is the anatomic response of the female vocal folds during menstruation (Chae, Choi, Kang, Choi, & Jin, 2001; Wadnerkar, Cowell, & Whiteside, 2006). An example of an extrinsic factor is exposure of the vocal folds to cigarette smoke, albeit primary or secondary. These intrinsic and extrinsic factors can have a negative impact on the vocal fold structure and the structures that support the vocal folds and help them to move.

Regardless of a patient's age, the case history process is the opportunity to engage in a dialogue with the patient to reach an understanding of the total life influences on the voice. To help ensure the development and implementation of a safe and effective voice recovery plan, it is critical for patients to understand which vocal fold behaviors are safe and which behaviors are unsafe. Safe vocalization, therapeutic exercises, and time-use restrictions should be discussed with the patient with regard to a variety of situations, always with the caution that there is no "one-exercise-cures-all" rehabilitative strategy to treating a voice problem. Although each voice disorder requires individual consideration and therapeutic plans may be similar from one situation to the next, they are by no means formulaic. As a clinician guiding the rehabilitation of a patient's voice disorder, an attitude of delicately balanced optimism and reality/truth, must be portrayed while carefully monitoring every stage of the process to ensure the best possible result.

Recovery Process

Voice recovery times can vary dramatically from person to person due to the numerous factors that are involved with the recovery process. Some of these factors cannot be con-

trolled; therefore, there can never be a guaranteed recovery outcome. These factors include each individual's ability to heal and/or to respond to medications, the patient's state of mind, the patient's previous level of vocal use, the current demands of the patient's vocal use, the patient's level of compliance with lifestyle and therapy demands, the choice of therapy, and the patient's "buy in" to the therapeutic process, as well as other factors.

Contributors to Poor Vocal Health

Nonprescriptive Drug Use

Certainly, the patient should avoid the use of nonprescribed drugs. It is important to be able to recognize when patients may be engaging in drug use and to approach questions about recreational drug use tactfully and professionally. Common symptoms of drug use, particularly marijuana and alcohol include the following.

- Impairment in thinking
- Acting inappropriately
- Smell on the breath and/or clothes
- Poor auditory judgments

Drugs may exert both a direct or indirect effect on the vocal folds. The most common substances that the patient may be exposed to are cigarette smoke, alcohol, or marijuana (Figure 3–1).

Cigarette Smoking

Cigarette smoke is toxic and contains nicotine, an addictive substance. Its largest effect is on the lungs, creating an increased possibility of upper respiratory infection, acute bronchitis, pneumonia and chronic lung diseases such

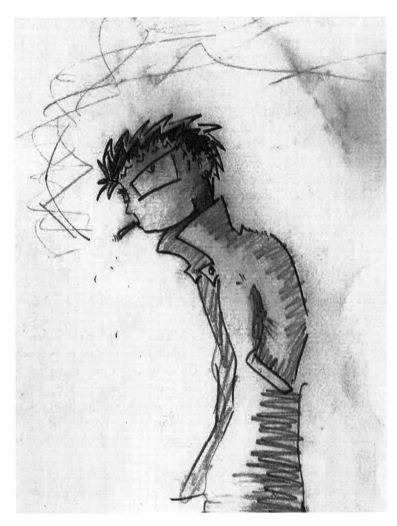

Figure 3–1

as chronic obstructive pulmonary disease and/or emphysema. Exposure to cigarette smoke is also a frequently cited cause of lung cancer. Smoking cigarettes may also contribute to an acceleration of the aging process due to poor oxygenation of tissues and exposure to other chemicals. Tobacco use also takes the form of smoking pipes, cigars, and use of chewing tobacco or snuff. Cigarette smoke is filled with tars that are packed with thousands of chemicals. These chemicals act directly on the cardiovascular system (heart and lungs) and the nervous system. The addictive nature of nicotine appears to be related to the "up feeling" associated with increased blood pressure, heart rate, steroids, hormones, or other neurotransmitters. The nicotine improves memory, alertness, and learning capacity and is highly addictive. Scientific results confirm the hypothesis that the role of nicotine in the compulsive use of tobacco is the same as the role of morphine in the compulsive use of opium derivatives or of cocaine in its obsessive use (Ventulani, 2001). It is the voice clinician's role to educate the patient about the addictive nature of nicotine and its negative effect of chronic chemical irritation on the vocal fold structure while discouraging those who do not smoke from starting. A referral to a psychologist or smoking cessation program may help. Simply telling the patient to stop smoking, although good advice, will likely not be enough, as over 50% of individuals who do try to quit can't and 75% of those who do quit go back to smoking within one year. It may help to explain to the patient that inhaling smoke results in irritation and inflammation of tissue in the nose, throat, and lower airway. The irritation comes from decreased action of cilia in the respiratory tract, decreased mucus production (i.e., drying of the respiratory tract), which can cause inflammation of upper and lower respiratory tracts, coughing and/or hoarseness of the voice.

Can the Adverse Effects of Cigarette Smoking Be Diminished?

Although there are nutritional supplements and behaviors that provide some immunity to the effects of smoking, these supplemental behaviors will never fully combat the effects of the irritation transferred on the body through smoking. The nutritional avenues followed by some to help combat against the act of smoking include taking vitamins, as mentioned above, and following a diet plan that is low in fats, and high in fruits, vegetables, and grains. Although these nutritional supplements may help diminish some of the adverse effects of smoking, there are no compensatory measures that can be taken to combat against the multitude of chemicals that are in cigarette smoke.

Increased water intake is important and should be encouraged. An average of 2 to 3 quarts of water per day is recommended to decrease the drying effect from the smoke irritation. Finally, although advertisements about low tar, low nicotine cigarettes may be an attractive alternative for the person who can't stop smoking, there are no safe cigarettes; all cigarettes damage and usually the "lighter" the cigarette, the deeper one inhales to satisfy the nicotine fix.

Effects of Secondary Smoke

What about exposure to secondary smoke? Is it an issue to caution patients about? It certainly is. The effect of secondary smoke has become a big area of concern over the last 10 years. Inhaled secondary smoke is unfiltered and actually contains more tar and nicotine than that ingested by the primary smoker (Glantz & Parmley, 1995; Howard et al., 1998). Common symptoms of those exposed to secondary smoke include an exacerbation of allergies, headache, cough, and/or hoarseness.

> The damage from secondary smoke carries about 40% of the effect of primary smoking.

Marijuana Use

Marijuana is one of the most commonly abused substances in the United States, with 3.3% of young adults, 19 to 28 years old, using it on a daily basis and 54% of all people between the ages of 25 and 34 years having used marijuana at least once (Nixon, 2006). Those smoking marijuana have a higher incidence of respiratory problems and other types of illness than those who do not smoke marijuana. What may be less apparent is the role marijuana plays in the development of head and neck cancer and problems in the respiratory, immune, and reproductive systems. Additionally, marijuana users also typically smoke cigarettes or engage in some other form of tobacco use as well as drink alcohol. It is becoming more common for individuals to use herbal incense (a.k.a Spice) due to its similar psychedelic and euphoric effects to marijuana yet is legal. Effects of Spice on laryngeal function are less known.

Because of the number of drugs a patient may be engaging in, difficulty arises teasing out what substance has caused the problem at hand, whether it is a diagnosis of respiratory tissue irritation or head and neck cancer. And, although some epidemiologic studies show that increased marijuana use leads to increased risk of head and neck cancer (Zhang et al., 1999), there are other studies not supporting this assertion (Hashibe, Ford, & Zhang, 2002). It is known that the compounds found in marijuana are of the same cancer-causing compounds as in tobacco, sometimes in higher concentrations. Daily cough and phlegm (chronic bronchitis) and upper respiratory infections are some common symptoms observed in individuals who use marijuana. Use of marijuana also increases the risk for pneumonia.

Chewing Tobacco

Chewing tobacco is primarily observed in high-school and college-aged males. Clinicians should advise patients to stop chewing tobacco as it is associated with increased risk of developing oral cancer (Gillison, 2007). Oral cancer has been shown to occur several times more frequently among snuff dippers than among nontobacco users, and the excess risk of cancers of the cheek and gum may reach nearly 50-fold among long-term snuff users. The addiction to nicotine is the other risk, as was discussed above.

Coughing and Throat Clearing

Initial evaluation of a patient with chronic cough (i.e., of more than eight weeks' duration) should include a focused history and physical examination, and in most patients, chest x-ray. The most common causes of chronic cough in adults are upper respiratory infection, asthma, and gastroesophageal reflux disease, alone or in combination. A diagnosis of asthma should be confirmed based on clinical response to inhaled bronchodilators or corticosteroids.

Patients should be counseled to avoid exposure to cough-evoking irritants, such as cigarette smoke. Further testing such as high-resolution computed tomography, and referral to a pulmonologist may be indicated if the cause of chronic cough is not identifiable. In children, a cough lasting longer than four weeks is considered chronic. The most common causes in children are respiratory tract infections, asthma, and gastroesophageal reflux disease. Evaluation of children with chronic cough should include chest x-ray and lung function testing (Benich & Carek, 2011).

Continual cough and throat clearing can have deleterious effects on vocal fold health due to the high expiratory pressures and shearing forces causing tissue irritation and damage to the vocal folds over time. Coughing and throat clearing may also be associated with secondary behaviors develop over time in response to perceived laryngeal sensation associated with laryngeal pathology. In some patients a perceived dryness, tickle, burning or lump in the throat sensation results in a cough or throat clear.

Cough can also be associated with a variety of different respiratory diseases including emphysema, asthma, chronic obstructive pulmonary disease and lung malignancies. In these examples cough is associated with a disease process that may be medically treated by a physician. When cough develops in response to laryngeal pathology the behavior is not always associated with an underlying disease process. When this is the case, behavioral strategies are provided by the voice pathologist to eliminate the behavior as part of the voice therapy plan.

Careful review of the patient's medication list should occur as the source of cough may be a side effect of certain prescriptions such as Albuterol, Zestril, and Diovan, Altrace (blood pressure medications) that create a dry irritating cough. Referral back to the patient's physician who prescribed this medication may be necessary in order to manage the cough severity and frequency.

Alcohol Intake

The most obvious signs of alcohol abuse or intoxication are deficits to walking, balance, and cognition. Alcohol use, even in the smallest doses causes a decrease in awareness, which undermines vocal discipline, and technique, all of which are designed to optimize and protect the voice Sataloff (1991). Consumption of alcohol can negatively affect adequate hydration levels and vocal behaviors. Some of the more common negative effects on vocal behaviors include increased vocal loudness, excessive pitch inflection and poor breath management. Furthermore, there is a synergistic relationship that exists between alcohol and smoking and when alcohol is consumed in large consumption along with cigarette smoking it has been implicated in the development of head and neck cancers. Also, note differences in life style and health characteristics are likely to be caused by the profession of choice with greater alcohol use in some occupations versus others. Careful questioning during the case history will help the clinician learn about the patient's patterns of alcohol consumption, which is equally important to

knowing the absolute number of drinks a person may have at one time (Rehm, Greenfield & Rogers, 2001). It is important to reiterate the deleterious effects of alcohol to the patient and counsel them about optimizing their vocal health.

Caffeine Intake

Caffeine is found in coffee, teas, sodas, chocolate, cocoa, and diet pills. One 5-ounce cup of coffee contains about 116 mg of caffeine. Sodas such as Jolt, Mountain Dew, and Coca Cola carry some of the highest concentrations of caffeine. Caffeine is a diuretic, meaning that it contributes to the elimination of water through the body, potentially contributing to dehydration. Dehydration is addressed therapeutically through reducing intake of diuretic substances (such as caffeine) or by increasing water intake (for example, drinking a glass of water for every cup of coffee that is consumed). Direct the patient toward enhancing their level of hydration and making them aware that their current hydration may be unacceptable from a vocal hygiene perspective. Like nicotine, caffeine is an addictive substance. As a stimulant it provides that extra little perk to get going in the morning. It does so by binding to adenosine receptors, a type of protein, at certain sites in the body. The result of this stimulation leads to heightened mental awareness, increased heart rate, and other effects. As the patient tries to cut back on their caffeine intake some of the symptoms they may experience include: headache, dry mouth, fatigue, and extreme sluggishness. Again, simply advising a patient to stop "drinking coffee" may be unrealistic as it may be part of their daily routine or a well-formed habit. One practical recommendation might be to cut back on the caffeine intake by brewing half decaffeinated coffee with the regular coffee.

An average cup of hot cocoa has 10 mg of caffeine and a 3.5-oz chocolate bar has 12 mg of caffeine, whereas Mountain Dew has 54 mg of caffeine in a 12-oz serving.

Sleep Deprivation

Normal sleep is an active state, essential for mental and physical restoration. Every person requires a specified amount of sleep but there is wide variability among people with regard to how much sleep they need to maintain their physical well-being. Most people require an average of eight to nine hours per night but this can vary from as little as six hours to as many as ten hours. The sleep requirement does drop with age. The more common sleep disturbances include restlessness, insomnia, and sleep apnea. Gastroesophageal reflux, obesity, anxiety, and stress lead to altered sleep patterns. Aggressive physical activity just before bedtime may affect the ability to fall asleep as can worrying about the next day's schedule. As Sataloff stresses (1991), general body fatigue is reflected in the voice. Optimal voice may not be achieved when a person is tired. Performers, in particular may be more susceptible to sleep problems because of the demands for time, travel, and the irregular hours of performance.

Vocal Load and Vocal Fatigue

Individuals who engage in prolonged periods of voice use are at increased susceptibility to the condition of vocal fatigue. Prolonged voice use most commonly occurs because of occupational demands (professional voice user). Symptoms of vocal fatigue include: odynophonia (soreness or pain in the throat following "prolonged" voice usage), dysphonia, and periods of voice loss. Vocal attrition (the wearing away of the voice) is also a condition associated with use of increased loudness levels for extended periods of time (Sapienza, Crandell, & Curtis, 1999). Muscle fatigue, a contributor to vocal fatigue, is characterized by repeated, intense use of a muscle (Allen, Lamb, & Westerblad, 2008). The repetitive nature of vocal fold vibration is potentially associated with muscle fatigue. Muscle fatigue affects the action potentialand the muscle's extra- and intracellular environment causing alterations to its contractile properties of the muscle. This in turn reduces the muscle force generation. Tissue fatigue is another component contributing to vocal fatigue, and results in inflammation as the body defends against invading pathogens. Common recommendations to reduce vocal inflammation include vocal rest and eating foods that do not sustain inflammation, such as those high in sugars and fatty acids, like doughnuts and other fried foods.

The Bogart-Bacall syndrome (Koufman & Blalock, 1988) is a particular condition characterized by vocal fatigue. This syndrome is commonly assigned to those professional voice users such as singers, actors, and radio or television personalities who use a low fundamental frequency or pitch of their voice. The term "Bogart-Bacall" syndrome (BBS) comes from the famous, low-pitched voice quality used by two historic actors, Humphrey Bogart and Lauren Bacall. Use of a low-pitch voice requires a change in the mechanical properties of the vocal folds. If an artificially low-pitched voice is used than more "physiologic work" is needed to produce that voice. Although this use of an artificially low-pitch voice may not initially cause problems for the user, its long-term use may result in a laryngeal pathology or vocal disturbance. Why some individuals choose to use this voice varies but it appears to stem from a psychological domain of wanting to sound more professional, authoritative or even male-like. Imaging of vocal fold movement in those deemed as having BBS usually reflects a pattern of muscle tension characterized by anteroposterior contraction of the larynx with the arytenoids cartilages being drawn or pulled forward toward the stem or base of the epiglottis (petiole) (Koufman & Blalock, 1988).

Talking Too Loudly

Use of voice amplification may help an individual avoid vocal fatigue. There is a direct positive relationship between the degree of elevated loudness level and the degree of vocal fatigue (Laukkanen, Ilomaki, Leppanen, & Vilkman, 2006). The louder a person needs to talk and the more they rely on their own system to self-amplify their voice, the greater the "wear and tear" on the vocal folds. The physiologic mechanisms one can use to self-amplify the voice were nicely summarized by Scherer (1991) and were discussed in Chapter 2. These mechanisms are the following: increased subglottal pressure, alteration of the glottal flow waveform, change in glottal geometry, and manipulation of vocal tract characteristics. Doubling the lung pressure from 5 to 10 cm H_2O increases sound pressure level by 9.5 dB. Increasing air particle velocity through the glottis raises sound pressure level by 3.5 dB, increasing glottal area and flow increases sound pressure level by 3 dB, increasing fundamental frequency provides a 1 dB increase, and increasing the speed of glottal closing increases sound pressure level by 2 dB. The vocal tract increases glottal intensity by 10 to 20 dB through impedance matching between the glottis and the space just in front of the lips. In voice therapy it is important to manipulate the patient's oral cavity and articulators appropriately to control upper airway resistance. If this is not done, an increased upper airway resistance can lead to a dampening or decreased output of the signal. Increased vocal fold adduction is one mechanism for increas-

ing the loudness level of the voice; however, too much vocal fold adduction can lead to irritation of the vocal fold medial edge and when this occurs the most common result is the development of vocal fold nodules.

Poor Nutrition

Nutritional deficiencies can affect an individual's ability to resist disease and infection or withstand stress. Nutrient deprivation, or protein-calorie malnutrition, can cause alterations in muscle and nerve function. Specific symptoms include general weakness, fatigue, and loss of respiratory strength, depression, irritability, mental confusion, inability to concentrate, and infection. Skeletal muscle wasting may occur in extreme cases.

Anorexia nervosa and bulimia nervosa are eating disorders that result in poor nutrition and/or malnutrition. Anorexia is associated with weight loss of more than 15% of ideal body weight. Bulimia is characterized by binge eating followed by vomiting or the use of laxatives. Both problems can lead to dehydration, fatigue, and gastrointestinal problems (Berkman et al., 2006). Specifically, episodes of repeated vomiting can cause chronic irritation of the esophagus and larynx. These disorders, most common in young females, can occur at any age with either sex. Voice disorders associated with bulimia are vocal fold edema, polypoid changes, posterior commisure hypertrophy, ventricular obliteration, and/or telangiectasia; see Chapter 6 (Rothstein, 1998).

> Telangiectasia means permanent enlargement of blood vessels.

Obesity

To maintain health, weight should be kept within 20% of the ideal weight. More than

20% over desirable body weight may be enough to constitute a health hazard, both physically and mentally. The body mass index (BMI) is used to determine if a person is above or below their expected weight. It is calculated by dividing weight by height squared. BMI should be between 10 and 50. Overweight is defined as a BMI above 27 with 30 to 40 as significantly overweight and over 40 extremely overweight. Additional weight can interfere with abdominal breath support for voice production. It may also affect endurance. Extra pounds contribute to general fatigue. In extreme cases, additional weight may affect vocal resonance as the extra pounds may significantly reduce the lumen (space) of the pharynx above the glottis. This same excess tissue also plays a role in sleep apnea, which also contributes to fatigue. Excess weight can exacerbate the effects of reflux. In fact, weight reduction is often highly recommended in reflux management programs. The effects of gastroesophageal reflux on the voice are well documented in the literature and are discussed in further detail in Chapter 5. Prevention, of course, is the best treatment for obesity.

Likewise, being underweight is not considered healthy. It can lead to poor circulation and psychological distress. Coupled with low and high body weight often comes low muscle tone and generally poor overall body conditioning which simply intensifies the symptoms described above.

Dehydration

The importance of hydration to combat the dehydrating effects of substances such as cigarette smoke and alcohol should not be underestimated. Increasing hydration is one of the most common and simplest recommendations made to patients who are suffering from a vocal disturbance. Strategies to increase hydration include recommending to an individual consuming more water or adding a humidifier to their environment so the humidity stays at 30% humidity or higher.

Typical recommendations for water intake are approximately six to eight 8-oz. glasses of water a day. Increased water intake is recommended because there is a growing body of evidence that indicates that vocal fold swelling and the size of vocal fold lesions such as vocal fold nodules are reduced with increased hydration (Verdolini-Marston, Sandage, & Titze, 1994). The effects of increasing water intake are systemic meaning that the whole body reaps the payoff of increasing water intake. The brain works more optimally and energy levels are higher with increased water intake (Maughan, Shirreffs, & Watson, 2007). Verdolini and colleagues (1994) completed a study on the effects of hydration and increased humidity on vocal fold function to determine whether increasing hydration/humidity made it less effortful to produce the voice. They determined effort through two measures, one being the minimum amount of pressure needed to vibrate the vocal folds for voicing, known as the phonation threshold pressure, and the other, the perception of voicing effort. Two humidity environments were created. The first was a dehumidifying environment (30 to 35%) and the second was an increased humidity environment (85 to 100%). Their work showed that dehydration resulted in the greatest perceived effort of voicing but when hydrated the perception of effort decreased. Further evidence of the effects of hydration is found in other empirical work (Jiang, Ng, & Hanson, 1999). Jiang et al.'s work on excised dog larynges showed again that increased hydration resulted in increased vocal fold efficiency and reduced phonation threshold pressures. In short, the vocal fold movement was more fluid and the degree of lung pressure to initiate vocal fold movement was decreased. Likewise both animal and human subject studies provide evidence that systemic and superficial dehydration are detrimental to vocal fold physiology. Dehydration challenges increase the viscous properties of excised vocal fold tissue. Systemic, superficial, and combined drying challenges negatively affect aerodynamic and acoustic measures of voice production in speakers. Certainly, the emerging theoretical and clinical evidence suggest that increasing both systemic and superficial hydration levels may benefit voice production, And although the evidence may not be as robust as it should be, recommendations for increasing hydration in the care of the voice remains high (Mahalakshmi & Ciara, 2010).

Use of Herbals

Herbal remedies have the advantage over prescriptive drugs in that they are easier to obtain and are usually thought of as having less significant side effects. It is not unusual for patients to look for alternative therapies to help enhance the voice or diminish adverse voice effects. Although use of herbal remedies represent a nonmedical treatment option, certain precautions should be taken as some herbal remedies may have negative side effects (see Chapter 11). The manufacturing of herbal supplements is largely unregulated and the potential risk of hepatotoxicity (chemically induced liver damage) is increased because the ingredients in herbal supplements are not standardized like prescriptive drugs (Seeff, 2007). During the case history interview, it is important to include questions regarding the use of alternative medicines or treatments, as some alternative treatments can cause significant side effects or drug interactions.

Allergies

An allergy is an overreaction of the immune system to a substance. Practically any substance can become an allergen or allergy-causing nuisance. Often, a patient will complain of having a runny nose or talk about the effects that certain seasons have on their voice quality. Seasonal allergies to pollens and the blooms

of certain flowers can cause allergic reactions. Allergies to cats and dogs are often common. As well, working in environments where there are molds, mites, and other particles in the air may create allergic reactions to the upper airway.

Some common symptoms of an allergic reaction include: headaches, runny nose, sneezing, sore throats, breathing (wheezing), skin rashes, stomach pains, watery, itchy eyes, persistent cough, diarrhea or constipation, recurring ear infections, a cold that won't go away, and/or a voice disturbance. An allergic reaction can be as mild as sneezing and sniffling, caused by house dust or seasonal pollens, to as severe as death. Allergic rhinitis is a term that is used by medical professionals to describe a wide variety of allergic symptoms all involving the eyes, ears, nose, and throat. It is typically caused by respiratory inhalants. The types of allergens can be plants, flowers and weeds (wind borne pollen), animal dander, shedding fur, and dust mites. These allergens typically result in nasal congestion, sneezing, clear drainage, watery itchy eyes, throat clearing, "scratchy" throat soreness, excessive coughing, pain and pressure in the ears, headache and fatigue. Persons with even the mildest symptoms may present with subtle vocal complaints such as occasional voice breaks or vocal fatigue that may result in drying in the vocal tract. These symptoms are typically seasonal; however, depending on your geographical location these may be issues year round.

Exposure to molds often creates cold-like symptoms which may be resistant to traditional therapies. Symptoms associated with allergic reactions to molds may include: postnasal drip, bloodshot eyes, headache, rhinorhea, and voice disturbance.

> Rhinorhea is the medical term for a runny nose.

These symptoms are indicative of possible exposure to allergens and the patient should be counseled to see an allergist. Inhalant allergy may be silent but the symptoms are overt and a common cause of laryngitis, either acutely or chronically.

Allergies to ingested substances including foods may affect patients by thickening secretions and causing congestion. The consequence of congestion and thickened secretions is excessive coughing and throat clearing. This can result in vocal fold swelling that may further lead to a vocal fold tissue lesion and/or breathy or hoarse quality.

The simplest and most obvious way to prevent an allergic reaction is to avoid contact with the allergen. But, with the exception of certain foods, animals, and drugs, this method is not very practical; dust, insects, pollen, and a variety of chemicals are present no matter where a person lives. If the history and physical examination suggest an allergy, the cause is determined by using either a skin test or a blood test. Once the diagnosis has been made, a course of treatment may include a combination of options including: avoidance, medication, or immunotherapy which would involve having injections that gradually help the body build up a tolerance to the allergen and minimize or prevent the symptoms.

Acute Sinusitis

Sinuses are spaces in the bones of the skull around the nose and the eyes. They create some of the resonance heard in the voice. If the sinuses get blocked with too much mucus, the voice quality may be perceived as muffled or "hyponasal." A short-term infection of the sinuses (less than 4 weeks) is called *acute* rhinosinusitis and can be caused by the following:

- Upper respiratory infection
- Hay fever or allergies
- Air pollution and /or cigarette smoke
- Swimming
- Pregnancy
- Aging
- Immune disorders, such as diabetes or Auto-Immune Deficiency (AIDS)

Summary

Poor vocal health (Table 3–1) contributes to vocal pathology and voice disorder. Educating patients about the deleterious factors that contribute to poor vocal health is an important step in the therapeutic process prior to initiating a voice therapy strategy. Monitoring a patient's compliance is recommended to track patient adherence to vocal health habits and is also vital to the successful outcome of therapy, as low adherence to good vocal health habits will result in maintenance of the vocal pathology/disorder.

Table 3–1. An Overview of the Factors and/or Behaviors That May Result in Vocal Fold Irritation, Inflammation, and/or Disease, Considered to Be Representative of Poor Vocal Health

Factors & Behaviors	Effect	Suggestion	Why
Exposure to Irritants (Smoking, Excessive Alcohol, Chemical Fumes)	Irritates the delicate mucous lining of the nasal passages, throat, and larynx	Avoid these irritants Do not use tobacco products	Minimizes vocal fold irritation and inflammation. Reduces potential incidence of cancer, emphysema, and other illnesses
Chronic Cough, Throat Clearing	Causes the vocal folds to adduct forcefully	Avoid overclearing the throat and excessive cough if possible. Use humming to clear the throat or soft swallow	Minimizes vocal fold irritation
Excessive Talking, Excessive Use of Vocal Loudness	Vocal fold irritation, inflammation, overadduction, excess subglottal pressure—increases vibratory amplitude and medial forces	Avoid forceful speaking. Use a soft voice or a comfortable effort level voice	Decreases the strain on the vocal folds
Excessive Strain Resulting From Talking While Lifting Weights, Moving Furniture, Engaging in Certain Sports or Aerobic Exercise	Excess pressure build up within the chest during these activities, talking will cause excess pressure on the vocal folds	Avoid overexertion or heavy lifting especially accompanied with talking	Reduces excess pressure on the vocal folds
Excessive Caffeine	Caffeine has a dehydrating effect on the vocal folds	Drink water or natural juice	Reduces the drying effect on vocal fold mucosa and subsequent alterations to vocal quality
Vocal Fatigue	Overstraining may occur to compensate for vocal fatigue	Take "vocal naps" during the day	Allows time to rest the voice, optimizing vocal function

continues

Table 3–1. *continued*

Factors & Behaviors	Effect	Suggestion	Why
Eating Rich Spicy Foods, Chocolate, Carbonated Beverages, etc.	May reduce pressure in the esophageal sphincter, allowing stomach acid to flow up into the esophagus*	Avoid spicy food, especially near bed time	Reduces reflux which is more active during sleep
Singing Without Warming Up	Minimizes vocal fold flexibility, reduces respiratory muscle activity, minimizes tongue and jaw flexibility and movement	Two octave pitch glides on /i/ or /u/ lip trill tongue trill Humming forward tongue roll messa di voce**	Increases blood flow to the vocal fold structure, activates intrinsic laryngeal muscle activity to encourage vocal flexibility loosens tongue and jaw

*Not everyone who eats spicy foods will suffer from heartburn or reflux. Heartburn is a common condition and affects over 40% of all Americans at least once a month. Kaltenbach, Crockett, and Gerson (2006) provide a review of the impact of lifestyle measures and the effects in patients with gastroesopageal reflux disease.

**These exercises were suggested by Dr. Ingo Titze and further information can be found on the National Center for Voice and Speech Web site http://www.ncvs.org/ncvs/info/singers/warmup.html

References

Allen, D. G., Lamb, G. D., & Westerblad, H. (2008). Skeletal muscle fatigue: Cellular mechanisms. *Physiology Review, 88*(1), 287–332.

Aronson, A. (1990). *Clinical voice disorders.* New York, NY: Thieme Medical.

Behrman, A., Rutledge, J., Hembree, A., & Sheridan, S. (2008). Vocal hygiene education, voice production therapy, and the role of patient adherence: A treatment effectiveness study in women with phonotrauma. *Journal of Speech Language and Hearing Research, 51*(2), 350–366.

Benich, J. J. 3rd, & Carek, P. J. (2011). Evaluation of the patient with chonic cough. *American Family Physician, 84*(8), 887–892.

Berkman, N. D., Bulik, C. M., Brownley, K. A., Lohr, K. N., Sedway, J. A., Rooks, A., & Gartlehner, G. (2006). Management of eating disorders. *Evidence Report/Technology Assessment, 135*, 1–166.

Blacklock, R. E., Rhodes, R. E., & Brown, S. G. (2007). Relationship between regular walking, physical activity and health-related quality of life. *Journal of Physical Activity and Health, 4*(2), 138–152.

Boone, D., McFarlane, S. C., & Von Berg, S. L. (2004). *The voice and voice therapy.* Boston, MA: Addison-Wesley.

Chae, S. W., Choi, G., Kang, H. J., Choi, J. O., & Jin, S. M. (2001). Clinical analysis of voice change as a parameter of premenstrual syndrome. *Journal of Voice, 15*(2), 278–283.

Colton, R., & Casper, J. (1996). *Understanding voice problems.* Baltimore, MD: Williams & Wilkins.

Gauffin, J., & Sundberg, J. (1978). Pharyngeal constrictions. *Phonetica, 35*(3), 157–168.

Gillison, M.L. (2007). Current topics in the epidemiology of oral cavity and oropharyngeal cancers. *Head and Neck, 29*(8), 779–792.

Glantz, S. A., & Parmley, W. W. (1995). Passive smoking and heart disease. Mechanisms and risk. *Journal of the American Medical Association*, *273*(13), 1047–1053.

Hashibe, M., Ford, D. E., & Zhang, Z. F. (2002). Marijuana smoking and head and neck cancer. *Journal of Clinical Pharmacology*, *42*(11), 103S–107S.

Howard, G., Wagenknecht, L. E., Burke, G. L., Diez-Roux, A., Evans, G. W., McGovern, P., . . . Tell, G. S. (1998). Cigarette smoking and progression of atherosclerosis: The atherosclerosis risk in communities study. *Journal of the American Medical Association*, *279*(2), 119–124.

Institute for Clinical Systems Improvement. *Acute sinusitis in adults*. Retrieved from http://www.guideline.gov/summary.aspx?view_id=1&doc_id=5449

Jiang, J., Ng, J., & Hanson, D. (1999). The effects of rehydration on phonation in excised canine larynges. *Journal of Voice*, *13*(1), 51–59.

Kaltenbach, T., Crockett, S., & Gerson, L. B. (2006). Are lifestyle measures effective in patients with gastroesophageal reflux disease? An evidence-based approach. *Archives of Internal Medicine*, *166*(9), 965–971.

Koufman, J. A., & Blalock, P. D. (1988). Vocal fatigue and dysphonia in the professional voice user: Bogart-Bacall syndrome. *Laryngoscope*, *98*(5), 493–498.

Kramer, A. F., & Erickson, K. I. (2007). Capitalizing on cortical plasticity: Influence of physical activity on cognition and brain function. *Trends in Cognitive Science*, *11*(8), 342–348.

Laukkanen, A.M., Ilomaki, I., Leppanen, K., & Vilkman, E. (2008). Acoustic measures and self-reports of vocal fatigue by female teachers. *Journal of Voice*, *22*(3), 283–289.

Mahalakshmi, S., & Ciara, L. (2010). The role of hydration in vocal fold physiology. *Current Opinions of Otolaryngology-Head and Neck Surgery*, *18*(3), 171–175.

Maughan, R. J., Shirreffs, S. M., & Watson, P. (2007). Exercise, heat, hydration and the brain. *Journal of the American College of Nutrition*, *26*(5), 604S–612S.

Nixon, P. J. (2006). Health effects of marijuana: A review. *Pacific Health Dialog*, *13*(2), 123–129.

Rehm, J. & Bondy, S. (1996). Risk functions, low risk drinking guidelines, and the benefits of moderate drinking. *Addiction*, 91, 1439–1441.

Rothstein, S. G. (1998). Reflux and vocal disorders in singers with bulimia. *Journal of Voice*, *12*(1), 89–90.

Sapienza, C. M., Crandell, C. C., & Curtis, B. (1999). Effects of sound-field frequency modulation amplification on reducing teachers' sound pressure level in the classroom. *Journal of Voice*, *13*(3), 375–381.

Sataloff, R. (1991). *Professional voice: The science and art of clinical care*. New York, NY: Raven Press.

Scherer, R. (1991). Physiology of phonation: A review of basic mechanics. In C. N. Ford & D. M. Bless, (Eds.), *Phonosurgery assessment and management of voice disorders*. New York, NY: Raven Press.

Seeff, L. B. (2007). Herbal hepatotoxicity. *Clinical Liver Disorder*, *11*(3), 577–596.

Stemple, J., Glaze, L., & Klaben, B. (2000). *Clinical voice pathology: Theory and management* (3rd ed.). Clifton Park, NY: Delmar Learning.

Ventulani, J. (2001). Drug addiction. Part I. Psychoactive substances in the past and presence. *Polish Journal of Pharmacology*, *53*(3), 201–214.

Verdolini, K., Hess, M. M., Titze, I. R., Bierhals, W., & Gross, M. (1999). Investigation of vocal fold impact stress in human subjects. *Journal of Voice*, *13*(2), 184–202.

Verdolini-Marston, K., Sandage, M., & Titze, I. R. (1994). Effect of hydration treatments on laryngeal nodules and polyps and related voice measures. *Journal of Voice*, *8*(1), 30–47.

Wadnerkar, M. B., Cowell, P. E., & Whiteside, S. P. (2006). Speech across the menstrual cycle: A replication and extension study. *Neuroscience Letters*, *408*(1), 21–24.

Zhang, Z. F., Morgenstern, H., Spitz, M. R., Tashkin, D. P., Yu, G. P., Marshall, J. R., . . . Schantz, S. P. (1999). Marijuana use and increased risk of squamous cell carcinoma of the head and neck. *Cancer Epidemiology Biomarkers Prevention*, *8*(12), 1071–1078.

Chapter 4

Evaluation

*W*hen a patient presents with a voice disorder it is accompanied by a change in the quality, pitch, or loudness of the voice that is different from what is expected for someone of the same age or sex (Smith, Verdolini, Gray, et al., 1996). More often than not, the patient is concerned over these changes and seeks professional help from a voice care team. During the evaluation process, the causes and/or mechanisms of the voice disorder are identified along with the severity of the impairment defined anatomically, physiologically, and functionally with regard to the disorder's impact on the patient's quality of life.

After reading this chapter, you will:

- Understand the components that make up a comprehensive evaluation of voice production
- Understand the contributions of instrumental assessment for examining voice production
- Understand the distinct imaging techniques available for examining laryngeal structure
- Understand the basic measurements used in aerodynamic and acoustic analysis of voice production
- Understand the purpose, pros, and cons of perceptual voice evaluation

A review article by Ma, Yiu, and Verdolini-Abbott (2007) described the application of the ICF model for persons with voice disorders. ICF stands for the International Classification of Functioning, Disability, and Health and was established to provide a standard mechanism for communicating the effects of impairments on body functions and structures, activities and participation, and the influence of environmental and personal factors on impairment.

Other resources with regard to topics on impairment, scope of practice in speech-language pathology and evidence-based practice research can be found at http://www.asha.org/members/ebp/.

Within the ICF model, environmental factors are defined as physical, social, and attitudinal features that voice patients are exposed to and describes which of these factors may shape the course of the impairment and treatment outcomes. Likewise, personal factors can be many and as described in the Ma et al. review, these factors are not acknowledged as co-occurring with the voice disorder, but rather may be existing even prior to the onset of the voice disorder (p. 346). A voice disorder according to Ma et al. (2007), within the ICF classification scheme, is described in terms of body structures and functional impairments.

Read more of this review to learn how to apply the ICF model to voice disorders.

Over the last 20 to 30 years, there have been vast changes in the field of laryngology, changes that have happened with the development of science and medicine, and sophisticated advances in voice research and evaluative equipment. For example, 30 years ago the tools physicians used to diagnose a voice condition were much simpler than those used today. Previous instruments were also less effective for detailing the course of a vocal injury particularly for the effects of a lesion on vocal fold function. With technologic advancements of laryngeal imaging, finer movements of the vocal folds can be imaged, allowing an injury's effects on voice production to be better defined and subsequently allowing for better prediction of the vocal recovery timeline for the patient.

Diagnosis (The 5 Ds)

Determine the etiologic factors related to the disorder

Determine the disorder severity

Determine the clinical course

Determine the likely response to treatment

Determine the actual response to treatment

The Specialty of Otolaryngology

Otolaryngology is the oldest medical specialty in the United States (http:www.entnet. org/healthinfo/about/otolar yngologist.cfm). The otolaryngologist or ear, nose, and throat (ENT) physician determines the structural condition of the vocal folds through a physical examination, which includes visualizing the vocal folds. An ENT physician is a special- ist who is concerned with the treatment and surgery of the ear, nose, throat, and related structures of the head and neck. In addition to treating voice disorders, the ENT treats benign and malignant tumors of the head and neck and manages patients with allergic, sinus, laryngeal, thyroid, and esophageal disorders. Not all ENT's specialize in voice care. There are subspecialties encompassed in this profession. For example, an otologist specializes in care of the ear and a laryngologist specializes in care of the larynx relating to its functions for voice production, breathing, and swallowing.

Even within the field of laryngology, physician specialty may differ. There are physicians who truly dedicate their education and research time to the study of the larynx and how it produces voice. These physicians understand the medical condition and the art and science of voice production. A voice care team working along with the laryngologist may include a speech pathologist (voice pathologist/therapist), voice scientist, singing specialist, physician's assistant, and nurse with consultants to such professionals as pulmonologists, neurologists, allergists, and psychologists. There is great power in the interchange of ideas that occurs when related disciplines converge on a clinical voice problem. The continuity of care that is provided with such a team ensures that all aspects of a patient's problem can be addressed, and that surgery, when necessary, will be followed with close monitoring and ongoing treatment of any aggravating factors in order to keep the condition from recurring. The next section describes the information to be gathered during the diagnostic interview by the voice pathologist.

Case History

The clinical case history is the clinician's time in which to explore the nature and time line of the patient's presenting symptoms (Appendix 4–1 gives examples). Although direct contact time with the patient varies among clinicians, the voice pathologist spends a substantially greater amount of time obtaining the diagnostic history from the patients. The outcome of this interaction is an extremely important one and sets the stage for the future relationship between the voice pathologist and patient. An overview of some of the important items gathered during the history and the tests performed during the case history data collection phase of the evaluation are listed below.

■ Collect information about the history of: surgeries requiring intubation, trauma, hospitalizations, medical problems being treated by another physician, and types of medicines or herbal supplements the patient is taking;

■ Obtain a list of the physicians currently treating the patient's condition or previous consultations the patient has experienced;

■ Document history of allergies and describe throat clearing coughing and eating activities;

■ Obtain information on any previous or present speech difficulties, history of difficulty breathing, history of stridor, and any history of upper respiratory infection, asthma, emphysema, cardiovascular and/or other respiratory conditions;

> Stridor is a high-pitch audible noise typically heard on inspiration.

■ Obtain a family history to help determine nature of the disorder;

■ Obtain a description of the patient's work and home environment;

■ Find out what the patient likes to do for fun and enjoyment;

■ Ask the patient about the physical and perceptual impressions of their voice disorder;

■ Document the main characteristics of the voice disorder including information about the pitch, loudness, and quality of the voice;

■ Gather a description of the voice disorder from the patient's perspective;

■ Determine the onset and course of the voice disorder;

■ Determine the consistency of the voice disorder symptoms and other associated symptoms;

■ Determine the contributory factors to the onset and course of the voice disorder;

■ Identify phonotraumatic behaviors, if present. Some examples include screaming, loud talking or engaging in substance abuse, smoking, alcohol intake, improper nutrition, lack of sleep, and so forth (see Chapter 3);

■ Determine if there is any pain, tightness, or fatigue associated with voice production;

■ Determine the functional impact of the voice disorder on daily living;

■ Pay attention to the stress or emotional anxiety the patient is reporting or displaying;

■ Perform a hearing screening to make a quick judgment of hearing status.

The Physical Examination

When a voice disorder is present it often means that there is vocal fold damage or some compensatory involvement of other vocal tract structures that are creating disturbances to the quality of sound production. Although the patient's main complaint may be sound production, a complete examination of the head and neck is necessary to assist in identifying conditions that may be causing or contributing to the voice disturbance. A routine examination of the patient's head and neck by the laryngologist often occurs after the patient provides the case history information to the voice pathologist. The laryngologist completes the physical examination and checks the head and scalp, the nose and sinuses, and the neck region by touching the area around the larynx. Palpation of the cervical lymph nodes near the carotid arteries is done along with palpation of the submaxillary and submental nodes under the inner surface of the mandible and the preauricular nodes in front of the ear and suboccipital nodes behind the ear. Checking for fullness over the thyroid region of the neck assesses the thyroid gland. A routine check of ears, nose, and sinuses is also completed.

Oral Peripheral and Cranial Nerve Examination

An oral peripheral examination, commonly performed by the voice pathologist, checks the anatomy and function of the head and neck structures with specific attention to the articulators including those of the face, within the mouth, and the larynx.

During the oral peripheral examination, lip, tongue, jaw, and soft palate mobility are assessed as well as the status of the dentition, and hard and soft palate. Sensory function of these structures is tested by touching the surface of the structure of interests. Judgments are made with regard to the normality of movement and sensation using a scale that commonly ranges from normal to hyperfunctional or adequate to inadequate. Additional assessment usually incorporates tests of speaking rate and articulatory dynamics. The oral peripheral examination is completed during

the voice evaluation to help determine if there is a generalized neurologic condition that may be involved in the voice disturbance. A cranial nerve examination is more comprehensive and is done to test the integrity of cranial nerves 1 to 12 (Table 4–1).

Visual Examination

The otolaryngologist can choose to complete a gross, initial examination of the vocal folds first by placing a mirror in the back of the patient's mouth about as far back as the soft palate. This is referred to as a mirror examination and is considered a traditional laryngeal examination to check for laryngeal structure abnormality (Figure 4–1).

The otolaryngologist completes the examination. A continuous light source is shone into the back of the patient's mouth and the physician can obtain an overall but gross view of the vocal folds to determine if the structure is abnormal. Vocal fold movement cannot be assessed with a mirror examination as the vocal folds move faster than the human eye can resolve.

Laryngoscopic Techniques

Oral Rigid Laryngoscopy

There are two methods used to obtain images of the vocal folds beyond the mirror examination. The first is with an oral endoscope (an endoscope is an instrument that is passed into the body) placed into the back of the mouth. The oral endoscope sits in the same position (near the soft palate) as the mirror but offers the advantage of increased magnification. Light is carried by a fiberoptic bundle and directed down onto the larynx. The light is then reflected back to the examiner providing

Table 4–1. Summary of Cranial Nerve Functions

Cranial Nerve	I	II	III	IV	V	VI	VII	VIII	IX	X	XI	XII
Motor			X	X	X	X	X	X		X	X	X
Sensory	X	X			X		X	X	X	X		

Major Function:

I. Olfactory nerve—smell

II. Optic—vision

III. Oculomotor—moves eyelid and eyeball

IV. Trochlear—moves eyeball (laterally and downward)

V. Trigeminal—innervates muscles for chewing, senses touch and pain to scalp, face, and mouth

VI. Abducens—moves eyeball (turns eye laterally)

VII. Facial—innervates muscles for facial expression, secretion of tears, saliva, and senses taste from anterior tongue

VIII. Vestibulocochlear—equilibrium sensation and hearing

IX. Glossopharyngeal—senses taste from posterior tongue, general sensation from pharynx and throat, and senses carotid blood pressure

X. Vagus—slows heart rate, senses aortic blood pressure, stimulates digestive organs, senses taste, and innervates laryngeal muscles

XI. Accessory—innervates muscles for swallowing, trapezius, and sternocleidomastoid muscles

XII. Hypoglossal—innervates tongue muscles

Innervate or innervation is how nerves make contact with muscles, stimulating them into action via muscle contraction.

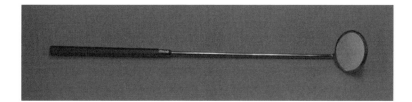

Figure 4–1. Schematic of a laryngeal mirror.

an image of the vocal folds. As the endoscope is used for specifically studying the laryngeal structures it is better to refer to this instrumentation as a laryngoscope. The oral laryngoscopic examination should not cause a great deal of discomfort for the patient, although some patients experience gagging as the scope is placed about two-thirds into the back of the mouth. If the patient cannot tolerate the oral endoscopic exam because of gagging, a topical anesthesia can be used to desensitize the reflex. Some clinicians do not advocate the use of an anesthesia because it may affect the normal function of the examined structures. If used, 20% benzocaine (Hurricane) is commonly sprayed into the back of the oral cavity (pharynx) to desensitize the structures, helping to reduce the gag reflex (Figure 4–2).

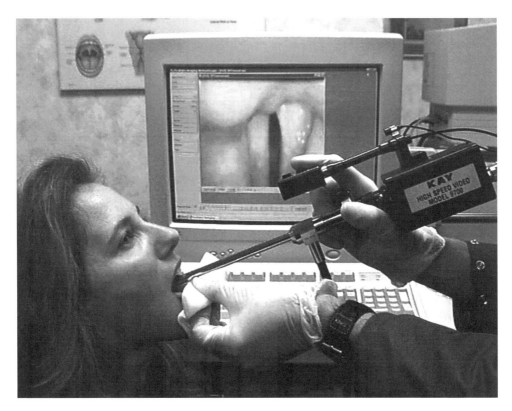

Figure 4–2. Oral rigid laryngoscopic technique. Courtesy of KayPENTAX.

Transnasal Flexible Laryngoscopy

The second imaging technique uses a flexible endoscope passed through the nasal cavity. The patient is awake for the procedure, just like during the oral laryngoscopic procedure. A water-based gel (such as KY Jelly) can be used to help ease the movement of the scope through the nasal passage. Patients typically do not experience pain, but rather a sense of mechanical discomfort as the scope passes through the narrow channels of the nose (nasopharynx). Additionally, an anesthetic spray to help minimize the discomfort associated with the scoping procedure can be used but this does not completely eliminate the sensation (Figure 4–3).

The benefit of using the transnasal laryngoscopic procedure is that it allows assessment of vocal fold function during more complex vocal tasks. Although the magnification is greater with the oral endoscope, and the quality of the image obtained with the oral scope is superior, only sustained vowel production can be produced because the position of the scope in the mouth hinders articulation. Connected speech and song production can be sampled while using the flexible scope, providing, perhaps, more functional behaviors associated with voicing that can be used in reaching a diagnosis.

Both the oral and flexible laryngoscopic techniques can be coupled with stroboscopic equipment if the vibration, referred to as mucosal wave, of the vocal folds requires assessment (Figure 4–4). Additionally, with laryngostroboscopy vocal fold opening and closure can be assessed, whether the vocal folds open fully and shut tightly, and whether

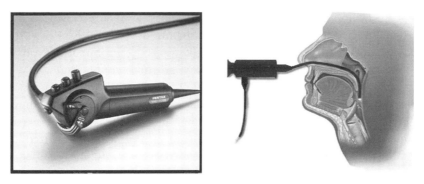

Figure 4–3. Transnasal laryngoscopic technique. Courtesy of KayPENTAX.

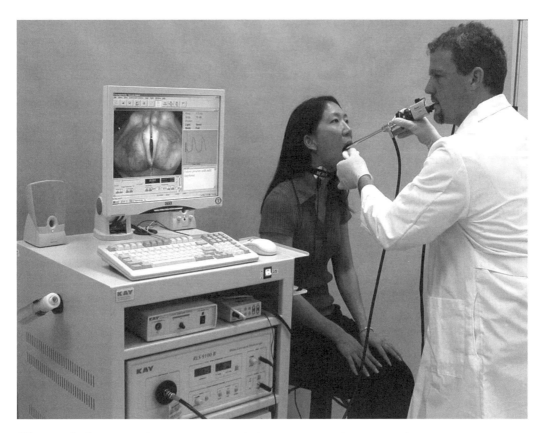

Figure 4–4. Indirect laryngoscopy and the KayPENTAX laryngostroboscopic unit. Courtesy of KayPENTAX.

the vocal folds move together as a unit. See the laryngostroboscopic rating form at the end of this chapter (Appendix 4–2).

Additional information that can be gained from the laryngoscopic exam is the presence or absence of compensatory behaviors. If compensatory behaviors exist, these can be documented and treated in the rehabilitation program. One compensatory behavior commonly exhibited during a laryngeal examination is ventricular (false) vocal fold movement during voice production. Typically, during voice production the false vocal folds do not participate in generating sound production. But when a vocal pathology/disturbance exists, the false fold movement may compensate for the impaired vocal fold movement. When this occurs the false vocal folds move toward the middle of the laryngeal structure during voicing. Unfortunately, in most cases, false vocal fold involvement is a sign of increased muscle tension and is therefore considered a negative compensatory maneuver. There is some disagreement that false vocal fold movement/compression is always associated with muscle tension. Stager, Neubert, Miller, Reganall, and Bielamowicz (2003) found increased false vocal fold compression with glottal stop production and speech initiation in females, activities that are not associated with disordered voice production. So, careful interpretation of the mechanism creating false vocal fold vibration is necessary for proper understanding of evaluation results.

The American Academy of Otolaryngology Voice and Swallow committee and the Special Interest Division on Voice and Voice Disorders of the American Speech-Language and Hearing Association (ASHA) developed a joint statement on the roles of the otolaryngologist and the speech-language pathologist in the performance and interpretation of laryngostroboscopy. More details of laryngostroboscopy follow below. Basically, laryngostroboscopy allows the structure and function of the vocal folds to be imaged and preserved digitally using specialized instrumentation. The position statement indicates "physicians are the only professionals qualified and licensed to render medical diagnoses related to the identification of laryngeal

pathology as it affects voice" (http://www.asha.org/docs/ html/RP1998-00132.html). Likewise, the examinations obtained with laryngostroboscopy should be viewed and interpreted by a laryngologist with training in the strobolaryngoscopic procedure. "Speech-language pathologists with expertise in voice disorders and with specialized training in strobolaryngoscopy are qualified to use the procedure for the purpose of assessing voice production and vocal function" (http://www.asha.org/docs/html/RP1998-00132.html). "Strobolaryngoscopy may also be used as a biofeedback tool for voice therapy" and this is discussed in Chapter 7 (http://www.asha.org/docs/html/RP1998-00132.html).

Instrumental Assessment

Quantifying parameters related to voice production requires some level of measurement sophistication. Inclusion of objective examination of voice is considered a valuable aspect of the voice evaluation. As voice is a product of multiple physiologic systems, it is important to quantify the function of the respiratory, laryngeal, and supralaryngeal systems as one or more may be impaired, creating the perceived disturbance in voice quality. Instrumentation is a collection of tools or devices used to measure data and it offers a controlled environment in which to do so. Today, instrumentation for measuring vocal fold function during voice production is currently available in research centers, major medical centers, and rehabilitation clinics.

The most important considerations in the selection of any instrument used to evaluate voice are that they meet the criteria of being reliable and valid. That is, the data the instrumentation yields should be repeatable when measured more than once (reliability) and the function that the device or tool claims to measure should be accurately reflected in the final data acquired (validity). Finally, the instrument should be responsive, that is, its sensitivity to change (pre- to post-treatment, for example) should be high. Uniformity, increased precision and increased accountability are some of the benefits if these criteria can be met.

There are several categories of instrumental assessment. These include imaging, aerodynamics, acoustics, and perceptual tools. Imaging techniques are discussed first, followed by aerodynamic and acoustic assessment, and then suggestions for using perceptual evaluation and rating scales conclude this section.

Imaging

Farnsworth in 1940 and other pioneers like Moore, White, and von Leden (1962), and Yanigihara and Koike (1967) helped define the physiology of vocal fold vibration by identifying specific parameters that could be measured from high-speed motion film. With the research of these scientists and others like Drs. von Leden, Van den Berg, and Timcke, details of the vibratory cycle were documented. In 1937, Bell Laboratories produced high-speed motion pictures of vocal fold vibration using a frame capturing rate of 2000 frames or pictures a second. It was scientists like von Leden, Timcke, and Moore who realized the capacity of such a tool and went on to examine the intricacies of vocal fold movement and then published the details of vocal fold physiology with and without disease (Moore et al., 1962).

Digital Laryngostroboscopy

As mentioned above, digital laryngostroboscopic systems are currently available for imaging the larynx. These are technologically advanced systems that allow the anatomic and physiologic characteristics of the vocal folds to be captured during sustained sound production. They provide excellent image quality; allow retrieval of the images for later examination, and pre- to post-comparison of the laryngeal image following treatment(s). As well, data management systems are available that allow the images to be exchanged between multiple institutions for the purposes of communicating research findings or collaborating on patient care.

The procedure of digital laryngostroboscopy (imaging the larynx using a strobe light) takes advantage of using interrupted light to make objects appear as if they are moving in slow motion. The light source is a very important part of the stroboscopic system and must be of high quality and able to flash at a rate of 5 microseconds, particularly when trying to freeze a frame of the video recording. The light source must flash less than 0.2 seconds between sequential images in order for the vibration to appear in slow motion. A throat microphone, placed near the thyroid lamina, detects the fundamental frequency of the patient's voice and emits a xenon light source intermittently, but at a slower rate than the fundamental frequency of the voice. The system samples a representative set of points along the vibratory cycles. The addition of these points represents different phases of each vibratory cycle such that the result is a full image but appearing in slow motion. The stroboscopic system takes advantage of Talbot's law, known as the persistence of vision (Kaszuba & Garrett, 2007). By using intermittent light flashes that are timed relative to the fundamental frequency, the motion of an object can be manipulated by altering the frequency of the intermittent light flashes.

The basic concept of laryngostroboscopy is very much like motion pictures or cartoons. If you draw separate sketches of a cartoon character walking in each position and flip the sketches in an orderly manner, the human eye will perceive a moving cartoon character. Along the same line, if several images of the vocal folds are obtained while they are moving at a certain point within the vibratory cycle and all of the pictures are put together at a certain rate, the result will be a slow motion movie (Figure 4–5). In order to obtain a still image of the vocal fold structure, the light source must flash at a rate that is equal to the fundamental frequency of the patient's voice.

There are several parameters that are rated from a laryngostroboscopic examination. These parameters are defined in Appendix 4–2 on the laryngostroboscopic rating form included at the end of the chapter for reference.

- Glottal closure: the degree to which the vocal folds close during maximum adduction during phonation
- Supraglottic activity: the degree of anteroposterior and lateral compression during phonation
- Vertical level of approximation: the degree to which the vocal folds meet on the same vertical plane during phonation
- Vocal fold edge: the smoothness of the vocal fold edges

- Vocal fold mobility: the degree of vocal fold movement during phonation
- Amplitude of vibration: the degree of movement from the medial to the lateral aspects of the vocal fold during phonation
- Mucosal wave: the assessment of the degree of traveling wave that is present on the superior surface of the vocal fold during phonation
- Nonvibration portion: identification of portions of the vocal fold that are not moving during phonation
- Phase closure: the degree to which the vocal folds move together during vocal fold closure during phonation
- Phase symmetry: degree to which the two vocal fold mirror each other's movement during phonation
- Periodicity: regularity of successive cycles of vibration during phonation
- Overall laryngeal function: assessment of the general impression of laryngeal function during phonation relative to a healthy laryngeal examination.

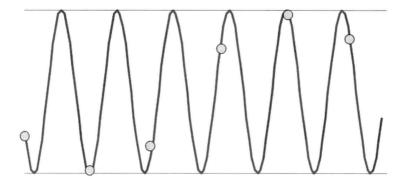

Figure 4–5. Illustration of stroboscopic flashing at different points in the vibratory cycle.

Videokymography

Clinically available since 1996, videokymography is another type of digital recording technique that provides visual information about vocal fold motion. It uses the standard rigid endoscope that is used for most laryngeal imaging procedures. It is distinct from laryngostroboscopy yet complementary in that it can provide high-speed images of vocal fold vibration, sampling up to 8000 frames per second (Svec & Schutte, 1996). By using a reference line that is located transverse to the glottis, the line images are portrayed in real time and vocal fold movement can be tracked, allowing for measurement of upper and lower vocal fold margin movement and time measurements of the open and closed phases (Figure 4–6). Svec, Sram, and Schutte (2007) provide an excellent review of the videokymographic technique, how it can be used in the clinical examination of voice disorders, and how it offers some distinct parameters for defining the vibratory aberrations associated with voice disorders as well as its ability to image aperiodic vibrations. Its use in everyday clinical practice has been marginal in the United States but it is available from KayPentax (http://www.kaypentax.com)

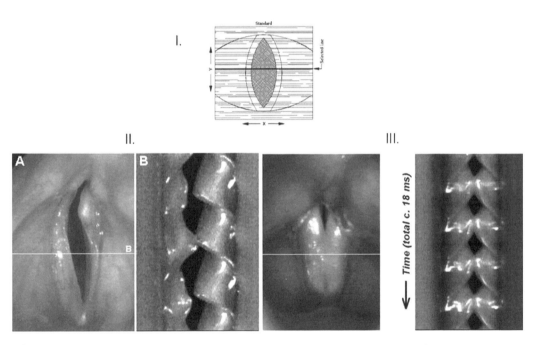

Figure 4-6. Plate I illustrates schematically the video image obtained from KayPENTAX's videokymography system using standard mode. Plate II shows videokymography used with a voice disorder characterized by asymmetric and perturbed vibration of the vocal folds in a male patient with a unilateral vocal fold paralysis. Plate III shows videokymography used with a normal voice indicating symmetric and regular vibration of the vocal folds in a female without voice problems. The videokymographic image on the right is obtained from the position marked by the line in the left image (i.e., the middle of the vocal folds) and covers a total time a 18 ms. From Svec and Sram (2002), used with permission of the authors. Adapted from Svec, Sram, and Schutte (2000) used with permission of the authors.

(Figure 4–7). Quantitative analysis of video-kymograms have been completed with a new software program called VKG-Analyser, which appears to be useful for objective evaluation of the vibratory pattern in normal and pathologic folds (Piazza et al., 2012).

High-Speed Digital Videoendoscopy

High-speed digital videoendoscopy can occur at a rate up to 2000 to 4000 frames per second (Hertegard, 2005) allowing the examiner to see the fine details of successive vocal fold vibration in real time rather than the illusion of successive vibrations as achieved with laryngostroboscopy. The standard capturing rate of video is 25 to 30 frames per second, so high-speed motion video captures the image at a rate approximately 1000 times the amount of standard video.

As stated earlier, the process of high-speed motion filming was first pioneered by Bell Laboratories in 1937. However, the use of high-

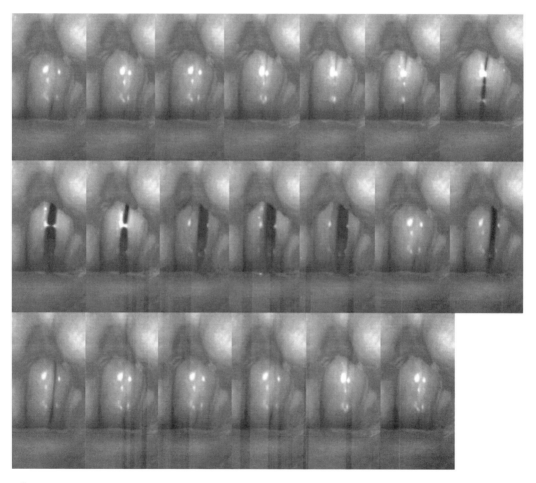

Figure 4–7. High-speed video images showing one cycle of habitual phonation from a male subject, 43 years old, recorded at 2000 fps using KayPENTAX HSV system, Model 9700, native resolution 120 × 256 pixels, 8-bit monochrome. This subject had no voice complaints, but a right vocal fold weakness/ paresis was diagnosed. Courtesy of Dr. Dimitar Deliyski.

speed film never quite made it into the daily clinical regime because its process was large and its analysis was time consuming. Yet, its use in the scientific world of voice has helped provide an understanding of the fine aspects of vocal fold vibration that can never be accomplished by laryngostroboscopic techniques.

Over the years, with advanced technology came high-speed digital video cameras providing a far less cumbersome and progressive technique compared to the equipment and analysis associated with high-speed film use. The accessibility to high-speed cameras has improved greatly over the last few years. They are used in many venues of research, not just the field of voice. High-speed cameras are used in the aerospace, automotive, security, defense industries and other disciplines concerned with high-level motion analysis.

The utility of high-speed videoendoscopy is certainly going to move our field further over the next 10 years and to date its use has already increased our understanding of the mechanisms of voice, the vibratory dynamics associated with artistic singing styles, and how vocal pathology alters vocal fold vibratory motion (Hertegard, 2005). Work by Patel, Liu, Galatsanos, and Bless (2010) describes the vibratory characteristics of adductor spasmodic dysphonia and muscle tension dysphonia using high speed imaging.

This advancement in technology has brought forth the ability to develop several experimental protocols, that when coupled with acoustic and aerodynamic sampling techniques, offers the examination of sound production at a variety of intensities, frequencies, and phonation modes (song, modal, fry, falsetto, etc.). Unlike laryngostroboscopy, which loses its ability to function validly when the sound production becomes aperiodic, high-speed digital imaging provides high precision in the analysis of voice disorders. Some truly interesting findings have emerged from the use of high-speed video. For example, one study showed that when the false vocal folds vibrate at a different frequency than the true vocal folds, a rough voice quality is produced and that the involvement of false vocal fold vibration plays a significant role in dysphonia. *But*, when the false vocal folds vibrate at a rate that is equivalent to the rate of true vocal fold vibration, the roughness is not perceived (Lindestad, Blixt, Pahlberg-Olsson, & Hammarberg, 2004). Looking forward to the future, analysis of other alterations to vocal fold vibration such as vocal tremor can be studied as could the application to the mechanisms involved in the aging voice and/or the differences between child and adult sound production may be discovered. Figure 4–7 shows the fine level of detail obtained with high-speed digital imaging during a vibratory cycle.

Aerodynamics

Aerodynamics is a branch of science that is concerned with the study of gas motion in objects and the forces that are created. Laryngeal aerodynamics is a specific field within this branch of science that studies the airflow and pressure that are produced during voice production and is considered an essential tool in the voice laboratory as part of the clinical voice evaluation (Dejonckere, 2000). Airway resistance, a byproduct of the relationship between pressure and flow, provide information about the impedance of the airway during voice production (Smitheran & Hixon, 1983). In a rudimentary physical model, the relationship between pressure, flow, and resistance is relatively straightforward. With an increased resistance, flow is restricted and greater pressure is needed to bypass the resistance. Likewise, with decreased resistance, air flows easily and less pressure is needed to generate the flow.

With regard to voice production, many aeroacoustic models have been developed to aid our understanding of the relationship between airflow, pressure, vocal fold vibration, and the acoustic output of the voice. The majority of previous aeroacoustic models of phonation have been based on Bernoulli's orifice theory that states that laryngeal airflow is quasi-steady.

> Most flow models are based on the Bernoulli equation and adjust the equation for pressure loses, viscosity effects, inertance of air, and so forth.
>   Flow models have evolved from simple one mass models, which allow one degree of freedom, to models allowing up to 16 degrees of freedom.

Mongeau, Franchek, Coker, and Kubli (1997) detailed aerodynamic measurements from a pulsating open jet model while modulating an orifice with a time-varying area. Their study provided insight on the aerodynamics of laryngeal airflow in order to refine the physiologic models of human voice production. Specifically, their experiments were designed to verify the legitimacy that flow phenomena within the larynx were quasisteady. Their results for airflow rate support the quasisteady assumption for most of the airflow cycle except for the early phase of flow development. This was again verified in Zhang et al.'s work (2002) across a range of frequencies, flow rates, and glottal orifice sizes.

Current aeroacoustic models, such as Mongeau et al.'s, are the basis for understanding sound generation in the larynx. However, many of these models do not account for variations in vocal fold vibration as a function of age (development) or sex or human compensation associated with disordered voice production. All are key factors that influence vocal output and should be incorporated into future models to broaden our understanding of normal and disordered laryngeal physiology.

With respect to the collection of aerodynamic signals from the human voice, there are several instrumental setups that can be used for collecting oral airflow and pressure data. The manufacturer and models used to collect the flow and pressure signals will vary depending on the aerodynamic measure of interest. For example, KayPentax, one of the leading manufacturers of voice and speech instrumentation, offer a system called the Phonatory Aerodynamic System (PAS), model 6600. The PAS is basically a fully integrated PC-based hardware/software system for measuring airflow and air pressure parameters during voice. It has software routines with which to calibrate the equipment and normative data bases built in the data management of its output for easy comparison. The PAS allows for the collection of oral airflow and oral pressure (Figure 4–8). Finer airflow measures can be sensed with other sensing equipment as discussed below.

General Methods for Collection of Aerodynamic Signals

Rothenberg (1973) introduced the circumferentially vented pneumotachograph facemask, a system that allows oral airflow to be collected at the mouth. The physical principle of this mask is similar to other pneumotachographs used with commercially available setup. The transduction system works on the principle of impedance to produce a measurable drop in pressure proportional to airflow. In the circumferentially vented design, the impedance is a wire cloth screen, made of a layer of fine-mesh stainless steel built into the mask. The mesh and the area of the screen (i.e., resistance) create an air pressure drop equivalent to flow that is approximately no more than 10% of the lung pressure used to produce the sound. The circumferential design mini-

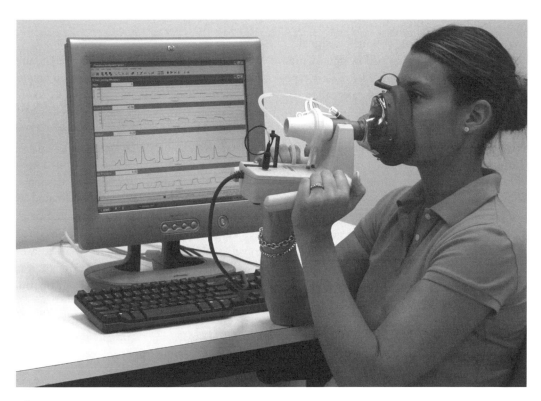

Figure 4–8. KayPENTAX PAS system. Courtesy of KayPENTAX.

mizes sound distortion and the loss of high frequency fidelity when compared to funnel type pneumotachographs (Figure 4–9).

There has been some debate regarding the use of facemasks for collection of oral airflow and its influence on voice production. One item of past discussion centered on the mask's effect on breathing and the accurate representation of the airflow signal during voice production. Huber, Stathopoulos, Bormann, and Johnson (2003), responded to that discussion and from their experimental study indicated that the resistance of the Rothenberg mask does not negatively impact rest breathing and breathing for speech when compared to a no mask condition. The implication of the Huber et al. (2003) findings is that the use of a facemask for collection of oral airflow should be considered noninvasive and noninfluential in modifying the normal aspects of

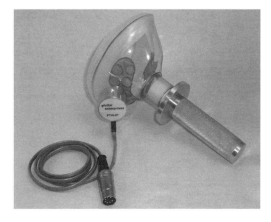

Figure 4–9. Glottal Enterprises, Inc. circumferentially vented pneumotachograph airflow mask. Reproduced with permission.

voice and breathing. However, the results are only applicable to the use of the Rothenberg circumferentially vented pneumotachograph mask. Mask types differ depending on which system is used to sample the airflow signal.

In order to acquire an airflow signal a pressure transducer is required. The easiest types of pressure transducers to use are called differential pressure transducers (Figure 4–10). A differential pressure transducer measures the pressure by calculating the difference between the pressure before a resistance and the pressure after a resistance. By measuring the pressure difference before and after a resistance, the flow velocity can be calculated.

Many of the commercial systems available for collecting laryngeal aerodynamic information gather data on average airflow produced during sustained vowel production. Systems like the KayPentax PAS (http://www.kaypentax.com), Glottal Enterprises system, and PERCI (Warren & Dubuois, 1964) allow for measurement of average airflow.

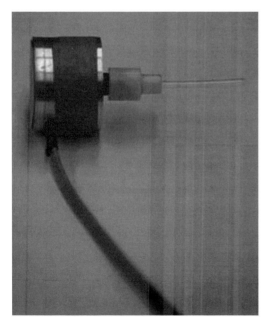

Figure 4–10. Glottal Enterprises, Inc. low-frequency pressure transducer (PTL). Reproduced with permission.

Average Airflow

With a healthy laryngeal condition, average airflow during sustained vowel production ranges from 40 to 320 cc/sec in men and 50 to 220 cc/sec in women with average data reported as 119 cc/sec and 115 cc/sec, respectively (Bless, Glaze, Biever-Lowry, Campos, & Peppard, 1993).

An average airflow signal provides a general idea of laryngeal function but does not give the detail about the flow modulated at the level of the glottis. When extracted from a voicing signal that is other than a sustained vowel prolongation, it not only estimates glottal airflow but also the airflow that is modulated by other articulators within the oronasal-pharyngeal cavities.

Therefore, by and large, the use of average airflow as a single independent variable for defining laryngeal physiology is not readily advocated.

Bielamowicz, Berke, and Gerratt (1995) exemplified the use of average airflow as an outcome measure in patients who underwent medialization procedures. They found a significant decrease in airflow from pre- to post-surgery. And, more recently, Kimura, Nito, Sakakibara, Tayama, and Nimi (2008) used mean airflow rate as an indicator of measurable improvement pre- and post-collagen injection of the vocal folds. There are other examples in the literature of using average airflow rate as a measure of pre-post outcome; however, caution should be used in interpreting its use as a fine measure of laryngeal function change. Rather, it should be interpreted as a gross measure of laryngeal function change.

Measures of average airflow can also be used in conjunction with measures of estimated subglottal air pressure for calculation of laryngeal airway resistance. Finnegan, Luschei, Barkmeier, and Hoffman (1996), estimated laryngeal airway resistance (subglottal pressure/average airflow) in those with spasmodic dysphonia. A pertinent finding from their study was that those with spasmodic dysphonia produced varying airflow. The authors cautioned that the use of average flow for calculating airway resistance in this population might be a source of error due to the variability in flow rate that occurs because of the chaotic nature of vocal fold vibration associated with spasmodic dysphonia. More recent work using average airflow as an outcome is scarce.

Before describing a finer measure of airflow, called glottal airflow, the measurement of estimated subglottal pressure and estimated laryngeal airway resistance are explained.

Estimated Subglottal Pressure

Subglottal air pressure (commonly measured in cm H_2O) is the amount of pressure directly below the vocal folds developed by the respiratory system for voice production (see Chapter 1). In order to directly measure subglottal air pressure, a pressure transducer is connected to a thin, relatively short piece of polyethylene tubing, which is then attached to a hypodermic needle inserted into the cricothyroid membrane. The issue with direct measurement of subglottal pressure has nothing to do with accuracy, as it is the most direct method, but rather with discomfort and anxiety during the data collection. Therefore, an alternative method for collecting oral pressure at the mouth for estimating subglottal pressure was developed by Smitheran and Hixon (1981).

Indirect measurement of subglottal pressure occurs by placing a small piece of polyethylene tubing between the lips, which is attached to a differential pressure transducer (Figure 4–11). With the pressure tube between the lips, the patient is asked to produce a string of bilabial syllables consisting of the voiceless stop /p/ followed by the vowel /i/, at a constant pitch and at a rate of 1.5 syllables per second. During the production of the /p/ segment, the vocal folds are open, yet the lips are

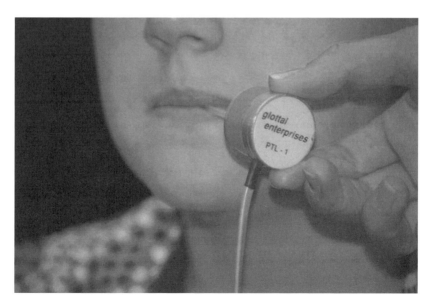

Figure 4–11. Depiction of oral pressure sensing tube and placement for making measurements of estimated subglottal pressure.

closed, offering an opportunity for pressure to reach a state of equilibrium throughout the upper airway. Maintaining the syllable rate is critical to allow the pressure to equilibrate. In fact, production of the syllable rate at a rate somewhat higher than 1.5 syllables per second would be all right but certainly no slower, if the data are to be valid.

> A differential pressure transducer measures the difference between two or more pressures. In the case of the differential pressure transducer described here, Pressure 1 = atmospheric pressure, Pressure 2 = pressure sensed in the oral cavity.

Estimated Laryngeal Airway Resistance

The measurement of estimated laryngeal airway resistance, also described by Smitheran and Hixon (1981) requires the accurate measurement of average airflow and estimated subglottal pressure as determined from the intraoral air pressure signal during the /pi/ syllable described above. It is calculated by dividing the value of estimated subglottal pressure by the average airflow value. Zhang et al. (2002) used resistance measures to differentiate muscle tension dysphonia from healthy adults.

Inverse Filtering

In order to obtain a useful estimate of the airflow modulated by the vocal folds during voicing, inverse filtering of the oral airflow waveform must be completed to obtain an estimate of glottal airflow. The inverse filtering procedure is complex but can be accomplished using either a digital or analog system and relies on the accurate identification of the formant frequencies from the oral airflow signal. The benefit of Rothenberg's circumferentially vented mask design, described above, is the preservation of the vowel quality because of the high bandwidth of the system, on the order of 3 kHz. Rothenberg (1973) outlined the following criteria for deriving accurate information using a pneumotachograph. These include:

- The output must be a linear function of the volume velocity
- The airflow resistance of the mask should be low enough so no negligible disturbance of the pressure and airflow occurs during speech. Adhering to the low airflow resistance criteria ensures that there is no distortion to the acoustic signal

Finally,

- The response time of the pneumotachograph should be small compared to the glottal period (see Rothenberg, 1973).

> A formant frequency is a peak in the frequency spectrum of a sound caused by acoustic resonance.

Many measures made from a glottal airflow waveform have been reported in the literature (e.g., Holmberg, Hillman, & Perkell, 1988). The clinical relevance of some of these measures is reported here. Figure 4–12 depicts an oral airflow waveform captured by the pneumotachograph facemask and the subsequent estimate of glottal airflow after the inverse filtering process is applied. From the glottal airflow waveform several measures can be derived (Holmberg et al., 1988; Stathopoulos & Sapienza, 1997).

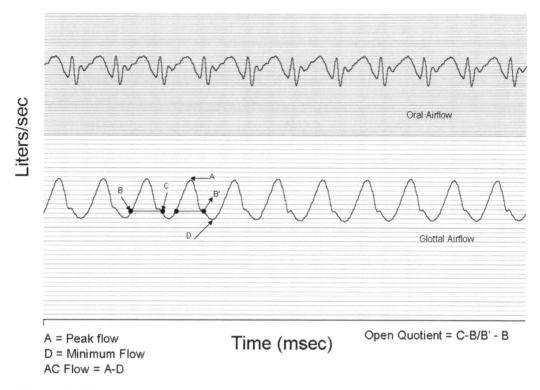

Figure 4–12. Depiction of oral and glottal airflow waveform. Glottal airflow waveform shows points related to peak (point A), alternating glottal airflow (A–D) and minimum glottal airflow (point D), and airflow open quotient (C–B/B'–B).

Airflow Open Quotient (OQ)

Clinically this measure provides duration information about the length of time the glottis is open relative to the duration of the entire cycle of vocal fold vibration. As glottal opening allows airflow to occur, this measure is useful for cases in which glottal closure is deemed inadequate or incomplete (hypofunctional vocal pathologies) or in cases where a high glottal resistance is suspected, that is, an obstruction, spasm, hyperfunction, or loud voice production (see Figure 4–12 [C–B/B'–B]). Open quotient, therefore, can help define the degree of glottal adduction from a pressed to a breathy voice; however, care must be taken to measure the subglottal pressure developed during the voice production as it

is influential on the measure of open quotient (Sundberg, 2008).

Maximum Flow Declination Rate

Scherer (1991) provided an excellent overview of the relationship between the glottal airflow signal and the mechanics of phonation, discussing how maximum flow declination rate represents the rate at which the glottal airflow shuts off and its relationship to perceptual differences in vocal quality, particularly vocal loudness. Maximum flow declination rate is measured as the maximum negative peak from the first derivative of the glottal airflow waveform (Figure 4–13). Maximum flow declination rate can be used

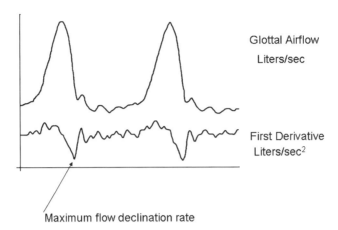

Maximum flow declination rate

Figure 4–13. Depiction of maximum flow declination rate derived from glottal airflow waveform.

to define hypo- and hyperfunctional glottal configurations. Assuming no compensatory strategies exist, hypofunctional voice cases would predictably yield a low maximum flow declination rate value because of the disability in completely closing the vocal folds and the slowness in the return of the weakened vocal fold toward midline. Maximum flow declination rate predictably would be higher in those with hyperfunctional voice disorders due to an increase in subglottal pressure and greater vibrational amplitudes. However, as those with hyperfunctional voice disorders can also have increased vocal fold stiffness, declination rates are not always predictable.

Peak Glottal Airflow

Peak glottal airflow relates to the maximum glottal area during vocal fold vibration. Increased stiffness, decreased mucosal wave, or any other pathologic condition or phonation type (pressed voice), which restricts the maximum displacement of the vocal folds, can alter the peak airflow during phonation (see Figure 4–12, point A).

Alternating Glottal Airflow

Changes in vocal fold tension and stiffness affect alternating airflow by altering the displacement of vocal folds during voicing. With increased stiffness of the vocal folds, alternating airflow typically decreases (see Figure 4–12, A–D).

Minimum Glottal Airflow

Minimum glottal airflow relates to the amount of airflow through the glottis during the closed phase of vocal fold vibration. Theoretically, a higher minimum airflow would reflect a greater degree of incomplete glottal closure. This measure provides a way to document the hypofunctional component of vocal pathologies such as adductor vocal fold paralysis or other cases where there is glottal incompetence. See Fisher, Scherer, Guo, and Owen's (1996) use of this measure for tracking glottal incompetence in patients with spasmodic dysphonia following botulinum toxin injection (see Figure 4–12, point D).

In summary, the glottal airflow waveform will be different depending on the phonation type. For a breathy voice, the glottal pulse will be more symmetric, with a higher OQ and higher peak airflow. With a creaky or pressed voice, the glottal airflow pulses are more irregular and the OQ will be low.

Laryngeal Aerodynamic Variations

Laryngeal Aerodynamics of the Developing Larynx

Stathopoulos and Sapienza (1997) studied the aerodynamic characteristics of voice production in children between 4 to 14 years and compared them to adults. They asked the children to vary the sound pressure level of their voice to determine the aerodynamic mechanisms of their developing structure. Obviously, children and adults are different with regard to laryngeal size (see Chapter 2). Children's smaller size limits glottal area and vocal fold vibrational amplitude, thereby affecting the aerodynamic to acoustic energy conversion (Hirano, Kurita, & Nakashima, 1981; Tang & Stathopoulos, 1995). Stathopoulos and Sapienza (1997) predicted that aerodynamic measures, as a function of development, would reflect the known changes in laryngeal anatomy. Their results revealed many functional differences between children and adults. Interestingly, 14-year-old boys and men showed comparable aerodynamic influence on voice whereas the women and all other children showed similar function. The researchers pointed out how these data correspond with the developmental anatomy of the larynx, which shows laryngeal size for women and children to be more similar than that of women compared to men.

Laryngeal Aerodynamics as a Function of Aging

Aging results in anatomic and physiologic changes to the larynx (see Chapter 2) such as degeneration of the cartilaginous framework, vocal fold tissue, and motor innervation to the larynx (e.g., Kahane, 1982). These anatomic degenerations with aging influence the biomechanical function of the larynx affecting laryngeal aerodynamics. In a study of 60 women (age groups 20 to 70 years), Sapienza and Dutka (1996) found no significant group differences, but did find increased variability for the 70-year-old group for the amount of airflow produced during maximum abduction. These results highlight the use of aerodynamic measures to document the variability in airflow that accompany the aging process. Since the 1996 study few have used glottal airflow measures to help understand how the anatomic and physiologic changes with age relate to alterations in vocal fold valving. Back in 1991, Higgins and Saxman recorded subglottal pressure and airflow and found sex differences in how the variables were affected for men and women with less age-related laryngeal degeneration in older women than older men. Goozee, Murdoch, Thompson, and Thompson (1998) found no age differences for the measure of subglottal air pressure in their study.

Laryngeal Aerodynamics Differences as a Function of Sex

There is literature that reports distinctions in aerodynamic parameters between young women and men (Goozee, et al., 1998; Stathopoulos & Sapienza, 1997). These studies document higher values for amplitude-based flow parameters, such as mean, peak and alternating flow, and maximum flow declination rate in men versus women and longer open phases of the airflow duty cycle in women versus men. The resultant aerodynamics is a reflection of the distinctions in glottal area and vibratory pattern differences documented between men and women (Titze, 1989) and relate well to the perception that the female voice is weaker and breathier than the adult male voice (Klatt & Klatt, 1990).

Laryngeal Aerodynamic Changes as a Function of Speech Task

The type of speech task chosen to sample laryngeal airflow makes a difference on the measurement outcome. That is, differences will occur depending on whether the data are measured from a sustained vowel task versus a connected speech task.

A few research papers in the past have addressed this topic but mostly with regard to acoustic measures. Sapienza, Stathopoulos, and Brown (1995) examined glottal airflow parameters during vowel production, syllable production, and reading and found statistical differences between vowels produced in isolation as compared to vowels produced in syllables and reading. Differences were found for airflow amplitude measures and time-based airflow measures. Although the differences were statistically significant the actual numeric differences were quite small causing speculation as to whether these differences would result in perceptually distinct voice quality. The relationship between aerodynamic differences in voice production and the role they play in perceptually distinguishing the voice still requires investigation. As well, the influence of different speech tasks on laryngeal aerodynamic information is still not resolved.

Clinicians should be cautious about overgeneralizing the results obtained from one phonatory task to another.

Using Aerodynamics for Examination of Voice Disorders

Raes and Clement's (1996) article reviewed measurement techniques, normative results, and clinical uses of aerodynamic measures but their measures were indirectly related to glottal aerodynamics. Measures such as maximum phonation time (MPT) and Phonation Quotient (PQ), a calculated variable based on MPT and vital capacity, were included in their study. Unfortunately, these measures are indirect with regard to defining phonatory physiology and are susceptible to variations in measurement procedures.

> Vital capacity is the total amount of air that can be exhaled after a maximum inspiration.

Dejonckere and Lebacq (1996) documented the relationship between glottal air leakage, high spectral energy and the perception of breathiness in 87 dysphonic patients. They found a positive relationship between glottal air leakage (high flows during the closed phase of vocal fold vibration), the presence of high frequency energy, and the perception of breathiness.

Ramig and Dromey's (1996) work addressed the aerodynamic mechanisms underlying treatment of voice/speech disorders. The purpose of their study was to document changes in aerodynamic aspects of vocal function in patients with Parkinson's disease that received two forms of treatment. The first treatment was the Lee Silverman Voice Treatment; the second technique was a respiratory breathing technique with no focus of training on the larynx. Measures included maximum flow declination rate and estimated subglottal pressure. LSVT resulted in significantly increased maximum flow declination rate and subglottal pressure but the respiratory training program did not alter these variables. They concluded that a combination of increased vocal fold adduction and increased subglottal pressure were key in generating posttreatment increases in sound pressure level (vocal loudness) in patients with Parkinson's disease.

Cantarella, Berlusconi, Maraschi, Ghio, and Barbieri (2006) analyzed the effects of botulinum toxin on airflow stability in spasmodic dysphonia by measuring mean airflow rate. Although not surprising, those with spasmodic dysphonia produced a highly unstable mean phonatory airflow patterns but the variability in the airflow signal became more stable following botulinum toxin injection. This study demonstrates a good example of using aerodynamic measures to document treatment outcome.

Finally, another clinical outcome study analyzed laryngeal aerodynamics in one patient with unilateral vocal fold paralysis under four different circumstances: before the onset of the paralysis, after two types of surgical vocal medialization procedures, and after the onset of the paralysis. This study design is an example of how objective measures can be used to compare treatment choices by defining the degree of improvement following surgical procedures (Hartl, Hans, Vaissiere, & Brasnu, 2005). And yet another study used laryngeal aerodynamic analysis to assist with the diagnosis of muscle tension dysphonia by determining if subglottal pressure, laryngeal airway resistance and maximum flow rate and maximum phonation time could differentiate muscle tensiond dysphonia from health control (Zhang et al., 2002).

The use of aerodynamic indexes for documenting changes in laryngeal status is relevant for reporting treatment outcome for a variety of populations with disordered voice production. Much more work in this area, however, is needed.

Acoustic Analysis of Voice

Much like aerodynamic measures, the ease of obtaining acoustic measures makes it ideal to monitor changes in voice over time, such as following therapy, before and after surgery, or with progression of a disease. Acoustic analysis is fast becoming a part of most voice evaluations by providing excellent measures of treatment outcome. This is due to the declining cost of necessary hardware and software, availability of more sophisticated algorithms for voice analyses and numerous research publications documenting normative data and may demonstrate the utility (and limitations) of various measures. The following section describes general considerations when making acoustic measurements of voice, along with a description of the most commonly employed measures, what information the measures provide, and the precautions necessary when obtaining and interpreting acoustic measures.

Goals of Acoustic Analysis

Efficient use of time while collecting the most pertinent information to differentially diagnose a voice disorder is the main goal of a voice evaluation. Acoustic analysis is one means used in the evaluation of voice, allowing clinicians to gather significant amounts of data in a noninvasive and cost effective manner. However, one must use prudence in choosing the tools that are most appropriate for assessing a particular patient's voice. Despite the many advantages of acoustic analysis of voice, it is necessary to take several precautions when using any acoustic measure for clinical decision-making. This is because acoustic measures, like most other behavioral tests, can easily be affected by variables other than the voice itself. These include factors such as recording procedures, elicitation instructions, and environmental interference. The accuracy of acoustic analysis will only be as good as the weakest link in the entire process. The acoustic tools used in the evaluation of voice must be guided by the nature of the information necessary for making a clinical diagnosis or to aid in rehabilitation for that particular patient. Clinicians generally use acoustic analysis of voice with the intent to obtain the following two kinds of information.

■ *Vocal fold physiology.* As voice disorders generally originate from some change in vocal fold structure or vibratory characteristics, any tool that helps identify and quantify these changes may help voice assessment and the development of rehabilitation goals. Although other tools such as laryngostroboscopy or aerodynamic assessment may also provide similar information, acoustic analysis may be the preferred approach because it is easy to quantify, less time-consuming, less expensive, and more comfortable to the patient.

■ *Perception of voice.* As perceptually healthy voice is often an important goal of voice therapy, any tool that helps identify and quantify changes in perceived vocal characteristics can help in the evaluation of voice disorders and for documenting the outcome of rehabilitation goals for patients with voice disorders. Again,

although similar information can be gathered by subjective evaluation of voice, such as through the use of rating scales, acoustic analysis of voice holds promise in standardizing the measurement tasks and in minimizing the variability associated with subjective evaluation.

Recording Voice for Acoustic Analysis

The accuracy of acoustic measures of voice is critically dependent on the fidelity of the recording equipment. A typical voice recording setup includes a microphone, a preamplifier, and a recording device such as a digital audio recorder or a personal computer. Each of these components must meet certain minimum standards for the acoustic measures to be accurate. These minimum standards have been described in a report by the National Center for Voice and Speech (Titze, 1994). In brief, one must be careful to use recording equipment that has a wide frequency response, high sensitivity, and good signal-to-noise ratio. Fortunately, many commercially available recording systems, those designed specifically for voice analyses as well as several others that are designed primarily for music, meet or exceed these minimum requirements. This makes it easier for clinicians to obtain recording equipment that can be used to obtain accurate acoustic measurements of voice.

Most modern instrumentation for acoustic recording relies on digital technology that represents the acoustic waveform as a series of numbers. In other words, digital recording devices represent acoustic signals by taking a snapshot (or a "sample") of the signal from time to time (Figure 4–14).

Because of this, the choice of recording parameters is critical to making proper acoustic recordings and analyses. Two important considerations when recording voices for acoustic

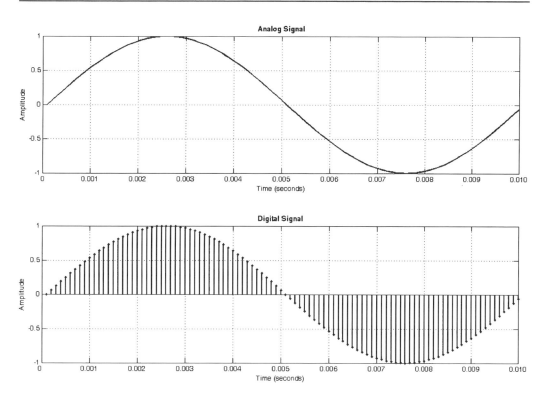

Figure 4–14. A sine wave and its digital representation.

analyses are the *sampling rate* and the *quantization level*. The sampling rate reflects how often the voice signal is sampled in time. One may think of this as the number of snapshots that one may take of the signal. The more snapshots taken (or higher sampling rates), the better the original signal can be approximated. It is recommended that for the purposes of acoustic analyses of voice, the sampling rate should be no less than 20 kHz (i.e., taking 20,000 snapshots per second). Similarly, the quantization level reflects the number of steps that may be used to represent changes in the amplitude of the signal. As shown in Figure 4–15, a 1-bit signal (*21*) can only have two possible levels (or steps); a 2-bit signal (*22*) may have four possible steps, and so on. Once again, higher *bit-rates* allow the acoustic signal to be more accurately reflected, thereby improving the accuracy of the acoustic analysis. It is

generally recommended that acoustic signals have at least 12-bit resolution (212 = 4096 steps), though many software packages now use 16-bit (216 = 65,536 steps) or higher quantization levels.

To obtain the best possible recordings for acoustic analyses, clinicians should be careful to avoid two possible errors. First, clinicians must be careful to avoid *peak clipping*. Peak clipping occurs when the signal intensity is so high that it cannot be correctly represented within the quantization levels available for recording (Figure 4–16). Peak clipping will damage the recorded signal and render it useless for many of the acoustic measures described later. To avoid peak clipping, the microphone gain needs to be adjusted such that the highest peaks in the signal do not exceed the maximum allowable input levels. A second kind of error arises when the recording

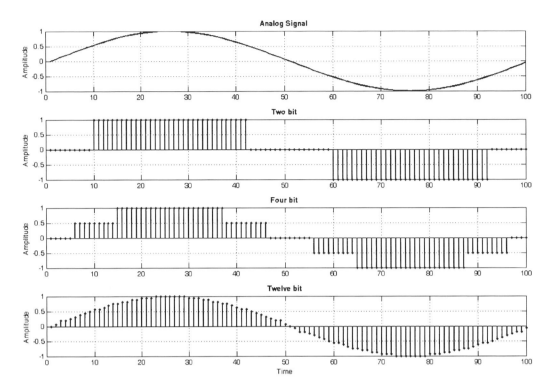

Figure 4–15. Digital representation of a sine wave with different quantization levels.

fails to use the available quantization levels adequately. For example, if the microphone gain is set too low, then the entire signal may only be recorded using a small number of quantization levels (see Figure 4–16). Although not as serious as peak clipping, this error fails to utilize the full amplitude resolution available and may limit the accuracy of specific acoustic measures (such as amplitude perturbation). Again, this may be avoided by making sure that the microphone gain is set to the highest values possible that does not result in peak clipping.

All voice recordings need to be obtained in a quiet environment. A special sound-treated room dedicated for voice recordings is ideal but is not essential for quality voice recordings. However, one must be vigilant and avoid external noise as much as possible. It is not uncommon for voice samples to be recorded in busy clinics where a patient's voice

signals may be contaminated by the sounds of other equipment, and the background noise of other people talking and/or ongoing activities. Much of this external noise tends to be in the lower frequencies and may overlap with the fundamental frequency in speech. Unfortunately, algorithms used for acoustic analysis of voice generally cannot distinguish such external noise from the patient's voice and this may lead to erroneous measurements. Therefore, it is imperative to choose an appropriate recording environment and to monitor the quality of the voice recording before submitting it to any analyses.

Acoustic Analysis of Voice

Once a voice sample has been recorded, it may be submitted for a variety of analyses. The last few decades have seen tremendous advances in

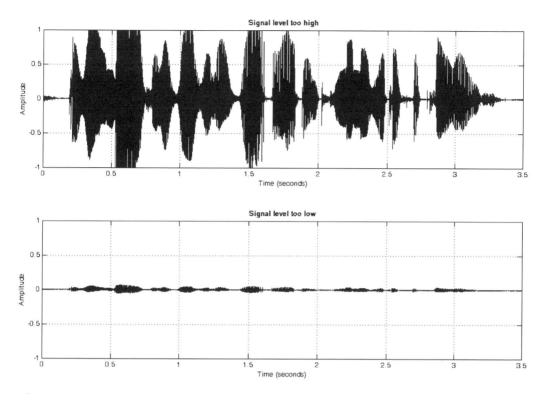

Figure 4–16. Two common errors during acquisition of the speech signal. The top figure shows peak clipping. The bottom figure shows failure to utilize all available quantization levels.

how the vocal acoustic signal may be analyzed and quantified. There now exist availability of numerous algorithms and procedures for voice analyses. However, most of these algorithms/procedures can be classified into six major categories. These include spectrograms, fundamental frequency, intensity, short-term perturbation, relative noise levels, and measures made from short- or long-term spectra. A brief description of auditory-based measures is also described, although these are still under development and are restricted to the research laboratory.

Spectrograms

When making acoustic measures of voice, it is generally a good idea to begin by carefully

examining its spectrogram. A spectrogram is not a specific measure; rather, it is a visual representation of the speech acoustic signal. It allows a clinician to inspect how the acoustic signal changes over time. A spectrogram represents speech in three dimensions: the ordinate or the horizontal axis shows time, and the abscissa or the vertical axis shows frequency and the intensity of various frequency, components typically shown by the darkness of the plot. Some programs also allow users to display differences in intensity by different colors on the plot.

Two types of spectrograms are commonly used for speech analyses. Using wider "windows" for analysis creates a "wideband" spectrogram, whereas a "narrowband" spectrogram is created using a shorter window size. These differences in computation offer certain advantages over the other. By averaging signals in wider windows, a wideband spectrogram gives very good time resolution, but lacks good frequency resolution. In other words, a wideband spectrogram can allow clinicians to clearly observe how the acoustic signal changes over time, but it cannot resolve neighboring frequency components distinctly. In contrast, a narrowband spectrogram gives a much better frequency resolution, but lacks the time resolution of the wideband spectrogram. Figure 4–17 shows the wide- and narrowband spectrograms for the same segment of speech.

Note how the wideband spectrogram can clearly distinguish the beginning and end of a consonant, but it fails to show individual harmonics in the vowel. On the other hand, the narrowband spectrogram for the same speech segment shows individual harmonics at the cost of losing the fine temporal structure.

Although wideband spectrograms are ideal for studying the formant structure or consonant-vowel boundaries, a narrowband spectrogram is an excellent way to inspect the vocal acoustic signal in patients with voice disorders. By inspecting changes in the harmonic structure of the voice, a clinician can observe the stability of the patient's vocal fold vibration.

> A harmonic is a frequency that is an integral multiple of the fundamental frequency. If the patient has a fairly stable vocal fold vibration pattern, the narrowband spectrogram shows clear and steady harmonics.

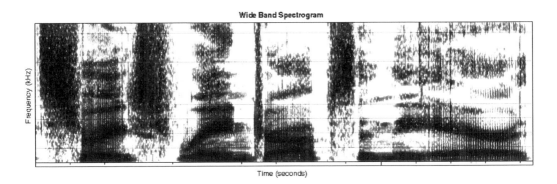

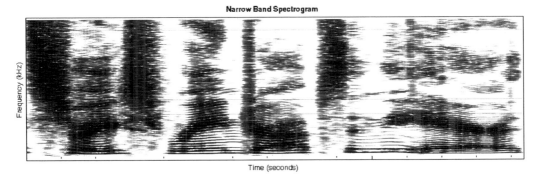

Figure 4–17. Wideband (*top*) and narrowband (*bottom*) spectrograms for the same speaker reading the "Rainbow Passage." The figures display the phrase " . . . strikes raindrops in the air . . . "

In contrast, a lack of stability in vocal fold vibration will result in frequent changes in this pattern. The vocal acoustic signal can be classified into three types of segments by observing the narrowband spectrograms (Titze, 1994). When the narrowband spectrogram shows clearly visible structure periods of the harmonic structure, these segments are classified as "Type 1." The narrowband spectrogram for some voice segments shows alternating dark and light horizontal lines. Sometimes, two or more light colored horizontal lines between each dark line may be observed. These lighter lines represent "subharmonics" in the vowel spectrum and voices that show subharmonics are classified as "Type 2." Finally, some segments in a patient's voice may show a complete lack of a clear harmonic structure. These segments are classified as "Type 3." Figure 4–18 shows examples of each of these three types of voice signals.

Classifying voices into these three types is an *essential* step in acoustic analysis of voices. This is because many of the acoustic measures will only be valid for signals that are classified as Type 1. For example, many acoustic measures, such as frequency and amplitude perturbation can be calculated from Type 1 segments but not from Type 2 or 3 segments. As Type 2 or 3 segments do not have a definite fundamental frequency, these measures do not convey any meaningful information. It is important to note that most acoustic analysis software cannot automatically distinguish between these three types of voice segments. Therefore, if a voice with Type 2 or Type 3 segments is submitted for computing such measures, the software nevertheless will

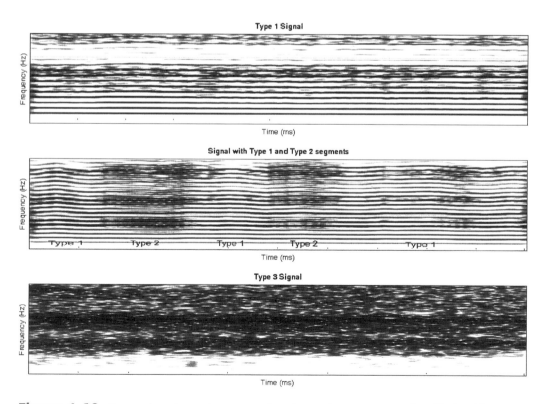

Figure 4–18. Narrowband spectrograms showing voice segments classified as Type 1 (*top panel*), Type 2 (*parts of the middle panel*), and Type 3 (*bottom panel*).

report some output. However, clinicians must interpret these numbers in light of the nature of the voice signal being analyzed. It is for this reason, that spectrograms are a good starting point for all further acoustic analyses.

Fundamental Frequency

The fundamental frequency of voice is one of the most basic measures made from the acoustic signal. Most software for acoustic analysis of speech will provide one or more algorithms for computing fundamental frequency. Most software packages typically display the fundamental frequency *contour* for the analyzed signal, and report the mean and standard deviation for that contour.

Physiologically, this measure typically reflects the number of vibratory cycles completed per second. However, this can only be clearly estimated for Type 1 signals. Care must be taken not to include measures from Type 2 and Type 3 segments when reporting fundamental frequency. Perceptually, fundamental frequency is related to pitch. In general, as the fundamental frequency of a sound increases, so does its pitch but this relationship is not linear. In other words, a doubling of fundamental frequency does not always lead to doubling of pitch. Unfortunately, the two terms, fundamental frequency and pitch, are often used synonymously in the literature as well as in common manner of speaking. *Remember* that the two terms refer to two distinct concepts, so choose the terminology appropriately.

A number of algorithms have been proposed to compute fundamental frequency from vocal signals. Although the earliest algorithms were relatively simple, more recently developed algorithms use much more sophisticated computations to estimate fundamental frequency in voice. Despite these advances in signal processing, none of the algorithms are perfect and some errors in estimating funda-

mental frequency can occur. One commonly occurring error is the *doubling* or *halving* of the fundamental frequency. In some instances, these algorithms may output values that are either double or half the actual fundamental frequency. Another error occurs when the algorithm accidentally reads the first formant frequency as the fundamental frequency. This typically occurs in vowels where the first formant frequency is close to the fundamental frequency. Always verify the accuracy of the measurement by visually inspecting the fundamental frequency contour. Any segments where the fundamental frequency contour shows abrupt changes should be matched against the time waveform to confirm the accuracy of the fundamental frequency output. These errors often are easily corrected by adjusting specific parameters of the algorithm. For example, many errors can be corrected by limiting the algorithm to search for candidate fundamental frequencies within a narrower range. Figure 4–19 shows the pitch contour for a vowel spoken by a female speaker. Note that there appear to be errors in estimating fundamental frequency for some segments.

More recently, algorithms have been developed that specifically attempt to predict *pitch* of various acoustic signals. Although it is not meaningful to compute fundamental frequency from Type 2 or 3 signals, it may be possible to compute the pitch of such voices. This is because even highly aperiodic signals may give rise to the percept of pitch. Although such algorithms have not yet been used with disordered voices, these have the potential to become important clinical tools in the near future.

Intensity

Along with fundamental frequency, vocal intensity is one of the most commonly reported measures obtained during acoustic

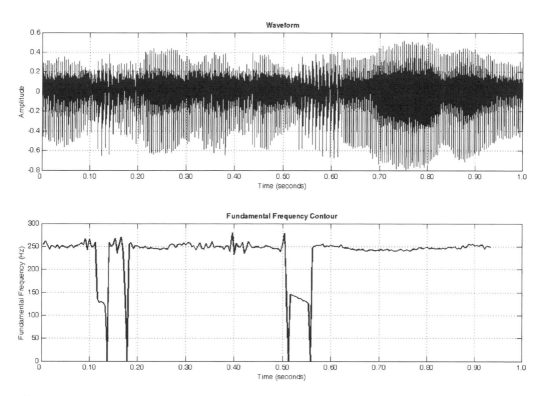

Figure 4–19. Vowel waveform (*top*) and its fundamental frequency contour (*bottom*). The fundamental frequency contour was estimated using the autocorrelation algorithm.

analysis of voice. Vocal intensity reflects the acoustic power in the voice and is related largely to a patient's ability to generate and maintain adequate subglottal pressure. Perceptually, vocal intensity is related to the loudness of the voice but once again the acoustic-perceptual relationship is not linear. Although greater intensity reflects greater loudness, the two do not increase proportionally. Most software for acoustic analysis will generate an intensity contour (as shown in Figure 4–20) and also provide some means for summarizing it statistically. Most often, these include the average intensity (measured in decibels) and its standard deviation.

From a signal-processing standpoint, measurement of vocal intensity is relatively straightforward and free of errors. However, measurement of vocal intensity is notoriously difficult to control because it is easily affected by numerous external factors such as ambient noise, microphone placement, and sensitivity, or the adjustments made on the analog/digital electronics such as a preamplifier. All of these variables can significantly alter the measured intensity and such factors need to be controlled meticulously. As stated previously, clinicians should take all necessary precautions to obtain voice recordings in a quiet environment, be consistent in keeping the microphone at a fixed distance and angle from the speaker, and be aware of the settings made on the preamplifier or other peripheral devices between the microphone and the recording equipment. Often the preamplifier gain will have to be adjusted to account for very low signals or to avoid peak clipping. These changes in gain must be accounted for if a

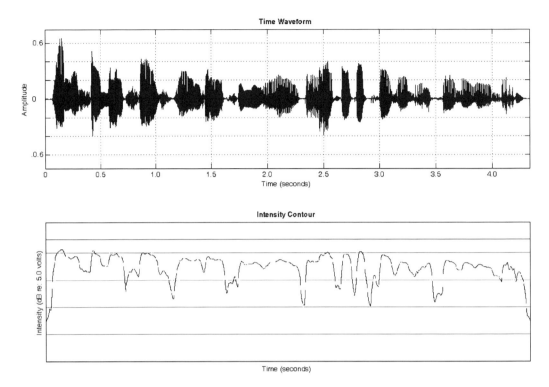

Figure 4–20. A speech waveform (*top*) and its intensity contour (*bottom*).

comparison of vocal intensity is made across different speakers or across different recording sessions for the same speaker. Many preamplifiers or recording devices have calibrated gain controls allowing the user to keep track of how changes in gain control may affect the intensity measured by the software.

Finally, it is important to remember that vocal intensity measures reported by most acoustic analysis software are made in decibels relative to some internal standard value (usually in millivolts). As such, these values do not reflect dB SPL, which has a standard reference value of 10 to 12 watts/m² of acoustic intensity. For this reason, the intensity (in dB) measured from one software package may not be exactly the same as that measured from another. However, as long as the measures are reported in decibels, the *change* in intensity

(measured in dB) should be similar across various software packages if the analysis parameters are adjusted appropriately.

Voice Range Profile

The voice range profile (VRP), also known as the phonetogram, is a method to gather comprehensive data about the entire range of fundamental frequencies and intensities that a patient can produce. The patient is asked to phonate at a wide range of fundamental frequencies, spanning the lowest to the highest note possible. Often an audio signal, such as a pure tone, is provided as a target to which the patient may match their fundamental frequency of phonation. The patient may also be provided real-time visual feedback to help them monitor their vocal output. At each of these fundamental frequencies, patients are required to vary the intensity from very low to as high as possible. Such systematic variation in fundamental frequency and intensity is then displayed on a frequency-by-intensity plot (Figure 4–21) and shows the patient's total range of phonation.

The VRP for a person with a healthy voice typically shows an elliptical shape, with the smallest range of intensity produced toward the lowest and highest fundamental frequencies. Patients with voice disorders may have an overall reduction in the range of fundamental frequency and/or intensity that

they can produce. Some patients may show a "notch" or specific areas within the VRP at which they are unable to produce voicing. Such differences are often monitored visually, but may also be quantified in terms of the total range of fundamental frequency and intensity that can be produced by a speaker or the total area of the VRP.

Generating the VRP requires some time and may be fatiguing to some patients. Some software packages simplify the task by requiring speakers to only phonate at a small number of fundamental frequencies and then interpolate the data at other fundamental frequencies. However, because of the greater time and effort required for generating the VRP, it

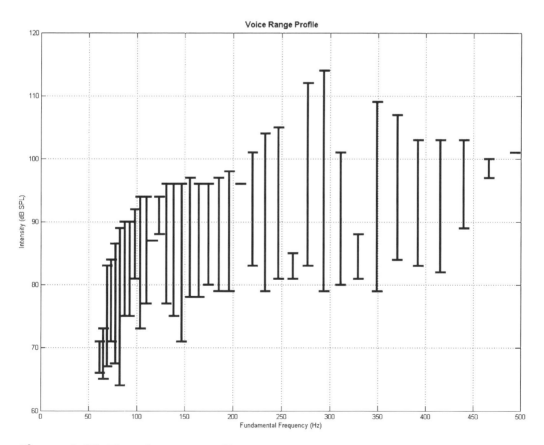

Figure 4–21. The voice range profile.

is not always included as a part of the clinical assessment. Nevertheless, the VRP can provide valuable information regarding the voice production capabilities for a specific speaker. VRP is often used when evaluating professional voice users such as singers.

> Interpolating data involves estimating missing values between real data points.

Short-Term Perturbation

Measures of short-term perturbation reflect the cycle-to-cycle variability in the speech acoustic signal. The sound generated by vocal fold vibration is not perfectly periodic and each cycle varies slightly from the ones preceding it. Successive cycles may differ in their amplitudes and in their time-period or fundamental frequency.

Figure 4–22 shows a few cycles of a vowel produced by a patient with a voice disorder. Notice how each cycle is slightly different from its neighboring cycles in terms of its time period and amplitude. A number of algorithms have been proposed to quantify each of these two aspects of the vocal acoustic signal and these are referred to as measures of frequency perturbation and amplitude perturbation, respectively. In common practice, amplitude perturbation is frequently referred to as "shimmer" whereas frequency perturbation is often labeled as "jitter." However, the two terms, shimmer and jitter, have a very specific meaning as these describe one particular

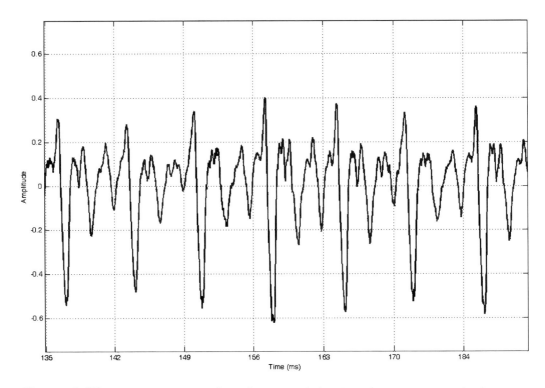

Figure 4–22. The acoustic waveform for a vowel showing short-term perturbation. Note that successive cycles vary in terms of their amplitude (amplitude perturbation) and time periods (frequency perturbation).

method for computing amplitude and frequency perturbation, respectively. Therefore, be careful when using these terms and avoid them for broadly describing short-term perturbation. Some examples of algorithms used to compute short-term perturbation include absolute shimmer (Horii, 1982), Amplitude Perturbation Quotient (Takahashi & Koike, 1976), Directional Perturbation Factor and Directional Shimmer Factor (Sorensen & Horii, 1984), and Least Mean Square Jitter and Shimmer (Milenkovic, 1987), and so forth.

Physiologically, it is believed that short-term perturbation reflects variability in the vocal fold vibration. Thus, speakers with highly aperiodic vocal fold vibration are likely to show greater perturbation values. However, note that perturbation values can only be correctly computed for Type 1 vowel segments. As Type 2 and Type 3 segments do not have a distinct fundamental frequency, it is not possible to compute *variability* in fundamental frequency or amplitude for each cycle. Therefore, perturbation values may be misleading if the type of signal being analyzed is not classified accurately. Again the algorithms for computing short-term perturbation will produce some output whenever *any* signal is analyzed, irrespective of whether it is of Type 1, Type 2, or Type 3. The user needs to interpret these values in light of the type of segment being analyzed and make sure the data being reported are valid.

It is often assumed that increased perturbation values correspond closely with a change in voice quality, such as an increase in breathiness or roughness. Although a number of studies have shown some degree of correlation between perceptual ratings of voice quality and short-term perturbation, these measures have not stood up to careful examination (e.g., Wolfe, Fitch, & Martin, 1997). Despite controlled experimentation, there is little evidence to show that an increase in short-term perturbation directly results in the perception of dysphonic voice quality. Therefore, these measures should not be regarded as a means to quantify a change in *voice quality*. Rather, these measures only help to quantify a specific change in the vocal acoustic signals and such changes may or may not have a clear perceptual correlate.

Despite these limitations, perturbation measures can be used clinically to monitor a change in voice production. For instance, these measures can be used to determine whether the voice changes over the course of voice therapy. Just keep in mind that several extraneous factors may affect short-term perturbation measures and care must be taken to control these adequately when employing these measures in the clinic. First, as discussed above, it is important to remember that different software packages offer different methods to compute perturbation. In fact, most programs will offer multiple measures of perturbation. As each algorithm uses different criteria for these computations, the values obtained from one algorithm are not directly comparable to that from another. When making any comparisons (for example, perturbation values before and after a period of therapy), users must ensure that they are comparing numbers from the same algorithm. Second, perturbation values are often affected by the type of microphone used, the distance and angle of microphone placement, as well as the recording environment such as noise and reverberation. Again, users can avoid erroneous measurements by controlling these factors adequately. Third, short-term perturbation values should only be measured from steady phonation and *not from running speech*. Conversational speech or reading tasks are not appropriate for estimating perturbation because these tasks typically involve a large degree of volitional changes in fundamental frequency and intensity, which will result in extremely high perturbation values. And finally, as described previously, perturbation values are only meaningful when a distinct fundamental frequency can be identified in the analysis segment. Thus, these measures can only be reported from Type 1 signals.

Relative Noise Level

Another acoustic measure commonly used in clinical voice evaluation is the level of noise relative to the level of the harmonics or the periodic signal generated by vocal fold vibration. As described previously, the vocal fold vibration does not result in a perfectly periodic acoustic signal. The departure from this periodicity is measured as noise and may arise from two factors. First, irregularities in vocal fold vibration (short-term perturbation) results in the presence of noise in the vocal acoustic signal. Second, an incomplete glottal closure results in the generation of turbulence at the glottis, which also adds noise to the vocal acoustic signal. Unfortunately, it is difficult to isolate the effects of short-term perturbation and incomplete glottal closure on the overall noise level. Hence, most measures of noise reflect a change in short-term perturbation as well as the presence of turbulence or aspiration noise in the vocal acoustic signal. Some researchers (i.e., Milenkovic, 1995) have attempted to develop algorithms that can isolate aspiration noise from the effects of signal perturbation, but even these cannot completely separate the two sources of noise.

Therefore, physiologically, measures of relative noise levels represent the overall stability of vocal fold vibration. The relative level of noise increases as the vocal fold vibration becomes irregular and/or if the vocal folds fail to completely close the glottis. Perceptually, relative noise levels have been associated with breathiness, roughness, as well as hoarseness. However, the perception of these vocal qualities appears to be more complex and is likely elicited by a combination of various acoustic changes in the vocal signal. Although the relative noise levels are correlated with the perception of dysphonic voice quality, this measure is neither specific to a particular voice quality type nor highly sensitive to changes in the vocal quality. Nevertheless, it has often been utilized clinically as a gross measure of change in vocal quality with greater noise levels generally reflecting a poorer voice.

Several precautions need to be taken when making and interpreting this measure. First, note that the relative noise level, much like signal perturbation measures, may be computed using a number of different algorithms. Some examples of commonly used algorithms include the Signal-to-Noise Ratio (SNR; Milenkovic, 1987), the Harmonic-to-Noise Ratio (HNR; de Krom, 1993), Normalized-Noise-Energy (NNE; Kasuya, Ogawa, Mashima, & Ebihara, 1986), Glottal Noise Energy (GNE; Michaelis, Frohlich, & Strube, 1998), and so forth. Each algorithm uses a different method to estimate noise levels. Therefore, the results from different algorithms are not directly comparable to one another. Second, as the absolute noise level in voice is highly variable and provides little information by itself, the noise level is typically reported by normalizing it to the harmonic or period energy. However, such normalization requires estimating the power of the harmonic part of the vocal signal. This computation is very difficult if the vocal fold vibration is highly irregular and does not result in a clear harmonic structure. Thus, measures of relative noise levels cannot be made accurately from Type 2 and Type 3 signals. Once again, users must remember that most computer algorithms will provide some numerical result even if the signal being analyzed is highly aperiodic. However, these results may not reflect the noise level in that voice correctly and the results can be invalid. Users should analyze signals and interpret results with the knowledge that the algorithms used for computing relative noise levels may not be accurate when the acoustic signal becomes highly aperiodic.

Spectral Measures

Another approach to analyze the vocal acoustic signal is through the study of its spectrum. A spectrum shows how energy is distributed across various frequencies in a signal. Modern computing makes it very easy to compute the spectrum of a signal and clinicians may quantify various aspects of the spectrum. These measures may be obtained either from a short-term spectrum (Figure 4–23) or from a long-term averaged spectrum (Figure 4–24). As the names suggest, the short-term spectrum is computed by analyzing a small part ("window") of the vocal acoustic signal, typically 30 to 50 msec in duration. In contrast, the long-term average spectrum (LTAS) is computed by averaging the energies in much longer utterances, ranging from a few seconds to a few minutes of speech.

Fast Fourier Transform (FFT)

Most software packages for acoustic analysis of speech allow users to generate a Fourier spectrum (FFT or Fast Fourier Transform) or a "Linear Predictive Coefficients" (LPC)

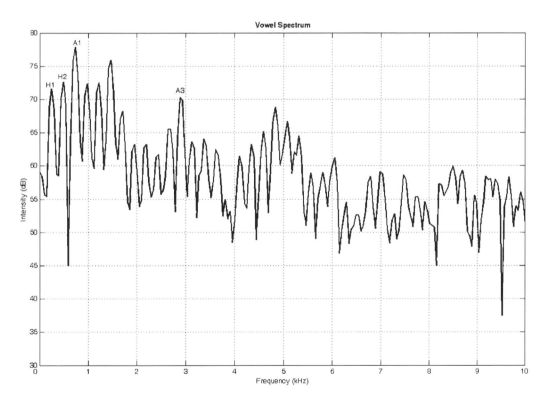

Figure 4–23. The FFT (Fast Fourier Transform) spectrum for the vowel /a/ computed from a 40-msec window. The first harmonic (H1), second harmonic (H2), the harmonic closest to the first formant (A1), and the harmonic closest to the third formant (A3) are marked.

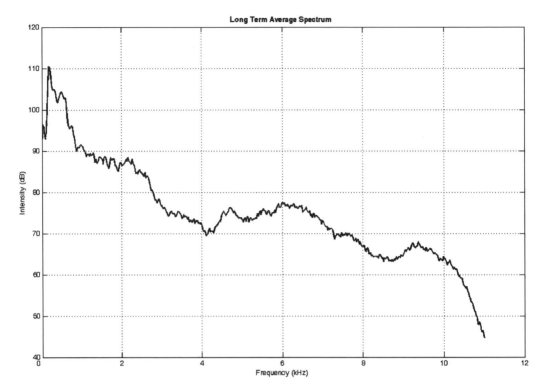

Figure 4–24. The long-term average spectrum (LTAS) for a speaker reading the "Rainbow Passage."

spectrum. Generally, FFT spectra are useful for voice analyses whereas LPC spectra are typically used to identify vowel formants.

Typically, a FFT spectrum for a vowel shows a series of equally spaced peaks on the horizontal frequency axis. Each of these peaks represents a harmonic component. As harmonics are multiples of the fundamental frequency, these occur at equal intervals when plotted on a linear frequency axis. Harmonic components that lie close to a formant frequency can be identified by their greater intensity. Otherwise, the intensity of the harmonics tends to decline with increasing frequency. However, the vowel FFT spectra for patients with voice disorders may not always look as clear. For instance, the higher level of aspiration noise observed in many patients tends to mask the harmonic structure, particu-

larly in the higher frequencies. In such voices, the harmonic structure is clearly visible at the lower frequencies, but is lost at the high frequency. Voices classified as Type 3 may show no harmonic structure at all, as these lack a clear fundamental frequency.

Aspiration noise generally refers to turbulent noise produced in the area of the glottis.

Vowel Spectrum

The vowel spectrum has been quantified using a variety of measures. Recent research (Hanson, 1997; Hanson & Chuang, 1999; Stevens

& Hanson, 1995) shows that certain changes in the vowel spectrum are related to specific aspects of vocal fold closure. By measuring the difference in the amplitude of the second harmonic relative to the amplitude of the first harmonic (H1–H2), one can estimate a change in the open quotient. A greater open quotient results in a greater H1–H2 ratio. Similarly, the amplitude of the harmonic closest to the third formant relative to the amplitude of the first harmonic (H1–A3) is associated with the spectral tilt. As spectral tilt is affected by the degree of abruptness during vocal fold closure, H1–A3 reflects the rate at which the vocal fold closure is achieved. In other words, H1–A3 is related to the speed of glottal closure within a cycle of vocal fold vibration. A greater H1–A3 reflects greater spectral tilt. Finally, the amplitude of the harmonic closest to the first formant relative to that of the first harmonic (H1–A1) is associated with the first formant frequency bandwidth. As the first formant bandwidth increases for incomplete glottal closure, H1–A1 may be used as a measure of glottal closure. Larger H1–A1 values reflect a lack of glottal closure. Perceptually, these measures have been associated with the presence of breathy voice quality. As breathy voice quality typically is observed when there is incomplete glottal closure, greater spectral tilt and longer open quotient, these voices have higher H1–A3, H1–A1, and H1–H2 values. In contrast, strained (or pressed) voices are typically generated with a very rapid adduction of the vocal folds, resulting in lower H1–H2 values.

These measures provide an excellent approach to make some conclusions regarding vocal fold vibratory characteristics. However, some precautions can help the user interpret these measures appropriately. First, these measures are most easily obtained for the vowel /æ/ because the formant frequencies for this vowel are fairly widely separated. In contrast, the low first formant frequency in high vowels may often be so close to the fundamental

frequency that it becomes difficult to separate the two. Second, these measures are difficult to compute from vowels that do not have clear harmonics or if there is a lot of aspiration noise. Lack of clearly visible harmonics makes it difficult for the user to select the appropriate peaks. Similarly, the presence of aspiration noise can *mask* specific harmonics, in particular, those close to the third formant region. In both these cases, these measures become difficult to obtain. Therefore, these measures are also typically restricted to voices classified as Type 1 signals. Finally, note that these values can be easily biased by the vowel formant frequency. As each speaker and vowel can have different formant frequencies, the user needs to correct for these differences before comparing data across speakers. A possible correction formula has been described by Hanson (1997).

Long-Term Average Spectrum

The long-term average spectrum has also been used in the study of voice. Unlike the vowel FFT spectrum, the LTAS is typically obtained from a reading or a conversational speech sample. The resulting spectrum can be used to study the distribution of energy across frequency. As the LTAS averages energy distribution across several vowels and consonants, it does not show the harmonic structure associated with the vowel FFT spectrum. Instead, it typically shows a smoother contour, with the greatest energy at the lower frequency regions. Some commonly used measures obtained from the LTAS include computing the ratio of energy within different frequency bands as well as computing various spectral moments. For example, users may calculate the ratio of energy between 0 to 1 kHz and 1 to 5 kHz or that between 0 to 2 kHz and 2 to 4 kHz. The former is often reported as "alpha-ratio" in the literature. Others may compute statistical *moments* of the LTAS. To compute spectral moments, the LTAS is treated like a bell-curve and its first four moments (mean, standard deviation, skewness, and kurtosis) are calculated. These ratios and moments are used to describe the overall energy distribution in the speech signal. Because all these measures are obtained by averaging a relatively long speech utterance, it is difficult to relate these to specific physiologic or perceptual attributes of voice. Instead, LTAS is best treated as an approach to describe and study the speech acoustic signal.

In many instances, the LTAS is simply used in a descriptive manner to compare two or more speech samples (for example, before and after therapy). Such use of LTAS is valid for all signal types, Type 1, 2, and 3, as the assumption of periodicity is not critical for this analysis. Nevertheless, clinicians must interpret the results with the knowledge that factors such as aspiration noise in voice can alter various LTAS measures to some degree. It is also important to note that the spectral characteristics, in particular the slope, is dependent on the overall intensity level and this must be controlled or accounted for when interpreting spectral measures.

Auditory-Based Measures of Voice Quality

As described above, most acoustic measures commonly used in voice clinic are not directly related to perceptual attributes of voice. The perception of vocal quality is believed to be highly complex, involving multiple acoustic cues that often have a nonlinear relationship with the percept they elicit. Some recent research (e.g., Shrivastav, 2003; Shrivastav & Sapienza, 2003) has attempted to develop acoustic measures that can be used to quantify

how a voice may be perceived by an average listener. These measures differ from traditional acoustic analyses primarily in terms of how the acoustic signal is represented prior to making any measurements. Conventional acoustic analysis uses a variety of algorithms to quantify various aspects of the signal recorded by the microphone. In contrast, the auditory-based measures are computed from the *auditory representation* of the acoustic signal. To accomplish this, the acoustic signal is recorded by a high-fidelity microphone and first passed through a computer program that simulates the transduction processes in the peripheral auditory system. The simulated output of the auditory system is then used to identify various features or cues that may reflect a change in voice quality. Because the peripheral auditory system involves several nonlinear processes, simulating these processes allows such measures to better reflect how voice may be perceived. Such auditory-based measures are currently under development and it is possible that these will become an important clinical tool in the near future, as they will allow clinicians to objective quantify changes in vocal quality. Briefly, this research suggests that the perception of breathiness may be related to the extent to which the harmonic components in a voice are masked or overshadowed by the noise in the same voice (Shrivastav & Camacho, 2010; Shrivastav et al., 2011). Another variable found to be highly correlated to the perception of breathiness was "pitch strength" (Shrivastav & Eddins, In Press). Pitch strength reflects the robustness of pitch sensation in a sound stimulus. For example, the same musical note produced by a stringed instrument (e.g., guitar) and a wind instrument (e.g., flute) differ in the strength of their pitch sensations. Likewise, voices with greater pitch strength are generally perceived to be less breathy than those with lower pitch strength. This ongoing research has also investigated the perception of roughness and observed that roughness is primarily related to the amplitude modulations or rapid changes in the intensity of the vowel waveform. However, amplitude modulations in a specific frequency region (20 to 50 Hz) appear to have the greatest impact on the perception of roughness in steady state vowels.

The dysphonia severity index (DSI) has been used to assist with describing the severity of a patient's dysphonia to augment perceptual assessment of voice and it is considered a more objective method of voice analysis. It is an index which provides an additional measure of noise components without being limited by the lack of identification of a fundamental frequency. The DSI is algorithm which combines a small subset of weighted acoustic variables. The variables included in the index were examined by Awan and include both time and spectral based measures which when used can accommodate the variability in the voice signal that is often presented by speakers with dysphonia. The more negative the index result after applying the algorithm to the patient's voice signal the more dysphonic the voice. The more positive the index result after applying the algorithm to the patient's voice signal the more nondysphonic the voice (Wuyts et al., 2000).

The most commonly used acoustic measures to study normal and dysphonic voices have been described. It is recommended that clinicians begin voice analysis by a careful study of the narrow-band spectrogram. This allows clinicians to classify the signal into three types of segments: mostly periodic (Type 1), signals with subharmonics (Type 2), or signals with no clear harmonic structure (Type 3). Type 1 segments may then be submitted for computing other measures, such as fundamental frequency, short-term perturbation, and relative noise levels. Type 2 and Type 3 signals may be best described using spectrograms or LTAS. Clinicians need to take adequate precautions when making or interpreting various acoustic measures.

Perceptual Rating Scales

An often intangible term to define, in the context of voice quality, perception may be described as the psychological representation of a physical stimulus. One's perception is difficult to define as it is often formed based on their world (influential factors include age, sex, language, culture, intrinsic and extrinsic bias, and so forth). With regard to voice production, a clinician listens and forms an impression of a patient's vocal quality, pitch, and loudness in order to describe the voice and to determine the baseline impression with which to compare a form of treatment, whether it be surgical, pharmacologic, or behavioral. One or more terms may be assigned by the listener to describe voice quality. The choice and definition of these terms have changed over the years as researchers attempt to depict voice quality as accurately as possible (Kreiman & Gerratt, 1999). More often than not, the physiologic process of the voice disorder does not match the perceptual description of the voice quality (Shrivastav & Sapienza, 2003) and more often than not listeners do not agree with each other very well, particularly when scoring in the midrange of an *n*-point rating scale (Kreiman & Gerratt, 1998). Therefore, systematic scaling techniques and specific strategies for completing perceptual analysis of voice have been developed to minimize the error in determining voice characteristics when listening to voice.

One organized manner for assessment of voice quality can occur using standardized rating scales and attending to specific aspects of vocal quality. The existence of rating scales for objectifying perception has been long standing and takes the form of an ordinal or visual analog scale. Which of the two scales is most desirable to use in terms of the best validity is mixed, yet the ordinal scale is often the preferred scale because it is easier to use (Yiu &

Chi-Yan, 2004). Ease of use, however, should not be the benchmark that defines a scale's accuracy.

> Ordinal Scale is where numbers are assigned to attributes: 1 = normal, 2 = mild . . . and so forth.
>
> Visual Analog Scale is a tool where a line is used with two defined endpoints and ratings can be placed on the line to define the magnitude of a sensation.

Ordinal scales like the Buffalo Rating Voice Profile (Webb et al., 2004) and the GRBAS scale use a 5-point and a 4-point rating system. The GRBAS Scale was introduced by a research society from Japan and its use as a voice quality evaluation tool quickly grew in popularity. It is still used widely in Japan and there is increasing interest in its use both in Europe and the United States (DeBodt, Wuyts, Van de Heyning, & Crouz, 1997).

To complete most rating scales, the patient is asked to produce a variety of stimuli. The stimuli most often elicited are a sustained vowel or a few short phrases. Using a sustained vowel allows the listener to focus on phonatory quality with less influence from articulatory dynamics that could influence the perception of the disorder. There are standardized passages that can be used as well for making judgments of voice quality pre- and post-treatment such as the Rainbow Passage (Fairbanks, 1960).

The GRBAS scale uses a 4-point rating system where "0" indicates a normal voice quality, "1" a mildly deviant voice quality, "2" a moderately deviant voice quality, and "3" an extremely deviant voice quality.

G = Grade or a judgment of how rough the voice sounds

R = Roughness is a judgment of how irregular and noisy the voice sounds; it should relate to aperiodicity in the vibratory cycle

B = Breathiness is a judgment of how much additional airflow is perceived; it should relate to higher minimum airflow during the glottal cycle

A = Aesthenia is a judgment of how weak the voice sounds; it should relate to the sound pressure level of the voice

S = Strain is a judgment of how compressed or hyperfunctional the voice sounds

Most recently, the American Speech-Language and Hearing Association's Special Interest Division 3, Voice and Voice Disorders organized a meeting to work toward a consensus on how to most reliably use perceptual rating scales and how to develop scales that would yield valid outcomes. The use of perceptual rating scales can be fraught with methodological difficulty yet their use remains popular for judging voice quality due to their ease of administration and time efficiency. From that conference a consensus document was produced by the working group and a scale was developed called the CAPE-V (Consensus on Auditory Perceptual Evaluation of Voice (see http://www.asha.org). As stated in the consensus document, the CAPE-V is *not* intended to be used independently of other means for determining the nature of a voice disorder, such as is the general case with other rating scale use. Rather, findings from the CAPE-V should be complemented by visual examination of the larynx and other tests of vocal function in order to arrive at the best evaluation and most comprehensive impression of the voice disorder (DeBodt et al., 1997).

Voice Handicap Scales and Quality of Life Scales

An emerging need in health care is the development of tools that can be used by a patient to communicate their feelings and impressions to clinicians about the impact a disorder(s) or disease(s) has on their lifestyle. The domains of lifestyle can be defined in terms of activities of daily living, communication ability, and quality of life, among others. A tool that defines these impacts on a patient and/or their family needs to also help the clinician understand the broader influence of the disorder(s)/disease(s) beyond the immediate impairment. It is not uncommon for clinicians to underestimate the difficulties their patients are having, so any means to improve clinician awareness of such problems will ultimately enhance communication and patient care.

It is important to ask patients to fill out handicap scales and quality of life scales at the time of the initial assessment in order to gauge the influence of the disease/disorder. It is also equally important is to have the patient fill out the questionnaires serially, during the course of treatment, as an indicator of improvement or deterioration in status. However, be mindful that if the voice therapy treatment time is going to be short then the use of handicap scales may not be useful. Likewise, be aware of the placebo effect whereby a patient may indicate perceived improvement in handicap while the disordered voice changes very little. To many, the utility of handicap scales is that they provide a better sense of a patient's perception of the voice problem. Patients with high scores and mild hoarseness, for example, are likely to be better candidates for therapy than a patient with a severe problem who is not hampered by voice quality.

As there are no "gold standards" in our field for which scale is best suited to collect this type of information, there are a number of tools available. The instrument ultimately selected by a clinician will depend upon the purpose for which the information is intended to be used. Like in the selection of any tool, validity, reliability, and practicality should all be considered. Ease of administration needs to be considered, not only from the clinician's perspective but from the patient's perspective. Is the tool readable? Is it tedious to complete? Does it ask the right questions of the presenting situation and condition? Does the tool require high cognitive functioning and memory of the patient? How might depression influence the patient's response? These are just a few examples of the many factors that require consideration when selecting the tool to help communicate the effects of a disorder or disease on patient life. Ultimately, the tools should highlight the functional problems, the severity of the difficulties and direct the clinician in finding mechanisms to improve patient outcome.

Voice Handicap Index

The Voice Handicap Index (VHI) measures how a voice problem influences a patient's quality of life. Three major areas are represented on this index. The first is referred to as a physical subscale, the second a functional subscale and the third a social subscale (Appendix 4–3). The physical subscale includes questions about how the voice disorder affects other physical functions such as breathing or breath control, how the voice sounds, and whether the sound quality is consistently impaired or varies throughout the day. The functional subscale includes questions related to how the voice disorder impacts other daily activities, such as work, family life, interactions with friends, and so forth. The emotional subscale represents questions related to how the patient feels about having the voice disorder.

Jacobson et al. (1997) developed the VHI. Initially, they produced an 85-item version of the VHI and gave it to 65 consecutive patients who were evaluated at a Voice Clinic at Henry Ford Hospital in Michigan. Following statistical examination of the initial 85-item version, the VHI was reduced to a 30-item final version. Test-retest stability was then completed, and shown to be very strong when administered to an additional 63 consecutive patients on two occasions. The authors indicated that a VHI test score difference of 18 points or more indicates a significant shift in psychosocial function. Therefore, when using the VHI to document a change in voice handicap following a treatment, a difference score of 18 points would be considered statistically significant and potentially clinically relevant.

In 2004, Rosen et al., developed and reported on the validation of the VHI-10. In this report no statistical differences were found between the original VHI and VHI-10. The VHI-10 therefore is a shorter scale to complete and can yield the quantification of a patient's perception of their voice handicap.

In 2007, an adaptation of the VHI occurred for use with the pediatric voice population known as the Pediatric Voice Handicap Index (pVHI). According to the authors (Zur et al., 2007), the adaptation involved altering the language of the original VHI statements to reflect parent responses about their child. The test results of Zur et al. on 33 guardians of children revealed good reliability between the VHI and pVHI.

In another study, the Voice Symptom Scale (VoiSS) and the VHI were compared on their structure and content using a factor analysis.

> A factor analysis is a statistical test that determines the smallest number of "fac-

> tors" required to "explain" a pattern of relationships. For example, the analysis helps to determine which factor makes the change in voice more positive or more negative and/or which factor has no role in changing the voice.

The VoiSS is a 43-item questionnaire that gathers data from patients about their voice severity (Deary, Wilson, Carding, & MacKenzie, 2003). Both the VoiSS and VHI scales were given to 319 people with dysphonia that came into a clinic for voice evaluation. The VoiSS is composed of three factors: impairment (based on 15 items within the questionnaire), emotional (based on 8 items within the questionnaire), and related physical symptoms (based on 7 items within the questionnaire), each with good internal consistency. The VoiSS was developed using 800 subjects in comparison to the 120 or so subjects tested for validating the VHI. To date, the VHI remains the more popular choice for patient administration.

Voice-Related Quality of Life Scale

The Voice Related Quality of Life index is a 10-item, patient-derived information gathering tool that is valid for its use with adult patients with voice disorders to measure both social-emotional and physical-functional aspects of voice problems (Hogikyan & Sethurman, 1999); see Appendix 4–4.

Pediatric Voice-Related Quality of Life Scale

The Pediatric Voice Related Quality of Life (PVRQOL) is also a 10-item instrument, adapted from the adult VRQOL instrument. As was the case for the pediatric adaptation of the VHI, individual items were changed to reflect parent administration. The domains of social-emotional and physical-functional effects are queried (Boseley, Cunningham, Volk, & Hartnick (2006).

> The role of the parent or guardian in the care of the pediatric voice problem should not be underestimated as they play a major role in monitoring their child, modifying their child's environment to promote vocal hygiene, practicing good vocal habits and homework exercises with the child, and providing the clinician with updates on progress or departures from the therapeutic goals.

Summary

Comprehensive evaluation of voice requires a sophisticated clinical skill set that is composed of intuitive and objective procedures. The accuracy of the clinical voice evaluation is critical in guiding the management decisions and the ultimate care of the patient's voice.

The next chapter presents structural pathologies of the larynx. The evaluation procedures presented here can be used to examine these conditions, describe their pathophysiology, and assist in their differential diagnosis.

References

AAO-HNS: American Academy of Otolaryngology-Head and Neck Surgery. (2008). *What is an Otolaryngologist?* Retrieved from http:www.ent-net.org/healthinfo/about/otolaryngologist.cfm

American Speech-Language and Hearing Association. (2008). *The roles of otolaryngologists and speech-language pathologists in the performance and interpretation of strobovideolaryngoscopy.* Retrieved from http:www.asha.org/docs/html/RP1998-00132.html

Awan, S.N., & Roy, N. (2009). Toward the development of an objective index of dysphonia severity: A four factor acoustic model. *Clinical Linguistics and Phonetics, 20*(1), 35–49.

Bielamowicz, S., Berke, G. S., & Gerratt, B. R. (1995). A comparison of type I thyroplasty and arytenoids adduction. *Journal of Voice, 9*(4), 466–472.

Bless, D. M., Glaze, L. E., Biever-Lowry, D., Campos, G., & Peppard, R. C. (1993). Stroboscopic, acoustic, aerodynamic and perceptual attributed of voice production in normal speaking adults. In I. R. Titze (Ed.), *Progress report 4* (pp. 121–134). Iowa City, Iowa: National Center for Voice and Speech.

Boseley, M. E., Cunningham, M. J., Volk, M. S., & Hartnick, C. J. (2006). Validation of the Pediatric Voice-Related Quality-of-Life Survey. *Archives of Otolaryngology-Head and Neck Surgery, 132,* 717–720.

Cantarella, G., Berlusconi, A., Maraschi, B., Ghio, A., & Barbieri, S. (2006). Botulinum toxin injection and airflow stability in spasmodic dysphonia. *Otolaryngology-Head and Neck Surgery, 134*(3), 419–423.

Deary, I. J., Wilson, J. A., Carding, P. N., & MacKenzie, K. (2003). A patient-derived voice symptom scale. *Journal of Psychosomatic Research, 54*(5), 483–489.

De Bodt, M. S., Wuyts, F. L., Van de Heyning, P. H., & Croux, C. (1997). Test-retest study of GRBAS scale: Influence of experience and professional background on perceptual rating of voice quality. *Journal of Voice, 11,* 74–80.

Dejonckere, P. H. (2000). Perceptual and laboratory assessment of dysphonia. *Otolaryngologic Clinics of North America, 33*(4), 731–750.

Dejonckere, P. H., & Lebacq, J. (1996). Acoustic, perceptual, aerodynamic and anatomical correlations in voice pathology. *Journal for Otorhinolaryngology and Its Related Specialties, 58*(6), 326–332.

de Krom, G. (1993). A cepstrum-based technique for determining a harmonics-to-noise ratio in speech signals. *Journal of Speech and Hearing Research, 36*(2), 254–266.

Eddins, D. A., Shrivastav, R., & Singh, S. (2010). Predictions of rough voice quality with a temporal modulation filter bank model. 39th Annual Symposium of the Voice Foundation: Care of the Professional Voice, Philadelphia, PA, June 2–6, 2010.

Fairbanks, G. (1960). *Voice and articulation handbook*. New York, NY: Harper & Row.

Farnsworth, D. (1940). High-speed motion picture of the human vocal cords. *Bell Telephone Laboratories Record*, *18*, 203–206.

Finnegan, E. M., Luschei, E. S., Barkmeier, J. M., & Hoffman, H. T. (1996). Sources of error in estimation of laryngeal airway resistance in persons with spasmodic dysphonia. *Journal of Speech and Hearing Research*, *39*(1), 105–113.

Fisher, K. V., Scherer, R. C., Guo, C. G., & Owen, A. S. (1996). Longitudinal phonatory characteristics after botulinum toxin type A injection. *Journal of Speech and Hearing Research*, *39*(5), 968–980.

Glottal Enterprises. Retrieved from http://www.glottal.com

Goozee, J. V., Murdoch, B. E., Theodoros, D. G., & Thompson, E. C. (1998). The effects of age and gender on laryngeal aerodynamics. *International Journal of Communication Disorders*, *33*(2), 221–238.

Hanson, H. M. (1997). Glottal characteristics of female speakers: Acoustic correlates. *Journal of the Acoustical Society of America*, *101*(1), 466–481.

Hanson, H. M., & Chuang, E. S. (1999). Glottal characteristics of male speakers: Acoustic correlates and comparison with female data. *Journal of the Acoustical Society of America*, *106*(2), 1064–1077.

Hartl, D. M., Hans, S., Vaissiere, J., & Brasnu, D. F. (2005). Laryngeal aerodynamics after vocal fold augmentation with autologous fat vs. thyroplasty in the same patient. *Archives of Otolaryngology-Head and Neck Surgery*, *131*(8), 696–700.

Hertegard, S. (2005). What have we learned about laryngeal physiology from high speed digitial videoendoscopy? *Current Opinions in Otolaryngology-Head and Neck Surgery*, *13*(3), 152–156.

Higgins, M. B., & Saxman, J. H. (1991). A comparison of selected phonatory behaviors of healthy aged and young adults. *Journal of Speech and Hearing Research*, *34*(5), 1000–1010.

Hirano, M., Kurita, S., & Nakashima, T. (1981). The structure of the vocal folds. In K. N. Stevens & M. Hirano (Eds.), *Vocal fold physiology* (pp. 33–43). Tokyo, Japan: University of Tokyo Press.

Hogikyan, N., & Sethuraman, G. (1999). Validation of an instrument to measure voice-related quality of life (V-RQOL). *Journal of Voice*, *13*(4), 557–569.

Holmberg, E. B., Hillman, R. E., & Perkell, J. S. (1989). Glottal airflow and transglottal air pressure measurements for male and females speakers in soft, normal and loud voice. *Journal of the Acoustical Society of America*, *84*(2), 511–529.

Horii, Y. (1982). Jitter and shimmer differences among sustained vowel phonations. *Journal of Speech and Hearing Research*, *25*(1), 12–14.

Huber, J. E., Stathopoulos, E. T., Bormann, L. A, & Johnson, K. (1998). Effects of a circumferentially-vented penumotachograph masks on breathing patterns of women as measured by respiratory kinematic techniques. *Journal of Speech Language and Hearing Research*, *41*(3), 472–478.

Jacobson, B. H., Johnson, A., Grywalkski, C., Silbergleit, A., Jacobson, G., Benninger, M. S., & Newman, C. W. (1997). The Voice Handicap Index (VHI): Development and validation. *American Journal of Speech, Language and Hearing Research*, *6*, 66–70.

Kahane, J. (1982). Growth of the human prepubertal and pubertal larynx. *Journal of Speech and Hearing Research*, *25*(3), 446–455.

Kasuya, H., Ogawa, S., Mashima, K., & Ebihara, S. (1986). Normalized noise energy as an acoustic measure to evaluate pathologic voice. *Journal of the Acoustical Society of America*, *80*(5), 1329–1334.

Kaszuba, S. M., & Garrett, C. G. (2007). Strobovideolaryngoscopy and laboratory voice evaluation. *Otolaryngologic Clinics of North America*, *40*(5), 991–1001.

KayPentax. Retrieved from http://www.kayelemetrics.com

Kimura, M., Nito, T., Sakakibara, K., Tayama, N., & Nimi, S. (2008). Clinical experience with collagen injection of the vocal fold: A study of 155 patients. *Auris Nasus Larynx*, *35*(1), 67–75.

Klatt, D. H., & Klatt, L. C. (1990). Analysis, synthesis, and perception of voice quality variations among female and male talkers. *Journal of the Acoustical Society of America*, *87*(2), 820–857.

Kreiman, J., & Gerratt, B. R. (1998). Validity of rating scale measures of voice quality. *Journal of the Acoustical Society of America*, *104*(3, Pt. 1), 1598–1609.

Kreiman, J., & Gerratt, B. (1999). Measuring vocal quality. In R. Kent & M. J. Ball (Eds.), *Voice quality measurement* (pp. 73–101). San Diego, CA: Singular.

Lindestad, P. A., Blixt, V., Pahlberg-Olsson, J., & Hammarberg, B. (2004). Ventricular fold vibration in voice production: A high-speed imaging study with kymographic, acoustic and perceptual analyses of a voice patient and a vocally healthy subject. *Logopedia Phoniatrica Vocology*, *29*, 162–170.

Ma, E. P., Yin, E. M., & Verdolini-Abbott, K. V. (2007). Application of the ICF in voice disorders. *Seminars in Speech-Language Pathology*, *28*(4), 343–350.

Michaelis, D., Frohlich, M., & Strube, H. W. (1998). Selection and combination of acoustic features for the description of pathologic voices. *Journal of the Acoustical Society of America*, *103*(3), 1628–1639.

Milenkovic, P. (1987). Least mean square measures of voice perturbation. *Journal of Speech and Hearing Research*, *30*(4), 529–538.

Milenkovic, P. (1995). Rotation based measures of voice aperiodicity. In D. Wong (Ed.), *Workshop of acoustic voice analysis: Proceedings* (pp. 1–10). Iowa City, IA: National Center for Voice and Speech.

Mongeau, L., Franchek, N., Coker, C. H., & Kubli, R. A. (1997). Characteristics of a pulsating jet through a small modulated orifice, with application to voice production. *Journal of the Acoustical Society of America*, *102*(2, Pt. 1), 1121–1133.

Moore, G. P., White, F. D., & von Leden, H. (1962). Ultra high-speed photography in laryngeal physiology. *Journal of Speech and Hearing Disorders*, *27*, 165–171.

Patel, R. R., Liu, L., Galatsanos, N., & Bless, D. M. (2011). Differential vibratory characteristics of adductor spasmodic dysphonia and muscle tension dysphonia on high speed digital imaging. *Annals of Otology, Rhinology and Laryngology*, *120*(1), 21–32.

Piazza, C., Mangili, S., Del Bon, F., Gritti, F., Manfredi, C., Nicolai, P., & Peretti, G. (2012). Quantitative analysis of videokymography in normal and pathological vocal folds: A preliminary study. *European Archives of Otorhinolaryngology*, *269*(1), 207–212.

Raes, J. P., & Clements, P. A. (1996). Aerodynamic measurements of voice production. *Acta Otorhinolaryngological Belgium*, *50*(4), 343–344.

Ramig, L. O., & Dromey, C. (1996). Aerodynamic mechanisms underlying treatment-related changes in vocal intensity in patients with Parkinson's disease. *Journal of Speech and Hearing Research*, *39*(4), 798–807.

Rosen, C.A., Lee, A.S., Osborne, J., Zullo, T., & Murry, T. (2004). Development and validation of the Voice Handicap Index-10. *Laryngoscope*, *114*(9), 1549–1556.

Rothenberg, M. (1973). A new inverse filtering technique for deriving the glottal airflow waveform during voicing. *Journal of the Acoustical Society of America*, *53*(6), 1632–1645.

Sapienza, C. M., & Dutka, J. (1996). Glottal airflow characteristics of women's voice production along an aging continuum. *Journal of Speech-Language and Hearing Research*, *39*(2), 322–328.

Sapienza, C. M., Stathopoulos, E. T., & Brown, W. S. (1995). Speech task effects on acoustic and aerodynamic measures of women with vocal nodules. *Journal of Voice*, *9*(4), 413–418.

Scherer, R. (1991). Physiology of phonation: A review of basic mechanics. In C. N. Ford & D. M. Bless (Eds.), *Phonosurgery Assessment and Management of Voice Disorders*. New York, NY: Raven Press.

Shrivastav, R. (2003). The use of an auditory model in predicting perceptual ratings of breathy voice quality. *Journal of Voice*, *17*(4), 502–512.

Shrivastav, R., & Camacho, A. (2010). A computational model to predict changes in breathiness resulting from variations in aspiration noise level. *Journal of Voice*, *24*(4), 395–405.

Shrivastav, R., Camacho, A., Patel, S. A., & Eddins, D. A. (2011). "A model for prediction of breathiness in vowels." *Journal of the Acoustical Society of America*, *129*(3), 1605–1615.

Shrivastav, R., & Eddins, D. A. (2011). The influence of amplitude modulation frequency on perceived roughness of vowels. 161st meeting of the Acoustical Society of America, Seattle, WA, May 23–27, 2011.

Shrivastav, R., Eddins, D. A., & Anand, S. (In press). Pitch strength of normal and dysphonic voices. *Journal of the Acoustical Society of America*.

Shrivastav, R., & Sapienza, C. (2003). Objective measures of breathy voice quality obtained using an auditory model. *Journal of the Acoustical Society of America*, *114*(4), 2217–2224.

Smith, E., Verdolini, K., Gray, S., Nichols, S., Lemke, J., Barkmeier, J., Dove, H., & Hoffman, H. (1996). Effects of voice disorders on quality of life. *Journal of Medical Speech-Language Pathology*, *4*(4), 223–244.

Smitheran, J., & Hixon, T. J. (1981). A clinical method for estimating laryngeal airway resistance during vowel production. *Journal of Speech and Hearing Disorders*, *46*(2), 138–146.

Sorensen, D., & Horii, Y. (1984). Directional perturbation factors for jitter and shimmer. *Journal of Communication Disorders*, *17*(3), 143–151.

Stager, S. V., Neubert, R., Miller, S., Regnall, J. R., & Bielamowicz, S. A. (2003). Incidence of supraglottic activity in males and females: A preliminary report. *Journal of Voice*, *17*(3), 395–402.

Stathopoulos, E. T., & Sapienza, C. M. (1997). Developmental changes in laryngeal and respiratory function with variations in sound pressure level. *Journal of Speech, Language and Hearing Research*, *40*, 595–614.

Stevens, K. N., & Hanson, H. M. (1995). Classification of glottal vibrations from acoustic measurements. In O. Fujimura & M. Hirano (Eds.), *Vocal fold physiology: Voice quality control* (pp. 147–170). San Diego, CA: Singular.

Sundberg, J. (2008, May). *Personal voice quality? Experiences from my forty years' attempt to catch it.* 37th Annual Symposium: Care of the Professional Voice. Philadephia, PA.

Švec, J., & Schutte, H. K. (1996). Videokymography: High-speed line scanning of vocal fold vibration. *Journal of Voice*, *10*(2), 201–205.

Švec, J.G. & Sram, F. (2002). Kymographic imaging of the vocal fold oscillations. In J. H. Hansen & B. Pellom (Eds.), *ICSLP-2002 Conference Proceedings, Vol. 2. 7th International Conference on Spoken Language Processing* (pp. 957–960), Denver, CO: Center for Spoken Language Research.

Švec, J. G., Sram, F., & Schutte H. K. (2000). Videokymography in 2000: The present state and perspectives of the high-speed line-imaging technique. In T. Braunschweig, J. Hanson, P. Schelhorn-Neise, & H. Witte (Eds.), *Advances in quantitative laryngoscopy, voice and speech research. Proceedings of the 4th International Workshop* (pp. 57–62), Jena: Fredrich-Schiller University.

Švec, J., Sram, F., & Schutte, H. K. (2007). Videokymography in voice disorders: What to look for. *Journal of Voice*, *116*(3), 172–180.

Takahashi H., & Koike, Y. (1976). Some perceptual dimensions and acoustical correlates of pathologic voices. *Acta Otolaryngologica Supplement*, *338*, 1–24.

Tang, J. & Stathopoulos, E.T. (1995). Vocal efficiency as a function of vocal intensity: A study of children, women, and men. *Journal of the Acoustical Society of America*, *97*(3), 1885–1892.

Titze, I. (1994). *Workshop on acoustic voice analysis: Summary statement.* Denver, CO: National Center for Voice and Speech.

Titze, I. R. (1989). Physiologic and acoustic differences between male and female voices. *Journal of the Acoustical Society of America*, *85*(4), 1699–1707.

von Leden, H., & Moore, G. P. (1961). Vibratory pattern of the vocal cords in unilateral laryngeal paralysis. *Acta Otolaryngology*, *53*, 493–506.

Warren, D. W., & Dubois, A. B. (1964). A pressure-flow technique for measuring velopharyngeal orifice area during continuous speech. *Cleft Palate Journal*, *1*, 52–57.

Webb, A. L., Carding, P. N., Deary, I. J., MacKenzie, K., Steen, N., & Wilson, J. A. (2004). The reliability of three perceptual evaluation scales for dysphonia. *European Archives of Oto-Rhino-Laryngology*, *261*(8), 429–434.

Wolfe, V., Fitch, J., & Martin, D. (1997). Acoustic measures of dysphonic severity across and within voice types. *Folia Phoniatrica et Logopaedia*, *49*(6), 292–299.

Wuyts, F. L., DeBodt, M. S., Molenberghs, G., Remacle, M., Heylen, L., Millet, B., . . . Van de Heyning, P. H. (The Dysphonia Severity Index: An objective measure of vocal quality based on a mulitparameter approach. *Journal of Speech, Language and Hearing Research*, *43*(3), 796–809.

Yanagihara, N., & Koike, Y. (1967). The regulation of sustained phonation. *Folia Phoniatrica (Basel)*, *19*(1), 1–18.

Yiu, E. M., & Chi-Yan, N. G. (2004). Equal appearing interval and visual analogue scaling of perceptual roughness and breathiness. *Clinical Linguistics and Phonetics*, *18*(3), 211–229.

Zhang, Z., Mongeau, L., & Frankel, S. H. (2002). Experimental verification of the quasi-steady approximation for aerodynamic sound generation by pulsating jets in tubes. *Journal of the Acoustical Society of America*, *112*(4), 1652–1663.

Zur, K. B., Cotton, S., Kelchner, L., Baker, S., Weinrich, B., & Lee, L. (2007). Pediatric Voice Handicap Index (pVHI): A new tool for evaluating pediatric dysphonia. *International Journal of Pediatric Otorhinolaryngology*, *71*(1), 77–82.

Case History Form—Voice

Name: _____   Date: _____

D.O.B. _____   Age: _____   Sex: _____

Parents' Name (if under 18): _____

Address _____   Phone:

_____ (Home)

_____ (Work)

_____ (Cell)

_____ (E-mail)

Occupation: _____

Who referred you to this clinic? _____

Please describe your voice problem. _____

_____

Have you seen a physician regarding this problem? _____   When? _____

If yes, please list the name and type of physician. _____

What was the result of the evaluation? _____

What treatment was recommended? _____

Please describe your general health. _____

_____

Have you had any serious illness? _____

Have you had any recent surgeries? _____

Please list all medications that you take. _____

_____

Please list all vitamins and herbal supplements you take. _____

_____

Do you smoke or use tobacco products? _____ If yes, how much? _____

For how many years? _____

How much water do you drink each day? _____

Do you drink alcoholic beverages? _____ How many of these per day? _____

Do you drink caffeine? _____ How many cups per day? _____

Do you do any weight-training or heavy lifting? _____ If so, how often? _____

How are you required to use your voice at work? _____

Please check all of the following that apply to you:

_____ Talk loudly and often   _____ Talk frequently in loud noise

_____ Clear throat often   _____ Voice sounds breathy

_____ Cough excessively   _____ Pain in throat while talking

_____ Run out of breath while talking   _____ Talk frequently with person who is
                                                            hard of hearing

_____ Trouble producing loud voice

_____ Trouble producing soft voice

_____ Voice gets tired quickly

Please answer the following questions if you are a singer.

Number of years of individual voice training. _____

What is your voice classification? _____

With how many voice teachers or vocal coaches have you worked? _____

How many hours do you sing per week? _____

Do you warm up consistently before singing? _____

Do you use amplification when you perform? _____

Please list styles of music that you sing. _____

_____

continues

Please check all that apply and provide other information under comments.

ILLNESS	CHECK	COMMENTS
Allergies		
Recurrent cold/Sore throat		
Dizziness		
Dental problems		
Frequent laryngitis		
Epilepsy/Seizure disorder		
Attention deficit disorder		
Vision problems		
High fevers		
Kidney problem		
Swallowing/Digestive disorders		
Respiratory difficulties		
Heart or circulatory problems		
Stroke		
Neurologic disorders		
Cancer		
Thyroid problems		
Diabetes		
Connective tissue disorders (lupus, arthritis)		
Frequent headaches		
Measles		
Mumps		
Chicken pox		
Meningitis		
Unusual fatigue stress		
Hormonal problems		
Hearing/Ear problems		
Mental illness		

Appendix 4-2

Videostroboscopy Rating Form

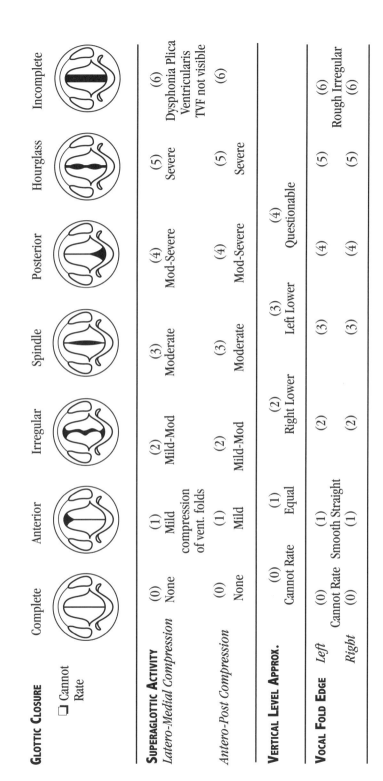

GLOTTIC CLOSURE

☐ Cannot Rate

Complete	Anterior	Irregular	Spindle	Posterior	Hourglass	Incomplete

SUPERAGLOTTIC ACTIVITY

	(0) None	(1) Mild compression of vent. folds	(2) Mild-Mod	(3) Moderate	(4) Mod-Severe	(5) Severe	(6) Dysphonia Plica Ventricularis TVF not visible
Latero-Medial Compression	(0) None	(1) Mild	(2) Mild-Mod	(3) Moderate	(4) Mod-Severe	(5) Severe	(6)
Antero-Post Compression	(0) None	(1) Mild	(2) Mild-Mod	(3) Moderate	(4) Mod-Severe	(5) Severe	(6)

VERTICAL LEVEL APPROX.

(0) Cannot Rate	(1) Equal	(2) Right Lower	(3) Left Lower	(4) Questionable

VOCAL FOLD EDGE

	(0) Cannot Rate	(1) Smooth Straight	(2)	(3)	(4)	(5)	(6) Rough Irregular
Left	(0)	(1)	(2)	(3)	(4)	(5)	(6)
Right	(0)	(1)	(2)	(3)	(4)	(5)	(6)

continues

127

Appendix 4–2 continued

VOCAL FOLD MOBILITY

	(0)	(1)	(2)	(3)	(4)
	Cannot Rate	Normal	Limited Adduction (mild) (mod) (sev)	Limited Abduction (mild) (mod) (sev)	Fixed (mild) (mod) (sev)
Left	(0)	(1)	(2)	(3)	(4)
Right	(0)	(1)	(2)	(3)	(4)

AMPLITUDE OF VIBRATION

	(0)	(1)	(2)	(3)	(4)	(5)	(6)	(7)
	Cannot Rate	Normal	Mildly Decreased	Mild-Mod Decreased	Mod Decreased	Mod-Sev Decreased	Severely Decreased	No Visible Movement
Left	(0)	(1)	(2)	(3)	(4)	(5)	(6)	(7)
Right	(0)	(1)	(2)	(3)	(4)	(5)	(6)	(7)

MUCOSAL WAVE

	(0)	(1)	(2)	(3)	(4)	(5)	(6)	(7)
	Cannot Rate	Normal	Mildly Decreased	Mild-Mod Decreased	Mod Decreased	Mod-Sev Decreased	Severely Decreased	Absent
Left	(0)	(1)	(2)	(3)	(4)	(5)	(6)	(7)
Right	(0)	(1)	(2)	(3)	(4)	(5)	(6)	(7)

NON-VIBRATION PORTION

	(0)	(1)	(2)	(3)	(4)	(5)
	None	20%	40%	60%	80%	100%
Left	(0)	(1)	(2)	(3)	(4)	(5)
Right	(0)	(1)	(2)	(3)	(4)	(5)

PHASE CLOSURE

☐ Cannot Rate

(-5)	(-4)	(-3)	(-2)	(-1)	(0)	(1)	(2)	(3)	(4)	(5)
Open Phase Predominates (Whisper dysphonia)					Normal					Closed Phase Predominates (Gottal fry-extreme Hyperadduction)

PHASE SYMMETRY

☐ Cannot Rate

(0)	(1)	(2)	(3)	(4)	(5)
Regular always symmetrical	Irregular during end or begin tasks	Irregular during extreme pitch or loud	50% asymmetrical	75% asymmetrical	Always asymmetrical

OVERALL LARYNGEAL FUNCTION

(0)	(1)	(2)	(3)	(4)
Normal	Hypofunction	Hyperfunction	Laryngeal tremors (sust.) (speech) (mild) (mod) (sev)	Phonatory spasm (add) (abd) (mild) (mod) (sev)

128

Voice Handicap Index

Instructions: These are statements that many people have used to describe their voices and the effects of their voices on their lives. Circle the response that indicates how frequently you have the same experience.

0 = Never   1 = Almost Never   2 = Sometimes   3 = Almost Always   4 = Always

Part I — F

1. My voice makes it difficult for people to hear me.

        0   1   2   3   4

2. People have difficulty understanding me in a noisy room.

        0   1   2   3   4

3. My family has difficulty hearing me when I call them throughout the house.

        0   1   2   3   4

4. I use the phone less often than I would like to.

        0   1   2   3   4

5. I tend to avoid groups of people because of my voice.

        0   1   2   3   4

6. I speak with friends, neighbors, or relatives less often because of my voice.

        0   1   2   3   4

7. People ask me to repeat myself when speaking face-to-face.

        0   1   2   3   4

8. My voice difficulties restrict personal and social life.

        0   1   2   3   4

9. I feel left out of conversations because of my voice.

        0   1   2   3   4

10. My voice problem causes me to lose income.

        0   1   2   3   4

continues

Part II — P

1. I run out of air when I talk.
   0   1   2   3   4

2. The sound of my voice varies throughout the day.
   0   1   2   3   4

3. People ask, "What is wrong with your voice?"
   0   1   2   3   4

4. My voice sounds creaky and dry.
   0   1   2   3   4

5. I feel as thought I have to strain to produce voice.
   0   1   2   3   4

6. The clarity of my voice is unpredictable.
   0   1   2   3   4

7. I try to change my voice to sound different.
   0   1   2   3   4

8. I use a great deal of effort to speak.
   0   1   2   3   4

9. My voice sounds worse in the evening.
   0   1   2   3   4

10. My voice "gives out" on me in the middle of speaking.
    0   1   2   3   4

Part III — E

1. I am tense when talking to others because of my voice.
   0   1   2   3   4

2. People seem irritated with my voice.
   0   1   2   3   4

3. I find that other people don't understand my voice problem.

        0   1   2   3   4

4. My voice problem upsets me.

        0   1   2   3   4

5. I am less outgoing because of my voice problem.

        0   1   2   3   4

6. My voice makes me feel handicapped.

        0   1   2   3   4

7. I feel annoyed when people ask me to repeat.

        0   1   2   3   4

8. I feel embarrassed when people ask me to repeat.

        0   1   2   3   4

9. My voice makes me feel incompetent.

        0   1   2   3   4

10. I am ashamed of my voice problem.

        0   1   2   3   4

Voice-Related Quality of Life Measure

Name: _____ Date: _____

We are trying to learn more about how a voice problem can interfere with your day to day activities. Below, you will find a list of possible voice-related problems. Please answer all questions based on what your voice has been like over the past two weeks. There are no "right" or "wrong" answers.

Considering both how severe the problem is when you get it, and how frequently it happens, please rate each item below on how "bad" it is (that is, the amount of each problem that you have).

Use the following scale for rating the amount of the problem:

1 = None, not a problem
2 = A small amount
3 = A moderate (medium) amount
4 = A lot
5 = Problem is as "bad as it can be"

Because of my voice,	**How much of a problem is this?**				
1. I have trouble speaking loudly or being heard in noisy situations.	1	2	3	4	5
2. I run out of air and need to take frequent breaths when talking.	1	2	3	4	5
3. I sometimes do not know what will come out when I begin speaking.	1	2	3	4	5
4. I am sometimes anxious or frustrated (because of my voice).	1	2	3	4	5
5. I sometimes get depressed (because of my voice).	1	2	3	4	5
6. I have trouble using the telephone (because of my voice).	1	2	3	4	5
7. I have trouble doing my job or practicing my profession (because of my voice).	1	2	3	4	5
8. I avoid going out socially (because of my voice).	1	2	3	4	5
9. I have to repeat myself to be understood.	1	2	3	4	5
10. I have become less outgoing (because of my voice).	1	2	3	4	5

Reprinted with permission: Hogikyan, N. D., and Sethurman, G. (1999). Validation of an Instrument to Measure Voice-Related Quality of Life (V-RQOL). *Journal of Voice, 13*(4), 557–569.

Chapter 5

Vocal Pathology

The accompanying DVD shows endoscopic and laryngostroboscopic samples of the majority of pathologies described below. Use the DVD to increase your familiarity in identifying vocal fold pathology from these examination(s).

Etiology of Voice Disorders

It is human nature to look for the cause and effect associated with your patient's voice disorders. That is, we become conditioned to decide what happened to cause this disorder, why did it happen and why is it not going away. Generally, there are multiple etiologies (causes) of voice disorders but the general classification scheme tends to group the cause of voice disorders into three main categories. These categories are functional, organic, and neurologic. And while, for many voice disorders there are well accepted causes and effects, for other the relationship is less clear with multiple factors contributing to the symptoms presented by a patient. For example, it is very common for a voice disorder to be caused by a variety of etiological contributions including physical, neurologic, neurodegenerative, voice use, and/or psychogenic influences. Moreover, psychological trauma or excessive emotional stress may exist in a patient who is newly diagnosed with spas-

modic dysphonia or poor vocal behaviors and excessive voice demand may cause resistance of organic pathology to behavioral intervention (Stemple, Glaze, & Klaben, 2000). Likewise, voice disorders can develop at the onset of an upper respiratory infection (URI) and progress into a pathologic condition long after the cold/flu symptoms have resolved because the person is using effortful phonation and/or maladaptive behaviors (as a compensatory technique) to produce voice (Stemple, Glaze, & Klaben, 2000). Another example is when edema (swelling) or granulomas (inflammatory tissue) caused by laryngeal pharyngeal reflux (LPR) cause patients to compensate and they adopt a back-focused voice production to help diminish throat pain. In addition, a patient with unmanaged or mismanaged allergy symptoms may experience postnasal drip (PND) resulting in frequent throat clearing which could, over time, cause swelling and/or contact ulcers to develop on the arytenoid complex. These few clinical examples exemplify the overlapping influences that etiologic factors can play in the development or maintenance of a voice disorder and highlight the complexity of determining causation. It is more likely than not that by the time a patient seeks care for their voice disorder, secondary behaviors have developed that may exacerbate these undesirable vocal symptoms. Because of this, the voice rehabilitation plan must be tailored to include management of all etiologic factors identified. This will ultimately lead to better treatment of the vocal symptoms. The importance of a careful evaluation was discussed in Chapter 4.

Common Etiologic Factors

Phonotrauma

See Chapter 3 for a definition of phonotrauma. This classification most commonly describes voicing behaviors that the patient is using that is creating harmful effects on the structure or function of the vocal folds.

Laryngeal Surgery

Chapter 9 reviews surgical outcomes related to head and neck cancer which is often the most common direct surgery to the laryngeal structure resulting in a subsequent voice disorder that may or may not respond to behavioral treatment.

Other Surgery Unrelated

It is not uncommon for patients with voice disorders to have undergone other surgical procedures. Procedures that may have an ensuing effect on voice production include intubation for anesthesia (often exacerbated by a current condition of untreated reflux), thyroid gland procedures that impact the integrity of the recurrent laryngeal nerve (see Chapter 2), procedures on the carotid arteries due to the proximity of the vagus nerves, and other cardiothoracic surgeries. Cervical spinal procedures have resulted in acute airway obstructions, and voice and swallowing difficulties (Jung, Schramm, Lehnerdt, & Heberhold, 2005; Otto & Johns, 2005).

Acute and Chronic Illness

Patients suffering from illnesses affecting the multiple physiological systems of the human body could have detrimental effects on voice production. Most common are illnesses affecting the respiratory system such as chronic obstructive lung disease and emphysema as well as gastrointestinal disorders like esophageal disease, stomach dysmotility, and acute and chronic abdominal problems. Hormonal imbalance due to menopause or hormone change with age may also be a contributing factor to voice change. Other endocrine disorders linked with voice disorders include hypothyroidism. Autoimmune disorders such as systemic lupus erythematous, celiac disease, Sjogren's symdrome, and rheumotoid arthritis may also contribute to voice change. Illness particular to pediatrics might be chronic tonsillitis, sinusitis and ear infections, and velopharyngeal insufficiency.

Psychological Stress

Historically, and in particular, women, were treated with anti-anxiety medications when voice changed occurred. Psychological states such as anxiety, depression, impaired insight, personality disorders may all contribute to the characteristics of a presenting voice disorder. At the same time many individuals with voice disorders do not have more significant emotional issues than other people, other than those arising from the voice disorder. It is the clinician's role to determine if the psychological aspects are primary, concomitant or secondary to the voice disorder.

Drug Side Effects

See Chapter 11 for more information on this topic.

Vocal Lesions

The vocal quality that results from a voice disorder is influenced by the extent of the lesion both in terms of its size and depth of penetration within the histologic layers of the vocal folds as well as the lesions' location relative to the membranous and/or cartilaginous region of the vocal fold. Also, as stated above, the existence of compensatory strategies used by the patient as they try to "cover" a poor voice quality or reduce the pain associated with generating sound production may eventually contribute to further alteration(s) in voice quality. This chapter presents a general description of differential diagnostic signs of the most common voice disorders and considers the underlying contributions from medical, surgical, behavioral, rehabilitative, and psychosocial components.

After reading this chapter, you will:

- Understand which vocal fold pathologies are classified as structural voice disorders
- Understand the contributing causes and/or factors associated with structural vocal fold pathologies
- Understand how to describe the visual, stroboscopic, and perceptual features associated with structural vocal fold pathologies
- Understand the management strategies used to treat structural vocal fold pathologies

---

Covering is a term to describe a mode of protection used by a patient either purposefully or subconsciously to prevent further injury of pain during voice production.

Diagnostic History

- Review head and neck exam completed by physician

- Ensure a normal cranial nerve examination
- Probe the patient for other symptoms/medical conditions not discussed with physician or voice pathologist
- Uncover whether any "non related" symptoms are being treated

---

Other organ systems where symptoms and/or treatments may require referral to another specialist:

- Allergic
- Endocrine
- Neurologic
- Hormonal
- Pulmonary
- Gastrointestinal

Pathology Classifications

There are several approaches used to organize and classify the increasingly broad range of voice disorders and laryngeal pathologies. One approach is to classify each disorder as either functional, organic or neurologic, as suggested above. Another approach is to classify the disorders categorically as either benign or malignant pathologies. We decided to categorize the disorders as structural (changes in the vocal fold), neurologic (caused or affecting the central or peripheral nervous system, see Chapter 6), systemic (organic) disease, functional, and idiopathic (disorders with an unknown cause). The categorization of vocal disorders/pathologies is outlined in Table 5–1. Color plates providing examples of these pathologies are on the media that accompanies this textbook. Color plates are also included in a later section of this book to provide a basic image of the vocal pathologic condition.

Table 5–1. Review of Vocal Pathologies

Name	Onset	Benign/ Malignant	Histologic Layer Originates in	Typical Location
STRUCTURAL				
Vocal Fold Nodules	Acquired	Benign	SLLP	Midmembranous
Vocal Fold Polyps	Acquired	Benign	SLLP	Broad spectrum of appearance; free edge of true vocal fold, inferior border of true vocal fold, or more diffuse pattern as in polypoid degeneration
Reinke's edema/ polypoid degeneration/ diffuse polyposis	Acquired	Benign	SLLP	Diffuse swelling of the laryngeal submucosa
Laryngitis: acute and chronic	Acquired	Benign	Epithelial SLLP	Diffuse
Contact Ulcers/ Granuloma	Acquired	Benign	Arytenoid Mucosa	Arytenoid complex; subglottic, supraglottic
Cysts	Congenital and acquired	Benign	SLLP	Attached to vocal ligament or epithelia basement membrane
STRUCTURAL/ ORGANIC				
Candida	Acquired	Benign	Epithelial	Oral, laryngeal, and pharyngeal cavities
Papilloma	Congenital and acquired	Benign	Epithelial	Musculomembranous region but may extend into arytenoid, ventricle, and subglottis
Granular cell tumor	Acquired	Benign	Epithelial	Originates from the muscle

Table 5–1. *continued*

Name	Onset	Benign/ Malignant	Histologic Layer Originates in	Typical Location
Webs	Congenital and acquired	Benign	Epithelial	Level of the true vocal folds, some subglottic or supraglottic
Sulcus Vocalis	Acquired	Benign	SLLP	Vocal fold edge
Presbylaryngis	Acquired	Benign	N/A	Glottal gap may be present anteriorly or posteriorly
Leukoplakia, Hyperkeratosis	Acquired	Benign (pre-cancerous changes)	Epithelial	Vocal fold surface and/or interarytenoid area
Cancer	Acquired	Malignant	Epithelial	Epithelial in origin, highly variable in terms of extensiveness
STRUCTURAL/ AIRWAY				
Laryngeal Trauma	Acquired	Benign	N/A	Affects laryngeal cartilages and mucosa
Ankylosis of the CA Joint	Acquired	Benign	N/A	Affects cricoarytenoid and/ or cricothyroid joint
Subglottic Stenosis	Congenital or acquired	Benign	N/A	Membranous or cartilaginous
Laryngomalacia	Congenital	Benign	N/A	Upper airway, glottis
Laryngeal Cleft	Congenital	Benign	N/A	Commonly posterior, submucosal
STRUCTURAL/ VASCULAR				
Varix/Ectasia	Acquired	Benign	Superior surface of the true vocal fold	Varies—vocal fold edge, medial surface, lateral surface

continues

Table 5–1. *continued*

Name	Onset	Benign/ Malignant	Histologic Layer Originates in	Typical Location
Hemorrhage	Acquired	Usually Benign	SLLP	Membranous vocal fold
FUNCTIONAL				
Puberphonia	Acquired	Benign	N/A	N/A
Hyperfunctional/ Ventricular Phonation	Acquired	Benign	N/A	N/A
Muscle Tension Dysphonia	Acquired	Benign	N/A	N/A
Transgender Voice	Acquired	Benign	N/A	N/A
Conversion Aphonia	Acquired	Benign	N/A	N/A
IDIOPATHIC				
Paradoxical Vocal Dysfunction	Acquired	Benign	N/A	N/A

Incidence of Voice Disorders

Literature that has data regarding the incidence of voice disorders are very difficult to cite. This is because incidence varies demographically by region, age, sex, race, and occupation, and is also influenced by the sampling technique used to collect the data and the statistical power. There simply are too few epidemiologic studies on the incidence of voice disorders to provide an accurate number. In order to perform a comprehensive epidemiologic study, huge numbers of individual subject groups need to be surveyed, and the demographic factors indicated above require consideration. There do exist some studies that have provided incidence data from their individual clinical sites but these reports are limited in generalization to that particular geographic area (Painter, 1989). These studies have included patient numbers in the thousands (Coyle, Weinrich, & Stemple, 2000; Herrington-Hall et al., 1988). One of those reports estimates between 5 and 10% of the United States workforce demonstrate clinical signs of a voice disorder (Roy, Merrill, Gray, & Smith, 2005) with the incidence rate of voice disorders higher within certain occupational groups. These occupations include teachers, factory workers, preachers, etc., (Preciado-Lopez, Perez-Fernandez, Calzada-Uriondo,

& Preciado-Ruiz, 2007). In general, teachers report a higher incidence of voice problems compared to the general population (Preciado-Lopez et al., 2007). Other high-risk occupations include telemarketers, TV and radio broadcasters, sports coaches at various levels, aerobic/fitness instructors, air traffic controllers, pilots, lawyers, stage performers (actors, singers, etc.), military personnel, ministers, sales personnel, and so forth.

An occupationally related voice disorder is defined as a voice disorder that occurs when the job demands of a given profession require the individual to use the voice above and beyond how it is normally used every day. The repetitive voice use causes a load on the voice and talking becomes consuming and fatiguing. As a result, the quality of the employee's voice suffers and can even cause pain. The result for the employer may be days lost at work and a diminishing productivity.

Preventive approaches may assist in reducing or eliminating the risk for a voice disorder in at-risk populations, such as those listed above. Primary care physicians can serve an integral role in education of vocal health and early identification of voice problems by helping direct patients to the appropriate specialty of otolaryngology. As a medical specialty, otolaryngology is responsible for the diagnosis and treatment of diseases related to the ear, nose, and throat. The role of family primary care physicians and the importance of their involvement in patient education can help to reduce the incidence of voice disorders in all groups (Golub et al., 2006; Hamdan, Sibai, Srour, Sabra, &, Deeb, 2007).

The responsibility of the voice pathologist is to work with the primary care and family physicians so they have current diagnostic and treatment information to share with their patients and/or parents of children with voice disorders. For example, with regard to voice problems in the elderly, a voice disorder may be a sign of age-related degeneration or could relate to a neurological condition that requires further referral to multiple subspecialties. Voice symptoms can be the first presenting symptom of several medical conditions including Parkinson's disease, myasthenia gravis, multiple sclerosis, and amyotrophic lateral sclerosis.

With regard to the pediatric population the family physician again is likely the first-order contact that can help direct the child and/or child's parents/caregiver to an otolaryngologist, so that early intervention and accurate diagnosis can occur.

Structural Pathologies of the Vocal Folds

Structural pathologies of the vocal fold include those that cause any alteration in the histological organization of the vocal fold. Visual inspection of the vocal folds is a first-order step in order to verify the presence of structural pathology on the vocal fold.

Vocal Fold Nodules

Vocal nodules are one of the most common benign vocal fold pathologies resulting from phonotraumatic behaviors. These phonotraumatic behaviors may include talking too much, talking too loudly, talking over noise, yelling/screaming, coughing, throat clearing, making unusual noises, and speaking/singing in a pitch outside the normal mode of phonation (too high or too low). Vocal nodules are common in women, children, singers, actors, teachers, cheerleaders, clergy, and people in the sales industry and many other professions where voice use occurs often (Roy, Holt, Redmond, & Muntz, 2007) (Figure 5–1).

A   B

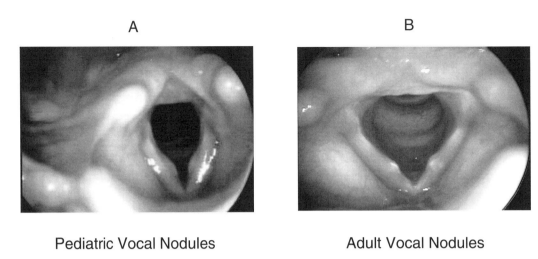

Pediatric Vocal Nodules   Adult Vocal Nodules

Figure 5–1. **A.** Broad-based bilateral pediatric vocal fold nodules in a 7-year-old female. **B.** Bilateral vocal fold nodules in an adult female with pachydermia in the interarytenoid space due to laryngopharyngeal reflux. Courtesy of The Ear, Nose & Throat Surgical Associates, Winter Park, Florida.

Description and Etiology

Vocal fold nodules are an inflammatory degeneration of the superficial layer of the lamina propria with associated fibrosis and edema (Hirano & Bless, 1993). They typically form bilaterally and develop at the margin or junction of the anterior and middle two-thirds of the vocal fold. This area of the vocal fold has high impact stress during phonation (Tao & Jiang, 2007). They can vary in size from very small, appearing as two small swellings to almost pea sized. They occur in children and adults with more common diagnosis occurring in young male children and female adults. The vibratory pattern of these groups is remarkably similar (Akif, Okur, Yildirim, & Guzelsov, 2004; Stathopoulos & Sapienza, 1997).

Three types of nodules have been described in the literature: (1) acute, (2) chronic, and (3) reactive nodular change. Acute nodules arise from traumatic or hyperfunctional voice use and appear gelatinous in nature. The gelatinous appearance arises from swelling in Reinke's space while the overlying squamous epithelium remains normal. Chronic nodules visually appear firm, callouslike, and fixed to the underlying mass of the mucosa due to increased fibrosis and thickened epithelium. Lastly, there is a condition called a "reactive nodular change." This occurs when a patient presents with a vocal fold polyp, vocal fold cyst, or other type of mass lesion which, because of its presence, creates a contralateral reaction on the otherwise healthy and opposite vocal fold. This reaction can develop over time into a larger and more discrete nodule.

Perceptual Signs and Symptoms

When vocal nodules develop, voice quality can be affected in several ways. In the early stages of nodular development, voice quality may be altered very slightly. As the nodular formation matures, more pronounced voice quality changes occur with the most severe changes occurring when the nodular formation becomes firm and fibrous. The most common voice quality associated with the presence of vocal nodules is a raspy, hoarse, slightly breathy voice that easily fatigues. Singers with vocal nodules typically complain of loss of vocal range (typically loss of their higher pitch range) and loss of vocal endurance. The main physiologic factors relating to these perceptual characteristics are increased glottal airflow, increased respiratory effort, overpressure of the vocal folds due to laryngeal hyperfunction and asymmetric vocal fold vibration (Sapienza & Stathopoulos, 1994).

Features of Visual Assessment

Laryngostroboscopic assessment of vocal fold nodules reveals increased mass and stiffness of the vocal fold cover as well as an hourglass closure pattern with decreased vibratory amplitude and mucosal wave. Mucosal wave can be absent at the nodule when the nodule is firm and fibrotic. If the nodule is edematous, soft, and pliable, then the mucosal wave may be observed on the nodule. Assessment of the mucosal wave can help describe the histologic characteristics of the nodule to a limited extent (Hirano & Bless, 1993). Furthermore, it is not uncommon to observe ventricular fold compression during phonation when viewing the results of the stroboscopic assessment due to compensatory behavior.

Management

The general management approach for treating vocal nodules is behavioral voice therapy (Boone, McFarlane, & Von Berg, 2005; Sulica & Behrman, 2003). A 16-item survey by Sulica and Behrman mailed to about 7,000 members of the American Academy of Otolaryngology-Head and Neck Surgery (16.5% response rate) indicated that voice therapy was an initial intervention for nodules. When nodules are removed surgically, without the benefit of vocal hygiene therapy and physiologic based vocal rehabilitation therapy, the nodular formation may reform. This is also the case with local injectable steroid injections (Lee et al., 2011). When vascular vocal fold lesions, such as hemorrhage, varix, or hematoma, accompany vocal nodules, a rapid course of oral steroids may help the healing response (Mortenson & Woo, 2006) and aid in avoiding a phonosurgical procedure. In general, nodules respond positively to behavioral voice therapy and medical therapies, and phonosurgery is most often not required.

Most recently a study examined the effectiveness of vocal hygiene education and voice production therapy in adult women with benign, bilateral phonotraumatic vocal fold lesions and the role of adherence in that perception (Behrman, Rutledge, Hembree, & Sheridan, 2008). Using the *Voice Handicap Index* (VHI) as a primary outcome measure, the findings indicated that the improvement in VHI scores was significantly greater for the voice production therapy group and that patients complied with a greater degree when involved in the voice production therapy group compared to the vocal hygiene only group. Current clinical trials testing behavioral treatment options for children with vocal nodules is currently underway at the Harvard Medical School, Massachusetts funded by the NIH/NIDCD.

Vocal Fold Polyps

Description and Etiology

A vocal fold polyp originates in the superficial layer of the lamina propria, usually in the middle one-third of the membranous vocal fold. Most polyps form from a working blood supply which may account for their sudden onset and rapid increase in size. Polyps can be present in a number of forms and effect voice quality differently depending on their relative size and location, as well as the compensatory strategies used by the patient to produce voice.

Polyps typically form unilaterally and can be sessile (blister-like) or pedunculated (footlike projection/attached to a stalk) in appearance. Sometimes a reactive nodular change on the contralateral vocal fold exists. As is the case with vocal nodules, the cause of polyps is thought to be from acute vocal trauma or from phonotraumatic behaviors, although polyps can also occur as the result of a *single* traumatic incident, such as yelling at a football game. This has a tendency to develop into a hemorrhagic polyp with sudden onset of hoarseness (Colton, Casper, & Leonard, 2006) (Figures 5–2, 5–3, and 5–4).

Perceptual Signs and Symptoms

The voice symptoms associated with having a vocal fold polyp vary from mild to severe dysphonia depending most on the size of the polyp (Cho et al., 2011) with other factors being color, location of the polyp and its interference with vocal fold closure. The most typical voice symptoms include hoarseness, roughness, or breathiness. In some cases a pedunculated polyp falls below the vocal fold edge during phonation and may not sub-

stantially alter voice quality but rather cause a sensation of difficulty breathing, particularly during the inspiratory phase of breathing. Other times, because of the mobility of the polyp, the voice changes quickly as the polyp changes position within the glottic space. Likewise, some patients may report a sensation of something in their throat, called a globus sensation, or effortful phonation and/or loss of vocal endurance.

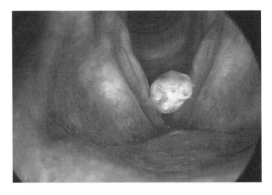

Figure 5–3. Right true vocal fold pedunculated polyp with leukoplakia. Note the feeder vessel supplying polyp on the right side. Courtesy of The Ear, Nose & Throat Surgical Associates, Winter Park, Florida.

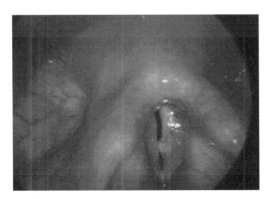

Figure 5–2. Left true sessile vocal fold polyp with mild bilateral ecstasia of the vocal fold. Courtesy of The Ear, Nose & Throat Surgical Associates, Winter Park, Florida.

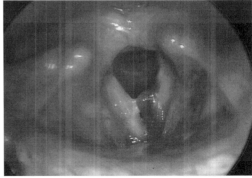

Figure 5–4. Left true vocal fold hemorrhagic polyp with left true vocal fold hemorrhage anteriorly and bilateral generalized edema. Courtesy of The Ear, Nose & Throat Surgical Associates, Winter Park, Florida.

Features of Visual Assessment

Visual examination of the larynx often reveals an hourglass vocal fold closure pattern with reduced vibratory amplitude and mucosal wave on the vocal fold with the polyp. Some polyps may appear firm with significantly reduced vocal fold vibration. In some cases the polyp can be quite large and obstruct the glottis. If the lesion is unilateral, which is most often the case, distinct differences can be observed in phase symmetry (Hirano & Bless, 1993) which has been cited as a distinctive visual feature of vocal polyps compared to vocal nodules (Rosen, Lombard, & Murry, 2000).

Management

Combined management approach of behavioral voice therapy, vocal hygiene, medical, and in many cases phonosurgery, is warranted in the treatment of vocal fold polyp(s). Physiologically based vocal rehabilitation is the optimal choice in attempt to intervene with the vocal fold polyp either as an independent treatment or following the resolution of the polyp by phonosurgery (Johns, 2003), see Chapter 7.

Generalized Edema/Reinke's Edema/ Polypoid Degeneration/ Diffuse Polyposis

Description and Etiology

Edema refers to a buildup of fluid that occurs primarily in the superficial layer of the vocal fold (Colton, Casper, & Leonard, 2006). Reinke's edema also called polypoid corditis, diffuse polyposis, or polypoid degeneration occurs when the superficial layer of the lamina propria (a.k.a Reinke's space) becomes filled with thick or gelatinous fluid because of long-standing trauma or chronic exposure to irritants, such as cigarette smoke or stomach acids due to laryngopharyngeal reflux (LPR) (Marcotullio, Magliulo, & Pezone, 2002). As severity increases, the entire membranous portion of the vocal folds becomes filled with the fluid. This extreme form of edema is referred to as polypoid degeneration (Figure 5–5).

Perceptual Signs and Symptoms

Typical voice symptoms associated with edema include a lowered pitch and varying degrees

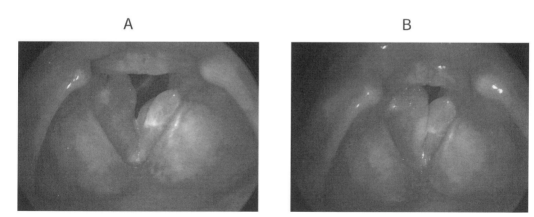

Figure 5–5. **A**. Bilateral Reinke's edema/severe polypoid degeneration creating reduced glottal space on abduction. Posterior erythema and pachydermia in the interarytenoid space. **B**. Adducted position. Courtesy of The Ear, Nose & Throat Surgical Associates, Winter Park, Florida.

of hoarseness (Colton, Casper, & Leonard, 2006). With Reinke's edema a very characteristic gravelly, low-pitched voice is heard. This is the result of the increased vocal fold mass. Because the voice is low in pitch, Reinke's edema is most noticeable in women, and may be overlooked in men, for whom a deep voice is not regarded as unusual. Sometimes, the swelling associated with Reinke's edema can become large enough to cause symptoms of dyspnea (breathlessness) because of impaired airway opening. Initially, dyspnea may only occur during strenuous exercise activity, but can ultimately affect breathing at rest, and based on clinical cases, can contribute to sleep apnea.

Features of the Visual Assessment

Visual assessment of the vocal folds commonly reveals bilateral swelling along the entire membranous length of the vocal fold, although the edema can be unilateral. There may be increased vocal fold stiffness of the most superficial layer of the vocal fold as well as increased mass of the vocal fold cover and depth of the vibratory edge. In cases of unilateral vocal fold edema, the edematous swelling often interferes with the vibratory movement of the contralateral vocal fold. Generally, glottic closure is complete. Vocal fold vibration tends to be asymmetric and successive vibrations are often aperiodic. The horizontal vibratory amplitude is often reduced. The appearance of vocal folds with Reinke's edema has been likened to water balloons. It is common for the swelling to shift with quiet respiration, and sometimes, the full extent of the swelling is visible only with a deep inspiration (Hirano & Bless, 1993).

Management

If the development of Reinke's edema is due to cigarette smoking, the initial step in its treatment is to quit smoking. For many patients this recommendation is easier said than done. In cases where Reinke's edema is detected early, improvement may occur with some reduction in smoking, by gradually decreasing the number of cigarettes smoked per day and by adhering strictly to a program of vocal hygiene.

More advanced cases of Reinke's edema generally do not respond to these strategies and continued smoking will ensure its recurrence following phonosurgical treatment, sometimes in a matter of weeks. For that reason, many laryngologists prefer that apatient stop smoking prior to surgical intervention for Reinke's edema. Phonosurgical procedures can include longitudinal incision, removal of the edema by suction, and resection of surplus vocal fold mucosa. The elimination of causal factors is highly significant in terms of the prognosis of those presenting with edema.

Laryngitis

Description and Etiology

Laryngitis is a general term that refers to a number of voice changes due to inflammatory conditions of the vocal fold mucosa. Other causes of laryngitis include reaction to a viral and/or bacterial infection (e.g. herpes simplex infection), traumatic conditions, autoimmune diseases (Ballenger & Snow, 1996), laryngopharyngeal reflux and allergic rhinitis.

Perceptual Signs and Symptoms

Laryngitis generally produces hoarseness that ranges from mild to severe; the more severe forms are typically due to continued or prolonged voice use during the bout of laryngitis. Often the acute phase of laryngitis is accompanied by a generalized sensation of a sore throat, cough and a fever, that lasts just a few days.

Features of Visual Assessment

In our experience, the most common visual features associated with acute and chronic laryngitis are generalized bilateral edema, reduced or absent mucosal wave, and slight reduction in vibratory amplitude of the vocal folds which will become more exaggerated when accompanied by chronic cough. In some instances the presence of ectasia and varix may occur. See description of ectasia and varix later in the chapter.

Management

Laryngitis often resolves with rest and hydration and, if indicated, the administration of an antibiotic. Yet, the treatment of laryngitis is highly dependent on causal factors. Therefore, it is important to try to pinpoint the cause of the inflammation, whether it stems from an infection or laryngopharyngeal reflux (LPR). Depending on the cause, highly different treatment strategies will be pursued. The goal is to remove the causative irritant or pathogen while considering the characteristics of the patient such as the lifestyle- or occupation-specific vocal demands. Adherence to vocal hygiene is a must during the acute phase of laryngitis to help prevent the development of further benign vocal fold lesions.

Contact Ulcers/Granulomas

Description and Etiology

Contact ulcers and granuloma are benign growths that can result from three causes: (1) laryngopharyngeal reflux (LPR) irritation, (2) intubation trauma, or (3) phonotrauma. They are usually found along the vocal processes and can form either unilaterally or bilaterally. Contact ulcers are raw sores that occur on the mucous membrane of the ary-tenoid processes. This area has little overlying tissue for protecting the vocal process, and is therefore prone to trauma from impact stress during phonation and even more so during forceful and louder phonation, singing, throat clearing, and coughing. Granulomas tend to grow over the area of the contact ulcer until the cause of irritation is addressed. Occasionally, a granuloma will become so large that it outgrows its blood supply and sloughs off. Granulomas are focused on next (Figure 5–6).

Laryngopharyngeal Reflux (LPR). There is a growing body of literature that provides strong evidence that LPR, a common source of irritation in the larynx, contributes significantly to the formation of granulomas (Lemos, Sennes, Imamura, & Tsuji, 2005). The mechanism of irritation from reflux occurs during the daytime because small amounts of reflux can occur when upright during the day. This causes damage to laryngeal tissues and produces localized symptoms. In the evening, the position of the body in the supine position (lying on one's back) allows for easier flow of the acid into the upper esophagus and airway.

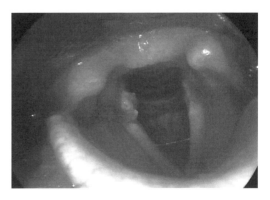

Figure 5–6. Right vocal fold process granuloma. Note the thin mucous strand bridging between vocal folds. Courtesy of The Ear, Nose & Throat Surgical Associates, Winter Park, Florida.

Reflux is acid backflow up from the stomach, into the esophagus. When the acid reaches into the upper pharynx and upper airway it is referred to as laryngopharyngeal reflux (LPR). Factors contributing to acid reflux include ingestion of fatty foods, chocolate, caffeine, alcohol, cigarette smoking, obesity, pregnancy, and delayed stomach emptying. The acid irritation directly affects the mucosal lining of the esophagus, pharynx, and upper airway and can give rise to granulation tissue as a reactive and protective mechanism to the acid irritation.

The larynx is very susceptible to the acid irritation as opposed to the esophagus which offers more protective lining (Farrokhi & Vaezi, 2007). Damage to the mucosal lining of the larynx can be minimized through aggressive management.

Intubation Trauma. Intubation is when a breathing tube is inserted into the trachea to aid ventilation. Intubation occurs during surgical procedures with general anesthesia and can occur in an emergency situation when a person's airway is significantly compromised. Granuloma formation related to intubation is rare (Lin, Cheng, & Su, 2008) but occurs because the mucosa overlying the arytenoids process becomes irritated by the placement of the endotracheal tube. As a reaction to the irritation, granulation tissue forms (typically within days or weeks of the intubation trauma). Granulation tissue forms in all parts of the body, including the mouth, sinuses, and lungs as a reaction to irritation. Laryngeal granulomas from intubation trauma can quickly and spontaneously resolve once the irritation is minimized.

Phonotrauma. Impact stress from shouting or repetitive arytenoid contact during high intensity talking can contribute to mucosal irritation of the arytenoid complex and subsequent development of a contact ulcer(s) or granuloma(s).

Perceptual Signs and Symptoms

A granuloma may commonly cause a globus sensation. The globus sensation is likely to provoke chronic throat clearing or coughing which simply creates more irritation to the already susceptible area. Other reported symptoms may include a bitter taste in the mouth (particularly in the morning), prolonged warm-up time needed to produce adequate voice, reduced pitch range, chronic throat clearing, cough. Discomfort or pain may be associated with the presence of the granuloma. The pain can be particularly sharp during coughing, swallowing, or throat clearing when the granuloma is directly irritated. Occasionally, the pain can be felt in the ear on the side of the mass. This phenomenon is known as "referred pain."

The mass of a large granuloma can prevent vocal fold closure. In such a situation, hoarseness and breathiness are typical with difficulty increasing vocal loudness. If the granuloma is small and unilateral it is possible that there will be minimal to no change in voice quality as the granuloma is not interfering with movements of the membranous portion of the vocal fold.

Features of Visual Assessment

Visual assessment of the vocal fold commonly reveals the granuloma to be located on the arytenoid complex or on the lateral wall of the posterior glottis. The growth of the granuloma is related to the extent and consistency of the irritant(s) creating the lesion. As stated above, larger granulomas can interfere with posterior glottic closure and sometimes cause phase asymmetry when unilateral. Smaller lesions often result in normal vibratory symmetry and no glottic incompetence.

Management

Intubation Granuloma. Intubation granulomas can resolve spontaneously (Harari, Blatchford, Coulthard, & Cassady, 1991) or be managed with a steroid injection. Lin et al. (2008) reported on several cases managed with potassium titanyl phosphate laser ablation which resulted in no re-occurrence of the lesion 14 months post follow-up.

> The properties of potassium titanyl phosphate make it a superior electro-optic modulator for laser treatment.

Granuloma Associated with LPR. Belafsky, Postma, and Koufman (2002) report that up to 50% of patients with voice disorders have LPR. Lifestyle management including diet modification in combination with medication prescription are two key components in the management of granuloma associated with LPR (Tsunoda et al., 2007). If the granuloma persists after a 3-month trial of behavioral modification and the use of anti-reflux drugs,

like proton-pump inhibitor medications for suppressing gastric acids, then further diagnostic testing and/or phonosurgery or more aggressive surgical approaches like fundoplication may be required (Figure 5–7).

> *Fundoplication* is a surgical procedure where part of the upper stomach is wrapped around the inferior aspect of the esophagus to correct the function of the lower esophageal sphincter. This will help prevent reflux by retightening the sphincter.

Drug Treatments for LPR. See also Chapter 11, special topic).

Antacids: Antacids are effective due to their acid neutralizing properties. They neutralize the pH of the reflux and can thereby prevent the tissue damage caused by bile salts and deactivate pepsin at the higher pH (Sontag, 1990). Antacids have been shown to

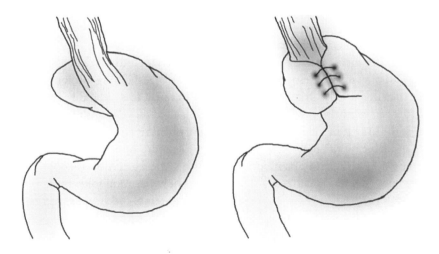

Figure 5–7. Schematic showing fundoplication procedure.

increase lower esophageal sphincter (LES) resting pressure (Sontag, 1990).

H2-blockers: Several H2-blockers are currently available by prescription and over the counter. These drugs act at the histamine type (H2) two receptor by competitive binding and reduce gastric acid secretion along with pepsin production (Gaynor, 1991; Sontag, 1990). Two doses (morning and evening) are generally recommended to control daytime and nighttime symptoms.

Proton-Pump Inhibitors (PPIs): Use of PPIs will help to prevent ulcers and assist in reducing the production of acid in the wall of the stomach. PPIs act against the enzyme hydrogen-potassium adenosine triphosphatase in the parietal cell thus blocking the final step in gastric acid production in the stomach (Gaynor, 1991). These drugs are more effective than H2 antagonists for the long-term reduction of basal and stimulated levels of gastric acid production.

Promotility Agents: Metoclopramide (Reglan) is a dopamine antagonist and is effective against reflux. It increases LES pressure, improves gastric emptying and may increase esophageal clearance (Gaynor, 1991; Orihata & Sarna, 1994). Metoclopramide (Reglan) is the only prokinetic agent currently available on the market. Unfortunately, up to a third of patients may experience adverse side effects (Gaynor, 1991).

Patients with diabetes mellitus, and anorexia nervosa may have significantly delayed gastric emptying and benefit from prokinetic agents (Orihata & Sarna, 1994).

Proton-pump inhibitors (PPIs) — some examples:

- Esomeprazole (e.g., Nexium)
- Lansoprazole (e.g., Prevacid)
- Omeprezole (e.g., Prilosec)
- Rabeprazole (e.g., Aciphex)
- Pantoprazole (e.g., Protonix)
- Zegarid (a rapid release form of omeprazole)

Common side effects associated with PPIs include headache, diarrhea, constipation, abdominal pain or rash. High does and long term use (1 year or longer) may increase risk of osteoporosis of the hip or spine.

H2-blockers — some examples:

- Cimetidine
- Tagamet
- Pepcid
- Ranitidine
- Zantac

> More detail about these drugs, their side effects, and interactions is in Chapter 11.

Granulomas Associated with Phonotrauma. Voice therapy should be employed to target the factors that are causing high impact stress to the posterior glottis/arytenoids mucosa, such as loud talking, shouting, prolonged talking time, and so forth. It is often difficult for patients to understand the relationship between these phonatory behaviors and the occurrence of a lesion. If patients are going to be asked to modify their existing vocal behaviors then they must understand how the vocal folds work, how and why impact stress occurs in the posterior glottis with loud talking, and the effects of prolonged voice use on vocal fold health. The closure pattern, in particular for men, has highest impact in the posterior glottis whereas for women and children the highest impact stress during phonation is located on the midmembranous portion of the vocal fold (Titze, 1984).

Cysts

Description and Etiology

A cyst is a benign mucous/fluid-filled lesion surrounded by a epithelial membrane and is located near the vocal fold surface (Hirano, 1981). The implicated causes of vocal fold cyst include phontraumatic behaviors as indicated for vocal fold nodules and polyps, and glandular blockage. Like other benign lesions, cysts appear at the midmembranous portion of the vocal fold, which in most persons is the most active segment during phonation. Vocal fold cysts can present congenitally but are very rare (Smith, Callanan, Harcourt, & Albert, 2000) (Figure 5–8).

Perceptual Signs and Symptoms

Vocal fold cysts generally result in mild to severe hoarseness as a consequence of vocal

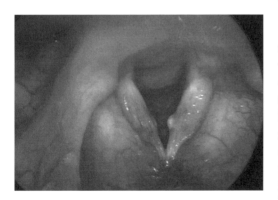

Figure 5–8. Left, midmembranous, mucous retention cyst with right reactive nodular change on true vocal fold. Bilateral ectasia, more prominent on the right true vocal fold. Courtesy of The Ear, Nose & Throat Surgical Associates, Winter Park, Florida.

fold asymmetry and irregular vocal fold closure. Variation in voice quality is a function of the size and shape of the cyst as well as its firmness. Depending on the size of the cyst, globus sensation may accompany a cyst, with the patient exhibiting throat clearing and cough.

Features of Visual Assessment

A cyst is a growth and can be found anywhere along the membranous vocal fold, in the laryngeal ventricle, or on the ventricular (false) folds. Cysts typically are *intracordal*, occurring underneath the mucosa of the vocal fold, located in the superficial layer of the lamina propria.

One study completed a retrospective review of laryngostroboscopic examinations carried out in a voice clinic between 1993 and 2002 and found the following distribution of cysts: out of 4,206 total cases, 42% were submucosal cysts and 10% were pseudocysts.

> A pseudocyst is a cavity that looks like a cyst but does not have an epithelial membrane like a true cyst.

Once the patient was taken into the operating room a correlation between what was identified from the laryngostroboscopic examinations and what was identified in the surgical suite was completed. The laryngostroboscopic to surgical correlation was positive for 78% of the cysts and 100% of the pseudocysts indicating that the laryngostroboscopic technique was very good at correctly identifying the diagnostic label (Hernando, Cobeta, Lara, Garcia, & Gamboa, 2007).

Management

Vocal hygiene therapy is often the first line of treatment prescribed for a vocal cyst. Voice therapy may function to improve the voice quality to some degree, but is not likely to make a cyst fully resolve. Voice rest and vocal hygiene are often prescribed to help reduce edema surrounding the cyst but the cyst itself does not diminish in size with these treatments. Because of this, phonosurgical removal of the cyst is the most common treatment choice. With any phonosurgical procedure, under and overexcision needs to be avoided to minimize reoccurrence and inadvertent damage to the vocal ligament. Microsurgical excision, as described in Chapter 8, is typically the surgical procedure of choice for removal of vocal fold cysts but can be quite a challenging procedure because cysts are often close to the vocal ligament and the risk of creating scar is high. The CO_2 laser assisted microsurgery technique has been shown to be reliable for treatment intracordal cysts (Mater et al., 2010).

Candida

Description and Etiology

Candida is a yeast normally present in the body. Candidiasis is a fungal infection that occurs as a consequence of weakness within the immune system. This weakness may occur because the person is sick, is on some medication that is suppressing the immune system (long term use of antibiotics), or is taking a chemotherapeutic agent. Cigarette smoking is a contributory factor as well. In persons with diabetes, candidiasis occurs more often as is the case with individuals using inhaled corticosteroids (Sulica, 2005). Many patients have more than one predisposing factor that is causing the candidiasis (Figure 5–9).

Perceptual Signs and Symptoms

Voice quality associated with candidiasis may be pressed, moderately hoarse, and breathy. Pain may be present in some cases (Sulica, 2005).

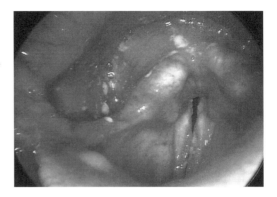

Figure 5–9. Fungal infection/*Candida* in the postcrioid space and superior surface of left true vocal fold. Bilateral hyperkeratosis. Courtesy of The Ear, Nose & Throat Surgical Associates, Winter Park, Florida.

Features of Visual Assessment

On visual examination, candidiasis often resembles leukoplakia of the true vocal folds, and it may be present on the arytenoids, and some supraglottic structures, as epithelial hyperplasia predominates and fungal pseudomembranes can be seen. Edema and erythema are often present. The vocal edges appear irregular and glottic closure is often incomplete. There can also be marked vocal fold stiffness, decreased mucosal wave, and an asymmetric weakness of the vocal folds.

Management

As Sulica (2005) pointed out, candidiasis is often misdiagnosed. In his presentation of 8 cases, Sulica found instances where no oral or oropharyngeal manifestation of candidiasis was present. In his case series, all patients responded to oral fluconazole (100 to 400 mg/day) and removal of predisposing factors where possible. The implementation of a good vocal hygiene program is recommended with the patient, with attempts to eliminate irritating factors such as gastroesophageal reflux while increasing hydration where appropriate. Voice therapy is often not necessary.

Laryngeal Papilloma

Description and Etiology

Laryngeal papilloma is caused by exposure to the human papilloma virus (HPV). HPV 6 genome and HPV 11 are the identified causative agents (Corbitt, Zarod, Arrand, Longson, & Farrington, 1988). Onset of laryngeal papilloma can occur during both child (called juvenile) and adulthood. Histologic evaluations from biopsied samples of both the juvenile and adults forms of papilloma do not appear to distinguish between the two (Corbitt et al., 1988), although the juvenile forms tends to be clustered and at multiple sites compared to single lesions in the adult form. The most common sites for papillomatosis are the true vocal folds, followed by the trachea, bronchi, palate, nasopharynx, and, in rare instances, the lungs (Kashima, Mounts, Levinthal, & Huban, 1993) (Figure 5–10).

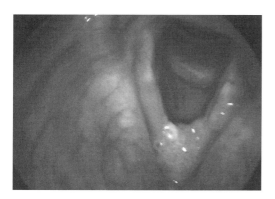

Figure 5–10. Laryngeal papilloma in the anterior commissure. Courtesy of The Ear, Nose & Throat Surgical Associates, Winter Park, Florida.

Juvenile papillomatosis typically occurs within the first five years of life from perinatal infection transferred by the mother. The mother carries condylomatous lesions in the genital tract. The condylomatous lesions are associated with the sexually transmitted HPV virus. HPV types 6 and 11, which are responsible for 80 to 90% of the condylomas in mothers, are documented in nearly 100% of the cases of juvenile papilloma (Gissmann, Diehl, Schultz-Loulon, & zur Hausen, 1982; Mounts, Shah, & Kashima, 1982). Identifiable as elevated growths on the surface of the genitals, the HPV in condyloma is very contagious and can be spread by skin-to-skin contact, usually during sex with an infected partner. And, although genital tract HPV is common, juvenile papillomatosis is rare. Children born to condylomatous mothers are at risk for developing juvenile onset papillomatosis, formally referred to as juvenile-onset recurrent respiratory papillomatosis. The papillomas may recur very rapidly in some cases, requiring surgery every 2 to 4 weeks to minimize threat to the airway. So, while a rare condition, the airway threat is very serious, the recurrence very fast after their removal and the impact on voice quality highly substantial because of the number of frequent surgeries and subsequent vocal fold scarring.

In the case of adult laryngeal papillomatosis, the recurrence rate is much slower than that experienced with juvenile papillomatosis and the papilloma tend to be more localized within the upper airway (Sharma, Gill, Kaur, & Hans, 2001). Kleinsasser and Cruz (1973) put forth a further differentiation for adult papilloma as precancerous versus nonkeratinizing lesions. The causative agents include sexual contact, a trigger that reduces the autoimmune system causing the dormant virus (present since birth) to flare up (Kuruvilla, Saldanha, & Joseph, 2008) or in rare cases severe gastro-esophageal reflux.

Perceptual Signs and Symptoms

Roughness is likely the best descriptor for the voice quality associated with laryngeal papilloma, as the lesion is irregular and results in vibratory asymmetry when present on the true vocal folds. If the papilloma interferes with glottal closure then breathiness may be a symptom. If the papilloma lesion(s) are diffuse and large then dyspnea and inspiratory stridor (noise on inspiration) become potential symptoms of airway obstruction. Chronic cough is not uncommon, and/or weak cry and periods of aphonia.

Features of Visual Assessment

Stroboscopically, papilloma tends to interfere with vocal fold closure causing incomplete glottal closure. The extent of interference with glottal closure is dependent on the relative size of the papilloma lesion. On examination, a "wart or raspberry" type appearance is seen. As mentioned previously, in the adult cases the papilloma can appear as a solitary lesion wherein the juvenile cases the papilloma tends to be spread diffusely throughout the upper and lower airway.

The increased stiffness created by the papilloma lesions on the vocal folds will impede vibratory amplitude of the vocal folds. Mucosal wave may be absent in the area of the lesions. When multiple surgical excisions have been required for vocal fold papilloma, the cover of the vocal folds may be stiff and interfere significantly with amplitude and vibratory behavior. Ventricular compression can be observed due to the loss of adequate vocal fold vibration.

Management

The first course of intervention for treating papilloma is to care for the airway obstruction and ensure that ventilatory support is adequate. Always with a case of papilloma, regardless of age, treatments must take precedent in successfully ensuring a patent airway over an improved voice quality. The surgical procedures only offer symptomatic relief and in the juvenile cases treatments try to stay ahead of disease recurrence; the treatments should not be considered a cure. There are several courses of management for laryngeal papilloma.

- Microsurgical ablation (Preuss et al., 2007) using a CO_2 laser. With any CO_2 excision care must be taken to not damage surrounding tissue.
- Microdebrider resection
- Surgical treatment and drug therapy using interferons are the most common treatment modalities at present. Interferons are naturally produced in the body and there are also synthetic interferons available to use in the treatment of papilloma. Side effects include as fatigue, dizziness, depression, body aches, headache, and fever, as well as a propensity for the papillomas to recur after the interferon has been stopped.
- In-office ablation using the pulsed-dye laser (PDL). No general anesthetic is needed. The laser specifically targets the papilloma without harming the normal laryngeal epithelium.
- Antiviral drugs including acyclovir, ribavirin, cidofovir, retinoic acic, indole-3-carbinole, and methotrexate.
  - Indole-3-carbinol, a natural offshoot of cabbage and broccoli, alters the growth pattern of papilloma. It appears to be safe and may prove to be a viable treatment for aggressive recurrent respiratory papilloma in certain

patients (Andrus & Shapshay, 2006; Coll, Rosen, Auborn, Potsic, & Bradlow, 1997).

- Methotrexate is a chemotherapeutic agent belonging to a class called antimetabolites. This medication blocks an enzyme needed by tumor cells to survive. Side effects may also occur with this intervention (blood, liver, or kidney problems, diarrhea, loss of hair, others). Additional study is needed to further define its therapeutic efficacy (Avidano & Singleton, 1995).

- Cidofovir is used to treat viral infections. Showing some promise in its outcomes, cidofovir is injected directly into the papilloma at the time of endoscopy. No serious side effects have been reported (Andrus & Shapshay, 2006; Coll et al., 1997; Snoeck et al., 1998).

- Celecoxib (Celebrex), a newly developed inhibitor of cyclooxygenase (COX)-2 is being tested to see if it can prevent papilloma from recurring.

- Cidofovir is used to treat viral infections. Showing some promise in its outcomes, cidofovir is injected directly into the papilloma at the time of endoscopy. No serious side effects have been reported (Andrus & Shapshay, 2006; Coll et al., 1997; Snoeck et al., 1998).

■ Photodynamic therapy. The details of photodynamic therapy are outside the scope of this chapter but it is a technique that allows targeted treatment to occur on the papilloma tissue. It uses a nontoxic dye, termed a photosensitizer, and low intensity visible light which, when in the presence of oxygen, combine to produce cytotoxic species. Studies show approximately 50% reduction, in the average rate of laryngeal papilloma growth following treatment. The response is especially pronounced in patients with the worst disease (Abramson et al., 2006).

Nonuseful treatments include the use of steroids, estrogens, ultrasound, irradiation, and cautery. See Bergler and Gotte (2000) for a more complete description of the management strategies listed before as their mechanism of action is outside the scope of this chapter.

Voice therapy may be a treatment option for either juvenile or adult papilloma but only when in a state of nonrecurrence. Voice therapy should focus on minimizing the compensatory strategies that may have developed as the patient tries to produce the best possible voice.

Granular Cell Tumor

Description and Etiology

Laryngeal granular cell tumors are uncommon but when they do occur they are more prevalent in women than men and evident in the third through sixth decades of life (White, Glade, Rossi, & Bielamowicz, 2007). They are benign tumors arising from muscle (myoblastomas) (Chiang, Fang, Li, Chen, & Lee, 2004), and are often associated with the presence of another granular cell tumor elsewhere in the body (White et al., 2007) (Figure 5–11).

Perceptual Signs and Symptoms

Voice quality is rough/hoarse and dysphagia may be present. The patient may complain of a globus sensation at rest or on swallow.

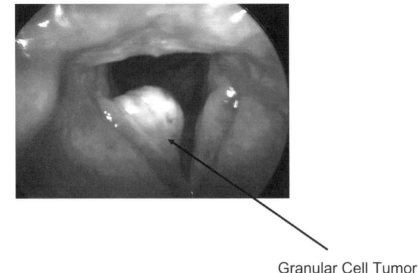

Granular Cell Tumor

Figure 5–11. Granular cell tumor, right true vocal fold in a 14-year-old male. Courtesy of The Ear, Nose & Throat Surgical Associates, Winter Park, Florida.

Dysphagia and inspiratory stridor may also be present.

Features of Visual Assessment

Laryngoscopy will indicate a moderately sized mass located on the arytenoids medial surface and/or within the subglottic region. Other locations can be on the anterior commissure, ventricular folds and posterior cricoid region (White et al., 2007). When a granular cell tumor is located in the posterior aspect of the larynx, it is most often confused with a laryngeal granuloma. Biopsy and histologic analysis will confirm the diagnosis. As with other types of posterior laryngeal lesions, vibration of the membranous portion of the vocal fold may not be affected resulting in a normal laryngostroboscopic examination.

Management

Granular cell tumors are removed with surgical excision typically using a combined modality of CO_2 laser and conventional surgical tools.

Laryngeal Web

Description and Etiology

Seventy-five percent of the laryngeal webs occur at birth (Bluestone & Stool, 1983). Congenital laryngeal webs occur when there is a failure of recanalization (restoration of the lumen) of the larynx during embryonic development. This occurs during the 4th to 10th week of gestation. Webs typically are located anteriorly, yet how much of the airway is blocked varies substantially. The more extensive the web, the greater respiratory distress exhibited by the patient. Webs can block up to 75% of the glottal airway in severe cases and the thickness can vary from very thin and translucent to very thick (Figure 5–12).

Acquired Laryngeal Webs. Acquired laryngeal webs can occur due to laryngeal trauma, particularly following emergency intubation or intubation during a surgical procedure that occurred for a prolonged period of time. They

A

B

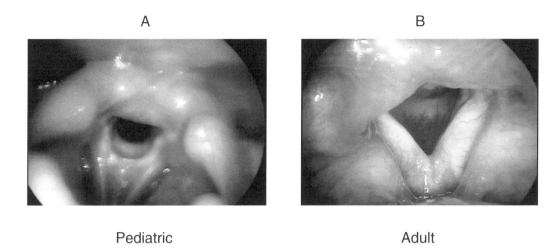

Pediatric   Adult

Figure 5–12. **A**. Laryngeal web of membranous vocal fold in a 7-year-old female.
B. Webbing of the anterior commissure status of multiple, postsurgical papilloma
removals. Courtesy of The Ear, Nose & Throat Surgical Associates, Winter Park, Florida.

often occur at the anterior commisure or anterior membranous portion of the vocal fold.

Perceptual Signs and Symptoms

Symptoms associated with laryngeal webs
include dyspnea and inspiratory stridor. Dyspnea and stridor occur as the glottal airway
resistance is increased and the amount of air
able to pass into the lower airway is limited
because of the decreased glottal space. Inspiratory stridor most often occurs when the web is
blocking the posterior glottis. Voice symptoms
range from hoarseness to difficulty sustaining
phonation, again depending on the extent of
the web.

Features of Visual Assessment

Office-based endoscopic procedures are satisfactory for identifying the presence of a web
but will not be able to define the extent and/
or thickness of the web. In order to determine
these parameters, direct laryngoscopy in the
operating room and bronchoscopy are necessary (Tewfik, 2006).

> Bronchoscopy is an endoscopic proce-
> dure that allows the trachea and bronchi
> to be examined.

Management

Management of laryngeal webs involves resection of the web using either a knife or laser
procedure. A keel may be placed between the
vocal fold edges to prevent rescarring of the
surgical site.

> A keel is a stent designed to keep the
> anterior commissure area from closing.
> It is typically made of silicone.

Sulcus Vocalis

Description and Etiology

Sulcus vocalis affects the superficial layer of the
lamina propria causing a thinning or loss/fur-
rowing to the vocal fold tissue. Sulci can occur

unilaterally or bilaterally. The etiology of sulcus vocalis is undefined but has been linked to history of smoking with a higher incidence in certain ethnic groups (Figure 5–13).

The Bouchayer theory (1985) states that there is a congenital cause of sulcus vocalis. This theory holds that an epidermoid cyst develops from faulty genesis of the 4th and 6th branchial arches. In time, the cyst ruptures and causes the sulcus. Van Canegham's theory, on the other hand, believes that the sulcus is acquired due to trauma or infection.

Ford (1996) offered a classification scheme identifying three types of sulci. The Ford Type I sulcus is when the depression or sulcus extends along the full length of the vocal fold into the lamina propria but does not affect the vocal ligament. There is little functional impact with a Type I sulcus. Ford Type IIa sulcus again extends the full vocal fold length up to the vocal ligament, leading to a moderate dysphonia. In Ford Type IIb sulcus, the sulcus is deep and has a cavity-like appearance because its focal nature extends into the vocal ligament and can even penetrate into the thyroarytenoid muscle. Severe dysphonia is associated with the Type IIb sulcus.

Perceptual Signs and Symptoms

Perceived voice quality associated with a sulcus vocalis is hoarseness, weakness, and increased effort. Vocal fatigue is also common complaint. The grade of dysphonia varies by the depth of the sulcus, as described above.

Features of Visual Assessment

Clinical examination rarely allows diagnosis of sulcus but it can establish suspicion (Giovanni, Chanteret, & Lagier, 2007). If visualized, a groove or furrow presents itself on the medial surface of the vocal fold. It can stretch the entire length of the vocal fold. The area of sulcus usually does not vibrate normally during voicing with reductions in mucosal wave and the tissue loss usually causes a spindle shaped glottic gap.

Management

Management of sulcus vocalis will often involve resection of the fibrous tissue and abnormal mucosa from the surface of the vocal fold. Following the dissection of the sulcus, a

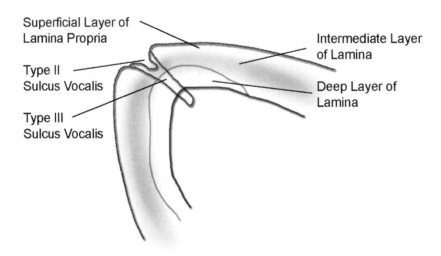

Figure 5–13. Schematic showing sulcus vocalis.

glottic gap will likely be present. Pinto and colleagues (2007) described augmentation in the treatment of sulcus vocalis using autogenous fat and/or fascia augmentation in 34 patients. One year after the procedure, improvements of vocal quality, glottal closure, mucosal wave excursion, and acoustic, perceptual, and phonatory functions occurred, thus affirming the usefulness of these augmentation techniques for the management of sulcus vocalis. Some results have been mixed with regard to the use of other phonosurgical procedures like medialization and the use of other types of injectables (see Chapter 8), (Kandogan, 2007). If considered a management strategy, the main materials used are fascia, fat, and collagen (Giovanni, Chanteret, & Lagier, 2007). Most recently hyaluronic acid was implanted and tested to determine its outcome on voice in those with glottal insufficiency including a few patients with sulcus vocalis and vocal fold scarring. Results were promising and safe for improving overall voice quality (Szkielkowska et al., 2011).

Presbylaryngis

Description and Etiology

Aging generally affects the physiological functions of the body resulting in deterioration in circulation, glandular, urinary tract, digestive, respiratory, joint, and muscle function, among others. (Dubeau, 2006; Paganelli et al., 2006; Ritz, 2000; Sharma & Goodwin, 2006) (Figure 5–14).

With regard to muscle function, all skeletal muscle in the aging human body, experiences sarcopenia, a wasting and thinning of muscle tissue (Johnston, De Lisio, & Parise, 2008) The vocal fold muscle, or thyroarytenoid muscle, is no exception. As the superficial connective tissue in the vocal fold begins to deteriorate with age, becoming thinner and

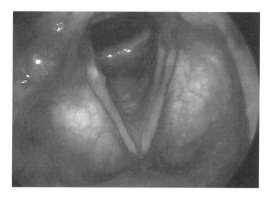

Figure 5–14. Presbylaryngis in an 84-year-old male, depicting bilateral vocal fold thinning. Courtesy of The Ear, Nose & Throat Surgical Associates, Winter Park, Florida.

less pliable, the collagen in the deeper portions of the vocal fold becomes dense.

Perceptual Signs and Symptoms

In general, for both sexes, a softer, altered pitch with some accompanying roughness might be present. Tremor may be associated with aging like that described in Chapter 6 (see essential tremor). And, although the pitch becomes altered with age, differences are observed between the sexes. Older men tend to have a higher pitch voice compared to their younger voice whereas women's voices tend to lower with age (Linville, 1996). Both sexes typically experience reduced vocal loudness as they age usually due to loss in tight glottal closure.

Features of Visual Assessment

The anatomic changes associated with aging result in physiologic changes to vocal fold vibration, such as reductions in vibratory amplitude, reduced speed of glottal closure and increased glottal gap. The vocal folds appear thin due to muscle atrophy and thinning of the superficial tissues. Bowing of the vocal folds may be present (Bloch & Behrman, 2001). Anterior and midmembranous gaps are more common (Linville, 1992) and often considered a classic sign of the aging larynx. Finally, the cartilages may be more prominent, particularly the vocal process of the arytenoid.

Management

Management of the aging voice with particular emphasis on improving glottal closure includes the following: voice therapy, medialization procedures, and the use of injectables in the vocal fold.

Voice Therapy. During voice therapy it is important to help the older individual understand the anatomic and physiologic changes occurring within the larynx and moreover to the respiratory, skeletal, joint, and muscular systems that may be affecting voice production. Unlike the apparent changes seen in the skin, weight, or even walking pattern, changes to the larynx and other associated systems are less apparent. As a clinician, offer explanation to the older patient about the relationship between respiratory and laryngeal structural changes and voice change. This will help older patients gain an understanding of their vocal limits and possibly ease anxiety about the potential of laryngeal cancer, a very common worry in older patients.

Although physiologic voice therapy techniques have the most obvious application for remediation of the aging voice, there is little published evidence to support its use (Ramig et al., 2001). One retrospective study of 54 patients with age-related dysphonia who sought voice therapy showed that voice therapy leads to statistically significant improvement in voice related quality of life as indicated by the results of the Voice-Related Quality of Life Index (Berg, Hapner, Klein, & Johns, 2008). Some group therapy programs may be helpful offering both social interaction and the ability to work on the vocal symptoms presented by older patients.

Medialization Procedures. The thinning of the vocal fold due to loss of connective tissue and muscle mass may result in glottal gap, particularly along the anterior and midmembranous portions of the vocal fold. As such, medialization procedures are used to help improve glottal closure including the use of the Isshiki Type 1 thyroplasty procedure (Isshiki, Shoji, Kojima, & Hirano, 1996); see Chapter 8.

Injectables. Injectables are used to restore lost bulk to the vocal folds with the intent to lessen the extent of glottic gap by improving vocal fold closure. Given the description of a thinning vocal fold that accompanies aging, the use of injectables can result in a stronger voice and less effort during voicing. However, injection does not remedy the changes have occurred in the vibratory tissues of the vocal fold, so a "perfect" voice is not typically obtained following these procedures. More recently, calcium hydroxylapatite for vocal fold augmentation was investigated for use in cases of vocal fold atrophy associated with aging. Of 39 vocal folds in 23 individuals injected with calcium hydroxylapatite, all individuals reported improvement on a self-administered disease-specific outcome which assessed speaking effort, throat discomfort and pain, vocal fatigue, and presence of voice cracks (Belafsky & Postma, 2004).

Leukoplakia/Hyperkeratosis

Description and Etiology

Leukoplakia is an abnormality change to the epitheliumwhite plaquelike formation occurring on the vocal fold surface. It is usually found at the anterior portion of the vocal fold but may extend into the interarytenoid area. Primary cause of leukoplakia is chronic irritation and the primary cause of that irritation is cigarette smoking. Other causes of irritation could be environmental exposure to irritants, LPR, alcohol use, or other inhaled drugs, like marijuana. It is considered a precancerous state and should be biopsied (Figure 5–15).

Perceptual Signs and Symptoms

Patients with leukoplakia/hyperkeratosis present with a rough and hoarse voice quality.

Features of Visual Assessment

Depending on the thickness of the plaque the vibratory behavior of the vocal folds will be affected to differing degrees. In most cases of leukoplakia there will be reduced vibratory amplitude, reduced mucosal wave, and increased vocal fold stiffness bilaterally.

Management

If the cells are not found to be atypical following the results of the biopsy, then vocal

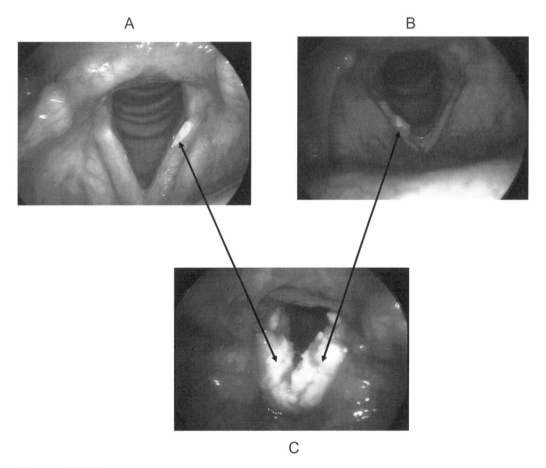

Figure 5–15. **A.** Leukoplakia of the epithelial layer of the left true vocal fold. **B.** Anterior web, right true vocal fold polyp with leukoplakia on the epithelial layer, endoscopic findings suggestive of LPR in the posterior larynx. **C.** Bilateral Reinke's edema, hyperkeratosis, and leukoplakia. Courtesy of The Ear, Nose & Throat Surgical Associates, Winter Park, Florida.

hygiene counseling needs to follow. The counseling should strongly indicate to the patient that unless the chronic irritation is minimized or removed the cell growth could reach a cancerous state. For small leukoplakias, surgical excision usually suffices. Again, counseling is highly recommended with the patient so the patient understands about the cause and effect relationship between chronic irritation and the risk of recurrence. Patients with leukoplakia should be followed for at least 3 to 6 months to monitor for recurrence and/or malignant transformation (benign to cancerous). Other treatments include retinyl palmitate (Issing, Struck, & Naumann, 1996) and proton-pump inhibitor therapy.

Dysplasia and Laryngeal Cancer

Description and Etiology

Dysplasia is pathologic tissue change in the vocal fold mucosa identified with biopsy, but the abnormal cells are not found to be malignant. It is, however, often indicative of an early cancerous process. Both dysplasia/atypia and early vocal fold cancer appears whitish or reddish in color due to hypervascularization. They can form a mass, plaque, or irregularity on the vocal fold edge (Figure 5–16).

Features of Visual Assessment

Endoscopically, the appearance of dysplasia, and early vocal fold cancer is not distinguishable from a malignancy; that is why the biopsy is necessary. Dysplasia is expressed as low grade or high grade. High-grade dysplasia represents a more advanced progression toward cancer formation and requires careful observation (Cotran, Kumar, & Collins 1999).

Laryngeal cancer, on the other hand, refers to a change of normal tissue that divides and grows uncontrollably. A diagnosis of laryngeal cancer can only be made from tissue biopsy. It is the most devastating laryngeal pathology due to the physical nature of the disease and the emotional consequences associated with the diagnosis. The cause of laryngeal cancer is multifactorial. Not all factors are currently known; however, smoking and heavy drinking of alcohol greatly increase the risk of development. Laryngeal cancer accounts for 2 to 5% of cancers diagnosed in the United States (http://www.cancer.gov). Also termed

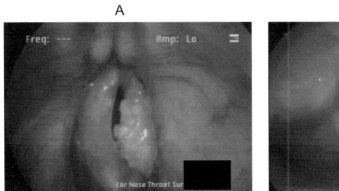 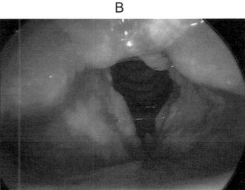

Figure 5–16. **A**. Left true vocal fold severe dysplasia. Fourteen months later second biopsy indicated squamous cell carcinoma. **B**. Laryngeal cancer. Courtesy of The Ear, Nose & Throat Surgical Associates, Winter Park, Florida.

laryngeal carcinoma or squamous cell carcinoma, these terms reflect the origin from the squamous cells which are flat, scalelike cells that form the epithelium of the vocal fold.

For the purposes of tumor staging, the larynx is divided into three anatomic regions (see Chapter 1). Chapter 9 describes the mechanisms and sites of cancer and tumor staging in detail. Most laryngeal cancers originate in the glottis. Laryngeal cancer may spread by direct extension to adjacent structures, by metastasis to regional cervical lymph nodes, or more distantly, through the bloodstream (Spaulding, Hahnn, & Constable, 1987).

Management of laryngeal cancer is typically prescribed and/or changed based on the stage of cancer and remains a powerful predictor of survival.

Perceptual Signs and Symptoms of Laryngeal Cancer

Symptoms can include the following:

- Hoarseness
- Change in pitch (typically lower due to the mass effect)
- Vocal strain
- Sore throat or globus sensation
- Persistent cough
- Stridor

Management

A combined modality treatment program typically includes surgery, radiation and chemotherapy. The ongoing management of laryngeal cancer requires continued cancer surveillance through regular laryngeal examinations. The role of the voice pathologist involves patient counseling, management of voice and swallowing issues, educating and facilitating alternative communication modes. See Chapter 9 for further detailed discussion on this topic.

Laryngeal Trauma

Description and Etiology

Laryngeal trauma is classified as either penetrating or blunt (O'Mara & Hebert, 2000) and can occur with gunshot and knife wounds, motor vehicle accidents, and other accidents such as a kick to the laryngeal area during karate and dropping a heavy object onto the neck during weightlifting. We have seen laryngeal trauma occur after a fistfight, as a sports injury following a soccer game, result of a flying trapeze artist hitting the trapeze bar, and in a case of attempted strangulation (Figure 5–17).

With laryngeal trauma the hyoid bone or cartilages may be crushed or fractured, the cricoarytenoid and/or cricothyroid joint may become dislocated and impaired, the tissues/mucosa may be torn, a hemorrhage, edema, or vocal fold paralysis may result, and a compromised airway may require management.

Perceptual Signs and Symptoms

With laryngeal trauma, hoarseness and inspiratory and expiratory stridor may be exhibited. The patient may report pain at rest or during voicing (odynophonia), along with dyspnea and possible dysphagia.

Features of Visual Assessment

In order to determine the extent of damage to the larynx, sub or supraglottis, imaging may need to occur beyond the endoscopic examination and include computerized topmography imaging. The endoscopic features are varied depending on extent of damage but can range from hematomas or lacerations to complete laryngotracheal separation (O'Mara & Hebert, 2000).

Management

Early surgical exploration and fixation for patients with dislocated joints, displaced

Displaced Structure

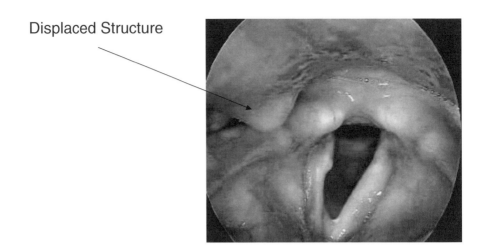

Figure 5–17. Blunt laryngeal trauma from a karate chop to the neck. Note the displaced anatomic structure. Courtesy of the University of Miami School of Medicine Center for Sinus and Voice Disorders.

laryngeal fractures, or mucosal lacerations exposing cartilage is recommended to avoid long-term complications.

Laryngeal Burn

Description and Etiology

Laryngeal burn can occur from exposure to chemicals either ingested orally or by smell or intense heat (150 degrees Celsius or higher). Each anatomical part of the larynx can be exposed to the irritant(s) and as such the laryngeal structures may suffer from swelling, blister formation or impaired laryngeal function. The most important concern is impairment to breathing due to extreme swelling of the airway.

Perceptual Signs and Symptoms

The dysphonia associated with laryngeal burn can range from hoarseness to weak voice to complete aphonia depending on the extent of the trauma. Pain may be reported by the patient during swallowing as well as dysphagia.

Features of Visual Assessment

Endoscopic examination may reveal caustic burn typified by ulceration, granulation tissue formation and/or necrotic eschar (black colored wound). The surrounding supraglottic structures, including the epiglottis, aryepiglottic folds, arytenoids, and ventricular vocal folds will likely appear erythematous and edematous. The piriform sinuses may be narrowed.

Management

Treatment for laryngeal burn with milder conditions is time for tissue to heal. For more moderate to severe cases treatment would include analgesics and cold steam inhalation. Intubation may be necessary for those patients suffering from a compromised airway.

Ankylosis of the Cricoarytenoid Joint

Description and Etiology

Resulting from injury after a traumatic dislocation (potentially from intubation) or from disease such as inflammation (i.e., rheumatoid arthritis), anklyosis results in stiffness and/or fusion of the cricoarytenoid joint.

Perceptual Signs and Symptoms

The dysphonia associated with ankylosis of the cricoarytenoid joint is characterized by a breathy or rough voice quality with difficulty prolonging a sustained vowel. Pain may be reported by the patient during swallowing.

Features of Visual Assessment

Immobility of the affected arytenoids will be observed and the appearance of the resulting vocal fold immobility will mimic a vocal fold paralysis. It is important to diagnostically differentiate vocal fold paralysis from ankylosis of the cricoarytenoid joint. The otolaryngologist may use laryngeal-EMG and place a small needle through the cricothyroid membrane and determine if there is activity within the intrinsic laryngeal muscle (thyroarytenoid). This will help to determine if the immobility is due to paralysis or fixation. During the stroboscopic examination use of pseudophonatory behaviors (i.e., whispering or coughing) can help determine if there is movement of the cricoarytenoid joint versus immobilization isolated only during voice production.

Management

Ankylosis is treated medically by performing vocal fold mobilization under direct laryngoscopy. If the joint cannot be mobilized during this procedure a medialization of one or both vocal folds may be performed to increase glottic closure for tasks such as speech or cough (see Chapter 8).

Subglottic Stenosis

Description and Etiology

Subglottic stenosis is either congenital or acquired and is defined as any narrowing of the tissue below the level of the glottis. As the third most commonly occurring congenital condition, there is no predilection for sex or race. Subglottic stenosis is associated with a malformed cricoid cartilage occurring in utero causing a smaller than normal cricoid and the presence of a thickening of the underlying submucosal layer. Acquired subglottic stenosis is most commonly caused by prolonged intubation (Baker et al., 2006). Prolonged intubation is often required following preterm birth in infants who suffer from respiratory distress syndrome or during medical management of patients requiring long-term ventilation. Acquired stenosis can also occur with other forms of mechanical trauma. Although a narrowing can occur at any point along the upper or lower airway, subglottic stenosis is the most common (Figure 5–18).

Perceptual Signs and Symptoms

With congenital subglottic stenosis, inspiratory and expiratory stridor is present, a low pitch cough, dyspnea, and significant chest-wall movements and nasal flaring during breathing denoting the effort associated with ventilation may be present.

With acquired subglottic stenosis all of the same symptoms can exist with the addition of an abnormal speaking voice characterized by hoarseness and/or breathiness. An associated vocal fold paralysis may exist if mechanical trauma was the cause of the stenosis.

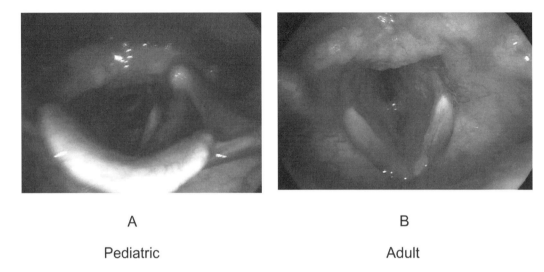

A

Pediatric

B

Adult

Figure 5–18. A. Pediatric subglottic stenosis secondary to intubation trauma. **B.** Subglottic stenosis in an adult female with sarcoidosis. Courtesy of Ear, Nose & Throat Surgical Associates, Winterpark, Florida.

Features of Visual Assessment

Due to the narrowness of the airway, there will be times when a complete view of the larynx is not possible with indirect laryngoscopy. Direct laryngoscopy then under anesthesia will be necessary to view the airway space and define the nature and extent of the stenosis. Myer, O'Connor, & Cotton (1994) developed a classification scheme for grading the degree of the stenosis based on the diameter of the lumen obstructed.

- *Grade I:* Obstruction of 0 to 50% of the lumen obstruction
- *Grade II:* Obstruction of 51 to 70% of the lumen
- *Grade III:* Obstruction of 71 to 99% of the lumen
- *Grade IV:* Obstruction of 100% of the lumen (i.e., no detectable lumen)

Management

Advances in surgical management of upper airway disorders have reduced the need for a tracheotomy in many patients (Bath et al., 1999; Myer & Hartley, 2000). In fact, decannulation (removal of tracheotomy tube) rates following airway reconstruction procedures in those with subglottic stenosis are approximately 80 to 95% (Monnier, Lang, & Savary, 2003; Rutter, Hartley, & Cotton, 2001). In less severe cases of subglottic stenosis, a reconstruction procedure called a laryngotracheoplasty is performed that involves the placement of an anterior and/or posterior costal cartilage graft in the cricoid lamina in order to increase the dimensions of the cricoid ring. In more severe cases of stenosis, a cricotracheal resection is completed which involves removal of the anterior half of the cricoid lamina as well as the first several tracheal rings. The two cut ends of the airway are then brought back together. Successful decannulation rates are reported to be as high as 80 to 90% following laryngotracheoplasty and as high as 95% following cricotracheal resection (Rutter et al., 2001). Restenosis of the subglottis may require additional surgical reconstruction, thus increasing the risk for further complications.

A clinical trial for behavioral management of subglottal stenosis in children is currently underway testing the outcomes of an inspiratory muscle strength training program for relieving dyspnea at Miami University of Ohio.

Laryngomalacia

Diagnosis and Etiology

The most common cause of inspiratory stridor in infancy is laryngomalacia, a congenital laryngeal condition of unknown etiology. Some proposed causes of laryngomalacia are neurologic hypotonia (low muscle tone) and laryngeal malformation during development. The symptoms associated with laryngomalacia are due to airway obstruction, as the laryngeal cartilages are susceptible to collapse (floppy) during the inspiratory phase of breathing. Diagnosis of laryngomalacia is by clinical manifestation of inspiratory stridor, evidence of immature laryngeal cartilages characterized by a floppy epiglottis, large aryepiglottic folds, which may occlude the glottis during inspiration, and large arytenoids process. If the cartilages are very soft the entire larynx may be seen to collapse during inspiration (Kay & Goldsmith, 2006).

Perceptual Signs and Symptoms

The predominant perceptual sign of laryngomalacia is intermittent inspiratory stridor which starts just after a few days or weeks following birth. The degree of stridor increases as the depth and rate of breathing is increased.

Features of Visual Assessment

During flexible fiberoptic laryngoscopy, collapse of laryngeal cartilages may be seen on inspiration, particularly during deep inspiration. The structures blow out again during expiration. There may be evidence of enlarged or floppy arytenoid cartilages, redundant arytenoid mucosa, short aryepiglottic folds, and an omega-shaped or elongated epiglottis.

Management

Aryepiglottic fold incision and CO_2 laser supraglottoplasty (surgical division of aryepiglottic folds) are needed in about 10 to 20% of cases of laryngomalacia. Most infants do not require treatment as laryngomalacia resolves with maturation. Less than 1% require a tracheotomy due to airway compromise (Benjamin, 1998).

When indications for surgery appear, such as severe stridor and airway obstruction, supraglottoplasty and surgical correction can be very effective for complicated cases and drastically reduce the need for tracheotomy (Olney et al., 1999). Treatment of esophageal reflux disease, and treatment of upper respiratory infections and any other associated illnesses, such as heart or lung disease or neurologic disease, are also recommended to ensure a positive outcome.

Laryngeal Cleft

Description and Etiology

Congenital laryngeal cleft is an extremely rare condition (1 in 20,000 births, Rabhar et al., 2006) of the cricoid cartilage, posteriorly resulting in a mucosal fold forming, which narrows the airway (Kleinsasser, 1990). More common in boys than girls, laryngeal cleft may be related to an autosomal dominant pattern of inheritance. Microlaryngoscopy is used to diagnose laryngeal cleft. Benjamin and Inglis (1989) presented a classification system "in which four types of cleft were described. Type 1 is a supraglottic interarytenoid defect that extends inferiorly no further than the level of the true vocal folds. In type 2, the cricoid lamina is partially involved, with extension of the cleft below the level of the true vocal folds. Type 3 is a total cricoid cleft that extends completely through the cricoid cartilage with or without further extension into the cervical trachea; and type 4 extends into the posterior wall of the thoracic trachea and may extend as far as the carina" (Rahbar, 2006, p. 1338).

Perceptual Signs and Symptoms

Due to the narrowing of the airway, inspiratory and expiratory stridor will likely be present. Complaints of dyspnea will occur in the more mild cases with severe aspiration, major respiratory distress and feeding difficulties existing in the more severe cases (Rahbar et al., 2006).

Features of Visual Assessment

See types of laryngeal clefts above.

Management

Management of laryngeal cleft is primarily surgical. Surgical procedures involve open reconstruction with or without interposition graft. Treatment following surgery may be for potential dysphagia and use of medications to reduce gastroesophogeal reflux and its irritation (Kleinsasser, 1990).

Vascular Lesions

Varix and Ecstasia

Description and Etiology

Originating in the superficial layer of the lamina propria, varices and ectasias area direct result of phonotrauma (Zeitels, 2006), and occur predominantly at the midmembranous portion of the vocal fold (Hochman, Sataloff, Hillman, & Zeitels, 1999) and are particularly related to high-pressure phonatory events like shouting and oversinging. More prevalent in women than men, their susceptibility may be related to the female hormonal cycle (Figure 5–19).

Perceptual Signs and Symptoms

Some patients presenting with a vocal fold varix or ecstasia have no perceptually abnormal phonatory symptoms. Others present

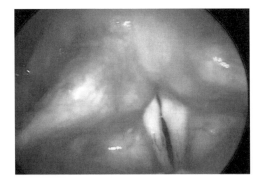
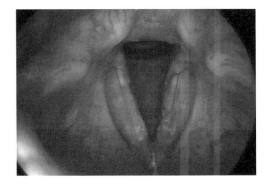

A   B

Figure 5–19. A. Right, superior surface varices. **B.** Prominent posterior, bilateral varices. Courtesy of The Ear, Nose & Throat Surgical Associates, Winter Park, Florida.

with a dysphonia characterized by a loss of vocal range, particularly in the higher frequencies and some hoarseness.

Features of Visual Assessment

A varix is a superficial, prominent vein that is enlarged and dilated. Ectasias are distinguished by a coalescent (fused) hemangiomatous (lesioning of the blood vessel) appearance (Schweinfurth, 2006). Reduced mucosal wave due to increased vocal fold stiffness is most often seen on the affected vocal fold.

Management

Voice rest is recommended until any blood, from a hemorrhage or bleed into the tissue, is reabsorbed. A program of vocal hygiene should be followed as well during the period of vocal rest. If surgery is necessary, cold instrument dissection is considered ideal in comparison to the CO_2 laser (Zeitels et al., 2006).

Vocal Fold Hemorrhage

Description and Etiology

Vocal fold hemorrhage is damage to the vocal fold tissues as a result of exposure to blood. The source of the bleeding is the network of extremely small and delicate blood vessels which traverse the various tissue layers of the vocal folds. When the superficial layer of the lamina propria is affected the ensuing voice effects can be devastating and include anything from dysphonia to complete *aphonia*, or absence of voice. The factor most commonly implicated in cases of vocal fold hemorrhage is phonotrauma or traumatic injury to the vocal folds themselves (Smith, Praneetvatakul, & Sataloff, 2005). This trauma can occur during surgical or medical procedures that involve some contact with the vocal folds as well as prolonged levels of high intensity voice use such as that frequently observed in professional voice users (Cotter, Avidano, Crary, Cassisi, & Gorham, 1995; Franco & Andrus, 2007). Excessive crying has also been observed as a potential cause of vocal fold hemorrhage (Murry & Rosen, 2000). The presence of microvascular lesions, including varices or capillary ectasias, may be indicative of past trauma to the vocal fold tissues and may increase the risk for vocal fold hemorrhage (Postma, Courey, & Ossoff, 1998). Use of anticoagulant (blood thinner) medications such as Coumadin or aspirin may also increase the risk for vocal fold hemorrhage as these medications reduce the ability of the blood to clot (Neely & Rosen, 2000) (Figure 5–20).

Perceptual Signs and Symptoms

Individuals with an acute vocal fold hemorrhage will typically present with hoarseness. The severity of this hoarseness can range anywhere from very minimal/mild to complete aphonia or loss of voice (Sataloff, Hawkshaw, Rosen, & Spiegel, 1996).

Features of Visual Assessment

Acute hemorrhage will typically present as an area of patchy redness on the vocal fold surface. Laryngostroboscopy may reveal impaired

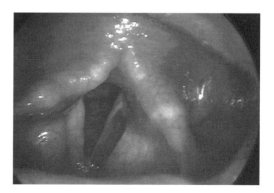

Figure 5–20. Right true vocal fold hemorrhage. Courtesy of The Ear, Nose & Throat Surgical Associates, Winter Park, Florida.

vibratory motion of the affected fold characterized by increased vocal fold mass and stiffness, both of which may contribute to reduced vibratory amplitude and reduced mucosal wave on the affected fold (Postma et al., 1998).

Management

Phonosurgical excision of microvascular lesions may prevent a vocal fold hemorrhage from occurring (Hochman, Sataloff, Hillman, & Zeitels, 1999). In the acute phase, meaning when the vocal fold is in the process of hemorrhaging, management typically consists of complete and total voice rest in order to eliminate mechanical forces against the vocal folds and allow the tissues time to heal. Once the hemorrhage has healed, residual dysphonia (brought about by scar tissue that remains following the hemorrhage) can be treated through a variety of augmentative procedures including injection of fat or collagen into the vocal fold to restore vibratory capacities (Ford, Staskowski, & Bless, 1995; Sataloff, Spiegel, Hawk-Shaw, Rosen, & Heuer, 1997).

Functional Voice Disorders

Puberphonia

Description and Etiology

Adolescent males who should have experienced a voice change with puberty may suffer from seemingly maladjusted growth of the larynx which results in maintenance of a high-pitched voice. Also termed mutational falsetto, pubescent falsetto, incomplete maturation, and persistent falsetto (among other terms), puberphonia has significant psychosocial repercussions for the male patient who is not past puberty. Several causes of puberphonia have been proposed with most including a psychological basis to the process

such as difficulty with acceptance of the new male voice, social immaturity, and male identity problems. Some physical reasons include presence of a hearing impairment, immature laryngeal maturation, and poor neuromuscular coordination.

Perceptual Signs and Symptoms

The pitch of the voice is higher than it should be for a postadolescent male. The voice quality may also be breathy and of a low vocal loudness.

Features of Visual Assessment

Indirect laryngoscopy commonly reveals normal male adult laryngeal size yet laryngeal function via laryngostroboscopy may reveal incomplete glottal closure, increased vocal fold stiffness, and decreased vibratory amplitude which are similar laryngeal function characteristics to high pitch phonation. In some cases, laryngeal hyperfunction, evidenced by high laryngeal position and ventricular fold compression, may exist.

Management

In the absence of a physiologic cause, such as endocrine disorder and/or a neurologic condition, management of puberphonia is typically behavioral, incorporating voice therapy techniques to reduce the higher than normal vocal pitch. Techniques can include biofeedback using the computerized software, such as the Kay Pentax Visi-Pitch, manual laryngeal massage therapy (see Chapter 7), and other relaxation techniques to help reduce muscle tension (Prater & Swift, 1984). Pau and Murty, (2001) described a case (2001) where surgical correction was used in attempt to remediate puberphonia in a 24-year-old male whereby the hyoid bone was lowered with sutures to the cricoid to reduce the cricohyoid space. The outcome of this procedure on swallow function was not discussed and raises question on the effects of the procedure on hyoid bone mobility for swallow.

Ventricular Phonation

Description and Etiology

Ventricular phonation is defined as use of the false or ventricular folds during voicing instead of, or along with, the true vocal folds. Long ago, ventricular phonation was attributed to central neurogenic causes (Jackson & Jackson, 1935). Today, two commonly occurring conditions appear to be associated with ventricular phonation: accompanying severe extrinsic laryngeal muscle tension or in the case of severe true vocal fold dysfunction (i.e., vocal fold paralysis, congenital true vocal fold anomaly) as a reliable, compensatory technique (Maryn, DeBodt, & Van Cauwenberge, 2003; Sataloff, 1997) (Figure 5–21).

Perceptual Signs and Symptoms

Due to more primitive make-up of the ventricular fold tissue, perceptually the voice sounds low pitched, with a reduction in vocal range, loudness, and pitch variability. Roughness and hoarseness are the predominant perceptual features (Maryn et al., 2003). Vocal fatigue, globus sensation, and pain in the ears may also be complaints expressed by patients.

Features of Visual Assessment

The primary visual feature is a relaxed "healthy" looking larynx on abduction yet abnormal adduction and vibration of the ventricular folds during voicing. If the ventricular folds have grown in size due to use (hypertrophy), it may be difficult to view the true vocal folds even during relaxed breathing.

Management

In order to determine the best management course for ventricular phonation a first step is to identify the function and capability of the true vocal folds. If the true vocal folds are unable to produce voice and their function cannot be intervened with, then ventricular fold phonation may serve as a suitable alternative source of voice production. If it is determined that the true vocal folds are capable of

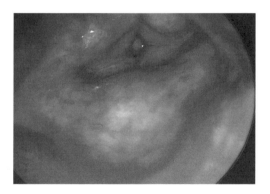

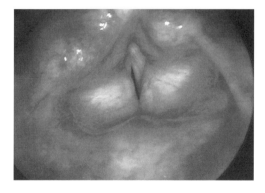

A   B

Figure 5–21. **A**. Severe anteroposterior compression, result was ventricular phonation. **B**. Hypertrophy of the ventricular folds with severe lateral compression. Courtesy of The Ear, Nose & Throat Surgical Associates, Winter Park, Florida.

meeting vocal demands, a variety of treatments might be tried to reduce ventricular phonation including voice therapy (i.e., inspiratory phonation, relaxation, EMG biofeedback, and labial contstriction technique), psychotherapy, pharmacological therapy (Botox injection), and surgical interventions (excision or laser surgery). According to Maryn et al. (2003), the combination of fiberoptic visual feedback and inspiratory phonation may be one of the best first steps to eliminate the behavior without more invasive techniques.

Muscle Tension Dysphonia (MTD)

Description and Etiology

Persons exhibiting MTD can show visible signs of increased muscle activity in the head and neck. Their responses on case history forms often relate to the occurrence(s) of stress, anxiety, depression, high vocal demand, issues with time management accompanying general complaints of being overloaded both physically and emotionally. Dietrich, Verdolini Abbott, Gartner-Schmidt, and Rosen (2008) cited depression and stress as two predominant features in a cohort of new patients with MTD seeking care at their voice clinic.

Although several mechanistic causes have been postulated about MTD, it is clear that in most cases, one single cause cannot be attributed to its onset or maintenance. For example, although it is apparent that the extrinsic muscles of the larynx are hypercontracted, and that the muscle activity controlling laryngeal adduction, abduction, and voicing seem uncoordinated, there is no specific neurologic or anatomic reason for these symptoms during voice production. Other conditions associated with MTD include laryngopharyngeal reflux. According to Altman, Atkinson, and Lazarus (2005) significant factors in their patient history included: excessive amounts of voice

use in 63%, gastroesophageal reflux in 49%, excessive loudness demands and voice use in 23%, and high stress levels in 18%, These results came from their chart review of over 150 patients diagnosed with MTD.

Perceptual Signs and Symptoms

The voice quality associated with MTD is most commonly strained and of high pitch. In some cases when the vocal fold tension appears to be very high, the vocal folds may never adduct causing a breathiness or weakness to the sound quality.

Features of Visual Assessment

MTD may take the form of excessive glottic and supraglottic medial contraction; anterior-posterior contraction of the supraglottal musculature including the arytenoids, epiglottis, and false vocal folds, decreased vibratory amplitude of the vocal folds, or psychogenic bowing of the vocal folds (Altman et al., 2005; Lee & Son, 2005). Glottic gaps range from anterior chink to incomplete closure along the entire membranous vocal fold length (Hirano & Bless, 1993).

Management

Voice therapy is the most common treatment for MTD and techniques have ranged from biofeedback, laryngeal relaxation techniques, resonant voice therapy, manual circumlaryngeal massage, and the Accent Method (see Chapter 7). Careful interpretation is necessary as many of the outcomes from these studies of therapy techniques are from one or two subjects or relatively small sample sizes ($N<10$). Yet the outcomes of these reports provide a window within which to evaluate their potential use for the remediation of MTD.

One technique popularized for treatment of MTD is circumlaryngeal massage.

The technique of manual laryngeal massage was first discussed by Aronson (1990) and involved delicate manipulation of the larynx. It is described in Chapter 7 in more detail but basically involves applying gentle pressure to the area of the hyoid bone, with continued manipulation of the thyrohyoid space and the posterior aspect of the thyroid cartilage with the goal of normalizing the laryngeal posture.

Following the use of circumlaryngeal massage as a treatment modality, Roy and Leeper (1993) indicated positive improvements in voice, both perceptually and acoustically. More detail about outcomes with circumlaryngeal massage were provided by Roy, Ford, & Bless (1996). More recently, Roy, Nissen, Dromey & Sapir (2009) manual circulmlaryngeal massage was shown to extend to creating positive improvements in vocal tract dynamics most likely related to the lowering of the larynx.

Transgender/Transsexual Voice Transition

Description and Etiology

Individuals seeking to move away from the gender role assigned to them at birth may seek voice treatment to assist in producing a voice pitch which is in agreement with their new gender identity. The transition may be from female to male (referred to as voice masculinization), or from male to female (referred to as feminization).

Perceptual Signs and Symptoms

Perceptually, the pitch of the person transitioning from female to male will be too high for the new gender identity and vice versa for the person transitioning from male to female. While pitch is not the single variable to work on during voice therapy with the person tran-

sitioning, it is a primary variable in gender identification. Other variables include resonance, intonation, rate, and vocal intensity (Adler, 2006).

Features of Visual Assessment

Laryngoscopic features are within normal limits for the gender assigned at birth.

Management

There are two major categories of intervention to accomplish a change in the voice for either masculinization or feminization. These include voice therapy and surgical intervention. The details of both of these are beyond the scope of this chapter, so the reader is referred to Adler, Hirsch, and Mordaunt (2006). Briefly, the voice therapy management focuses on reducing the fundamental frequency/pitch for those seeking masculinization and increasing the fundamental frequency for those seeking feminization. The strategies for accomplishing this elevation or reduction include biofeedback, the use of a hierarchical approach starting with vowel production and progressing to conversational speech, the use of homework exercises, and real-world tasks to help achieve generalization of the therapeutic target (Adler, 2006). Modification of loudness level may also be achieved with biofeedback techniques and/or Vocal Function Exercises. Resonance might best be achieved with frontal focus therapy or the use of the Lessac Madsen Resonant Voice Therapy Program (see Chapter 7).

Conversion Aphonia

Description and Etiology

Conversion aphonia is thought to relate to a manifestation of stress, depression, or anxiety (Bhatia & Vaid, 2000; Willinger, Volkl-

Kernstock, & Aschauer, 2005). It is considered a psychogenic voice disorder that tends to emerge very quickly and like other types of conversion disorders, conversion aphonia can be associated with a traumatic event associated with severe stress. With conversion aphonia there is no evidence of a physical or neurologic cause and the patient is not malingering (faking it) to attract attention, money, or some other form of material gain. Conversion aphonia has significant functional and social impact on the patient and the patient's family/spouse/partner.

Perceptual Signs and Symptoms

With conversion aphonia there is either no voice on attempted phonation or if voicing does emerge it is often high pitched and very strained. Often, pain in the neck area is reported by the patient and extrinsic laryngeal muscle tightness is exhibited by the patient when attempting to phonate.

Features of Visual Assessment

Nonphonatory movements of the vocal folds are most commonly normal. That is, vocal fold abduction on inspiration and vocal fold adduction on cough or throat clearing indicates normal mobility. When voicing is attempted, the vocal fold movement becomes irregular and the vocal folds are not able to adduct enough to produce a sufficient vibratory cycle.

Management

First, a physical examination needs to be completed to rule out physical and/or neurological cause to the voice disorder. If the results of these assessments are negative, then psychiatric treatment may be necessary, in isolation or simultaneous with voice therapy. In many cases, patients will respond quickly to the voice therapy, but if the issues are significant the symptoms may re-emerge if the stress cannot be resolved. Butcher recommends the use of cognitive-behavioral therapy in these cases (Butcher, 1995). In more serious cases, hypnosis may be a treatment consideration and/or the use of antidepressants (see Chapter 11).

Idiopathic

Paradoxic Vocal Fold Dysfunction

Description and Etiology

Paradoxic vocal fold movement (PVFM) is a complex disorder where vocal fold adduction occurs on inspiration. The result is obstruction of the airway. A synonymous descriptor for paradoxic vocal fold motion (PVFM) with dysphonia is episodic paroxysmal laryngospasm (EPL). Although PVFM describes intrinsic laryngeal abnormal activity, EPL describes the laryngeal dysfunction as episodic. It is paroxysmal in that a sudden attack or intensification of symptoms recurs periodically. Once the episode of EPL has started during inspiration, the forceful vocal fold adduction/spasm, sometimes likened to a "cramp of the larynx," may carry over transiently into the expiratory phase of breathing. PVFM/EPL can masquerade as asthma, vocal fold paralysis, laryngeal edema, voice disorder with diminished phonatory intensity during a sudden attack, and anatomic airway obstruction, for example, stenosing lesions of the upper airways. The intermittent inspiratory/respiratory distress of EPL may precipitate emergency clinical maneuvers, resulting in unnecessary endotracheal intubation, cardiopulmonary resuscitation (CPR), or tracheostomy (Andrianopoulos, Gallivan, & Gallivan, 1999; Gallivan, Hoffman, & Gallivan, 1996). PVFM/EPL has also been associated with chronic cough (Murry, Tabaee, & Aviv, 2004).

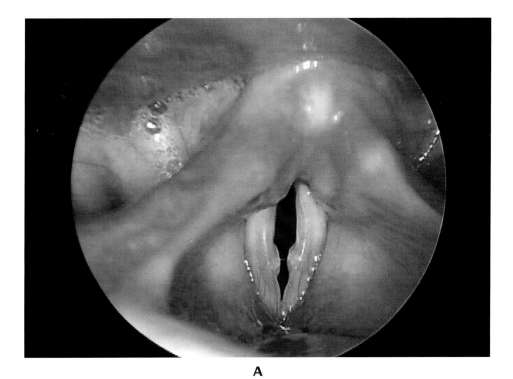

Plate 1. **A.** Vocal nodules in the abducted position. **B.** Vocal nodules in the adducted position during phonation.

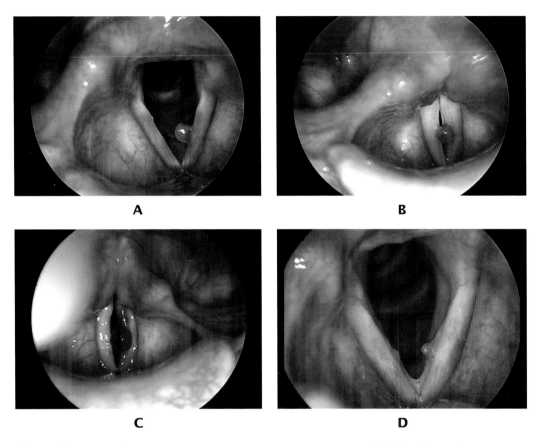

Plate 2. A. Vocal fold polyp in the abducted position. **B.** Vocal fold polyp in the adducted position during phonation. **C.** Hemorrhagic polyp. **D.** Left true vocal fold polyp, right true vocal fold reactive nodule, and anterior microweb.

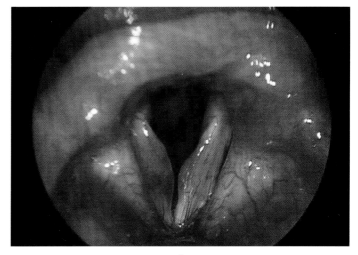

A

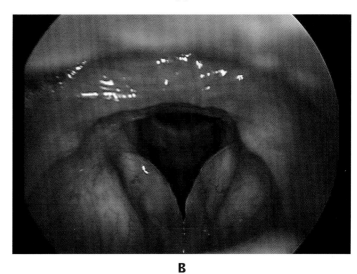

Plate 3. **A** and **B.** Reinke's edema. **C.** Severe Reinke's edema with leukoplakia and hyperkeratosis vocal folds positioned during inspiration.

B

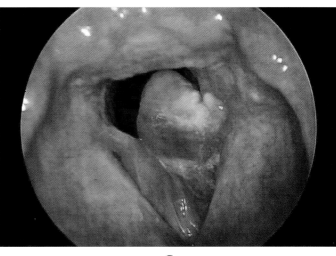

C

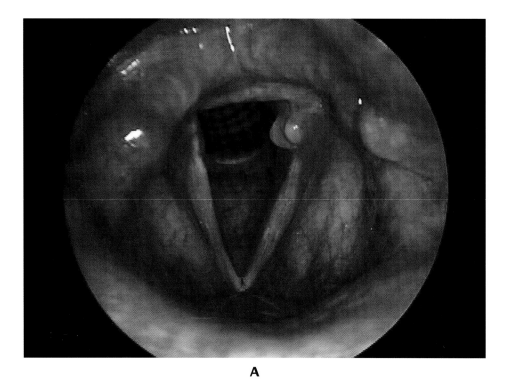

A

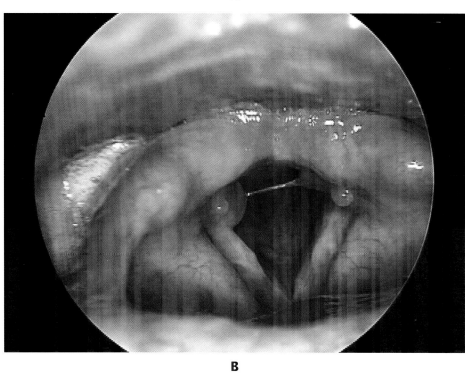

B

Plate 4. **A.** Unilateral granuloma. **B.** Bilateral granuloma.

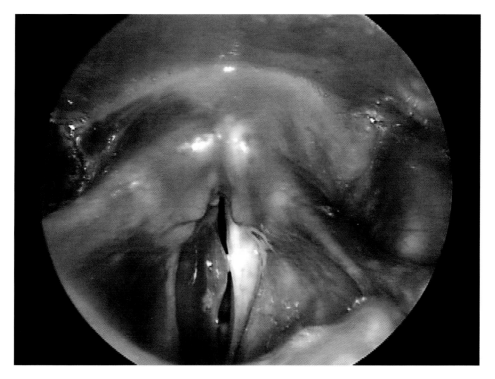

Plate 5. Unilateral vocal fold hemorrhage.

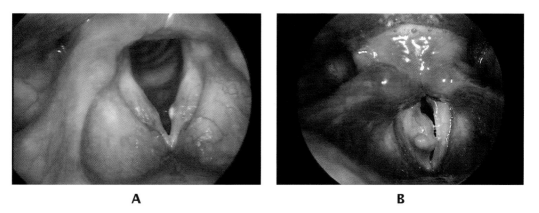

A   **B**

Plate 6. **A.** Left true vocal fold cyst with reactive edema and vascular change on the right true vocal fold. **B.** Right true vocal fold multilobed cyst.

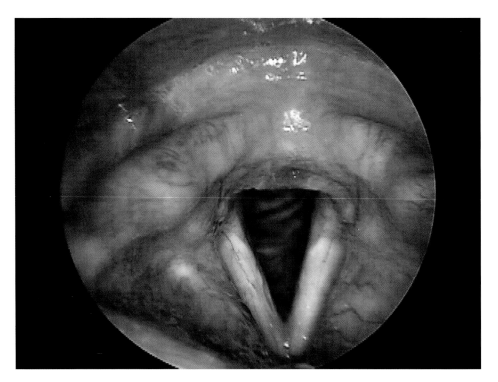

Plate 7. Right true vocal fold sulcus.

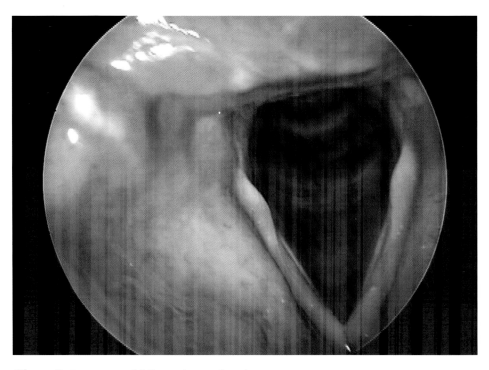

Plate 8. Bowing and bilateral pseudosulcus.

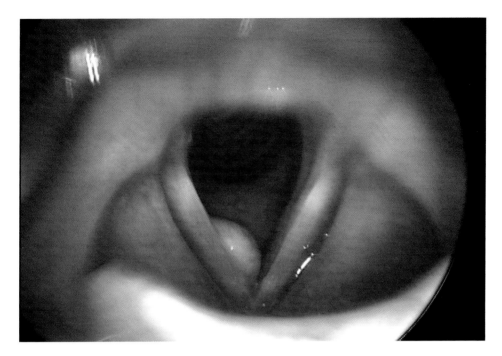

Plate 9. Right true vocal fold granular cell tumor.

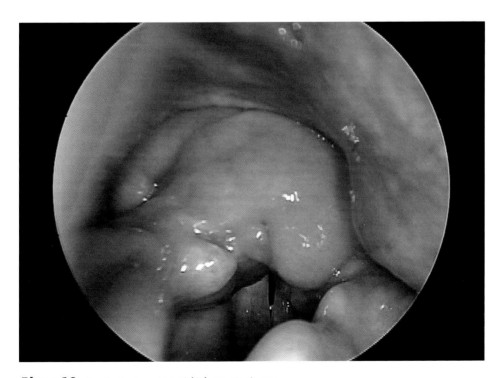

Plate 10. Posterior arytenoids hemangioma.

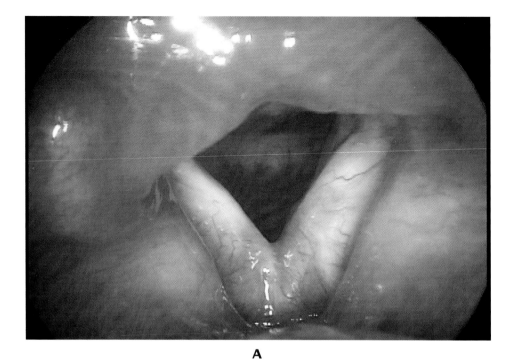

A

B

Plate 11. **A.** Anterior web. **B.** Pediatric anterior web and subglottic stenosis.

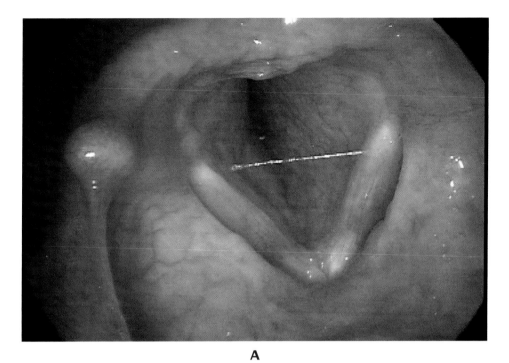

A

B

Plate 12. **A.** Subglottic stenosis. **B.** Subglottic stenosis from unknown etiology.

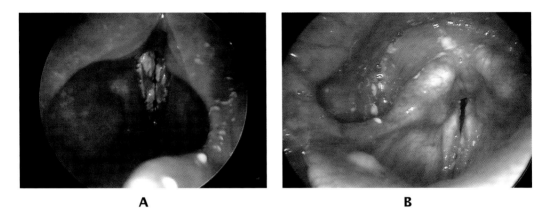

Plate 13. A. Candidia of the true vocal folds, aryepiglottic fold and supraglottic tissue. **B.** Candidia of the true vocal fold, right pyriform sinus and posterior arytenoids area.

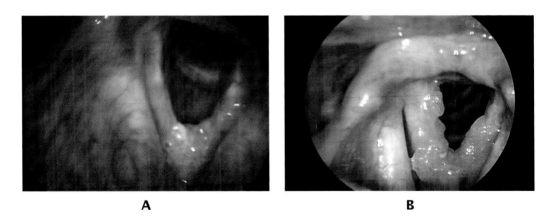

Plate 14. Papilloma.

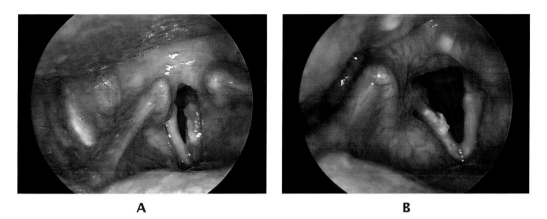

A   B

Plate 15. **A.** Leukoplakia on the left true vocal fold. **B.** Leukoplakia and hyperkeratosis of the right true vocal fold.

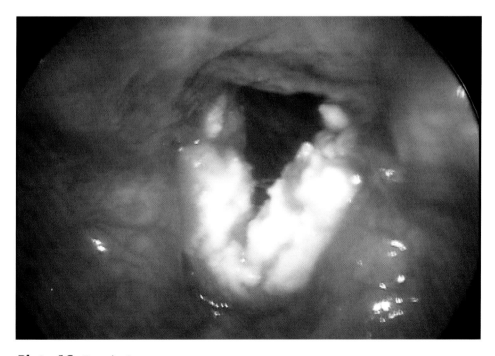

Plate 16. Dysplasia.

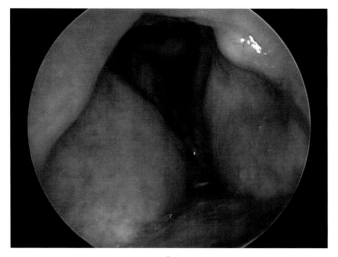

A

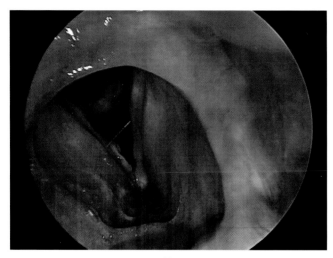

B

Plate 17. **A.** Right true vocal fold cancer. **B.** Right true vocal fold cancer (reoccurrence of Plate 17A, 10 months later). **C.** Supraglottic cancer.

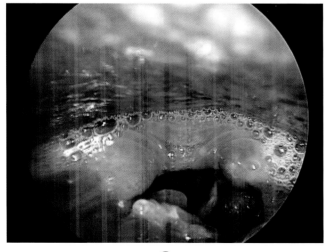

C

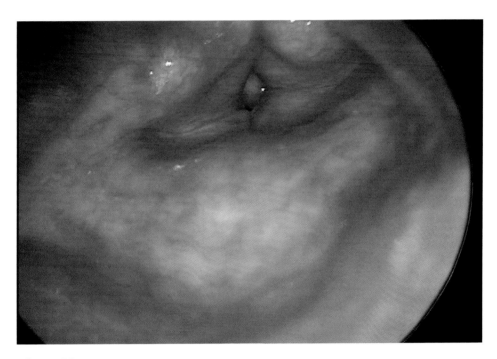

Plate 18. Ventricular compression.

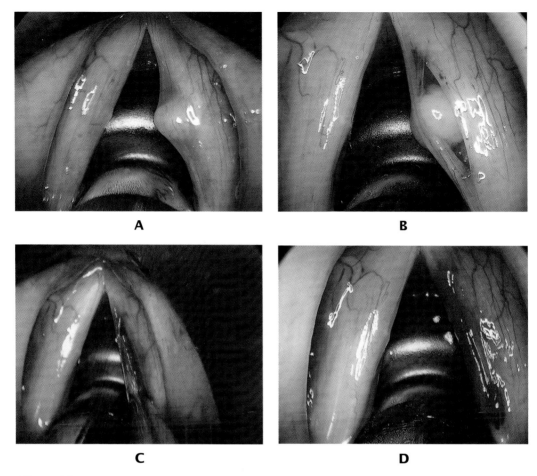

A   B

C   D

Plate 19. Vocal cyst removed by microflap approach. Courtesy of The Ear Nose Throat and Plastic Surgery Associates, Winter Park, Florida.

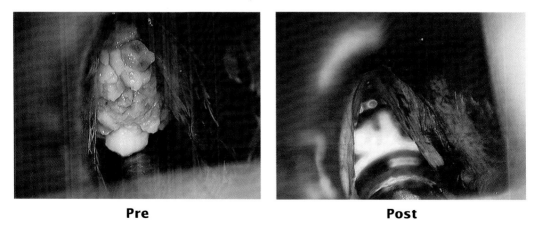

Pre   **Post**

Plate 20. Surgical removal of laryngeal papilloma by microdebrider approaches. Courtesy of The Ear Nose Throat and Plastic Surgery Associates, Winter Park, Florida.

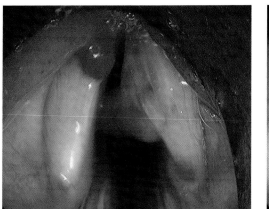

Plate 21

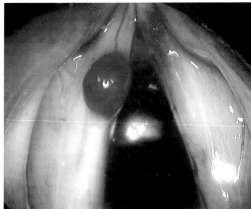

Plate 22

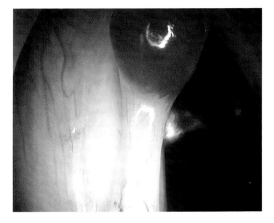

Plate 23

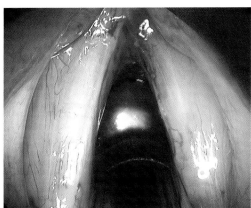

Plate 24

Plates 21 through 24 show surgical removal of left hemorrhagic polyp based within a mucosal band isolated by an underlying sulcus vocalis. Courtesy of The Ear Nose Throat and Plastic Surgery Associates, Winter Park, Florida.

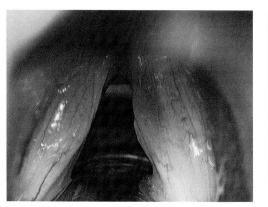
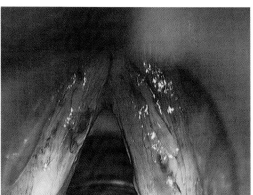

Pre   **Post**

Plate 25. Microflap dissection of moderate polypoid degeneration. Courtesy of The Ear Nose Throat and Plastic Surgery Associates, Winter Park, Florida.

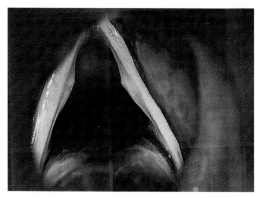
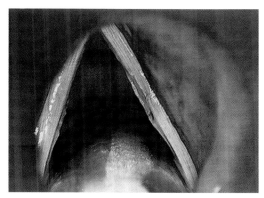

Pre   **Post**

Plate 26. Pre- and postsurgical removal of bilateral vocal fold nodules. Courtesy of The Ear Nose Throat and Plastic Surgery Associates, Winter Park, Florida.

Perceptual Signs and Symptoms

Perceptual signs and symptoms include evidence of audible airway obstruction/limitation causing inspiratory and/or expiratory stridor/wheezing, dyspnea, choking episodes, muscle tightness (neck, chest, generalized), intermittent or chronic cough, aphonia, dysphonia, hoarseness, strained-strangled voice, breathy voice, weak voice, and/or diplophonia. Other symptoms may incude dysphagia, heartburn, or globus sensation.

Features of Visual Assessment

During a nonepisodic EPL/PVFM event the laryngeal anatomy and function is normal. During an event, inspiratory adduction of the anterior two-thirds of the vocal folds with a posterior glottal gap is identified (Morris, Deal, Bean, Grbach, & Morgan (1999).

Management

Andrianopoulos et al. (1999) described a three-phase management approach to EPL/PVFM. Phase I involves the differential diagnosis process and recommends developing an inventory of the following variables to assist in establishing probable cause and effect sequelae: (a) psychological-emotional issues, (b) phonotraumatic behaviors, (c) medical factors, (d) muscle tension patterns, (e) triggers and exacerbating stimuli, and (f) phonatory and respiratory system involvement. Phase II uses established principles and guidelines of symptomatic-behavioral techniques and psychoeducational models within the Neurolinguistic Programming (NLP) model (e.g., Andrianopoulos et al., 1999; Duffy, 1995; Rosen & Sataloff, 1997). Phase III emphasizes carryover of optimal function. The patient should be trained to employ effective strategies to manage emotional stressors, physiological and sensory triggers that exac-erbate upper airway obstruction, muscle tension patterns, and laryngospastic symptoms. In Phase III, self-awareness and independence in controlling exacerbating stimuli and aberrant respiratory and phonatory behaviors are also encouraged.

Pitchenik in 1991 first described the panting maneuver as another respiratory-based behavioral treatment. Improvement of symptoms and the measures of pulmonary function testing were reported with this maneuver. According to the author, when panting at functional residual capacity, there is significantly greater EMG activity in the posterior cricoarytenoid muscle and a sustained increase in the width of the glottis compared to peak values of these measurements made during tidal breathing. Other treatments emphasizing the respiratory mechanism have been proposed, including Sperfeld et al.'s) suggestion for a rapid change to an upright position and slowed breathing as maneuvers to shorten the duration of laryngospasm.

Respiratory training has also been used including abdominal breathing with nasal inhalations and slow and prolonged exhalations, nasal inhalation and exhalation through rounded and pursed lips, inhalation and exhalation through pursed lips, and inhalation and exhalation while prolonging the /s/ sibilant (Blager, 1995). Vocal hygiene protocols should also be implemented.

Autoimmune

Systemic Lupus Erythematosus

Description and Etiology

Symptoms of lupus vary widely from individual to individual. predominantly in women of child bearing age. The symptoms are due to a hyperactivity of the immune system that can result in inflammation, damage to joints, skin, kidneys, blood, the heart, and lungs. Those with lupus cannot fight against viruses and bacteria and with lupus the immune system can't tell the difference between healthy tissue and unhealthy tissue. As a result the normal antibodies in the body start attacking the healthy tissue causing swelling, pain and damage to the tissue. Laryngeal abnormalities can include arthritis, inflammation with the most common sites involving the glottis and cricoarytenoid joints (Smith & Ferguson. 1976; Teitel, MacKenzie, & Stern, 1992).

Perceptual Signs and Symptoms

Perceptual signs and symptoms include hoarseness, throat pain, and/or dyspnea.

Management

Treatment may include nonsteroidal anti-inflammatory drugs, topical and systemic corticosteroids, antimalarial agents, and low-dose methotrexate. In severe cases, immunosuppressive agents, such as azathioprine and cyclophosphamide, can be used.

Rheumotoid Arthritis

Description and Etiology

Rheumotoid arthritis is a relatively common autoimmune disease which involves inflammation of the synovial tissue. Women are 2 to 3 times more likely to develop the disease. Laryngeal involvement is reported in 25 to 30% of cases.

Perceptual Signs and Symptoms

Perceptual signs and symptoms include globus sensation, hoarseness, dyspnea, stridor, or dysphagia.

Features of Visual Assessment

During a visual examination the vocal fold mucosa often looks normal. In a more chronic state of rheumatoid arthritis the cricoarytenoid may be anklosed and deformed. In more severe cases, nodules may appear on the vocal folds, referred to as rheumatoid nodules.

Management

Systemic treatment includes corticosteroids or other immunosuppressive agents. If the airway is compromised then a tracheotomy is performed and in more milder cases voice treatment may be beneficial with techniques focused on reduction in vocal fold inflammation. In cases where rheumatoid nodules are present phonosurgical excision is an option.

Sjogren's Syndrome

Description and Etiology

Sjögren's syndrome is an autoimmune disease characterized by dryness of the mouth and eyes. Autoimmune diseases feature the abnormal production of extra antibodies in the blood that are directed against various tissues of the body. There is no known cause but it is actively being studied (Theander & Jacobsson, 2008).

Perceptual Signs and Symptoms

Perceptual signs and symptoms include evidence hoarseness, and cough caused by thickening mucus.

Features of Visual Assessment

According to Belafski and Postma (2003), those with Sjögren's syndrome are prone to laryngopharyngeal reflux . Visual signs associated with reflux were previously covered.

Management

Treatment may include voice rest and/or guafenesin products to help thin mucus in the lower and upper airway to help relieve symptoms.

Fibromyalgia

Description and Etiology

Fibromyalgia is a disorder characterized by widespread musculoskeletal pain accompanied by fatigue, sleep, memory, and mood issues.

Perceptual Signs and Symptoms

Perceptual signs and symptoms may include hoarseness, pain on swallowing, and pain with voice.

Features of Visual Assessment

Limited information exists regarding the endoscopic or laryngostroboscopic findings associated with this disease.

Management

There is no cure for fibromyalgia. Some medications can help control symptoms such as Lyrica and Cymbalta. Exercise, relaxation, and stress-reduction measures are also typically recommended.

Scleroderma

Description and Etiology

Scleroderma is an autoimmune disease of the connective tissue featuring skin thickening, spontaneous scarring, blood vessel disease, varying degrees of inflammation, associated with an overactive immune system The occurrence of scleroderma of the larynx is rare.

The cause of scleroderma is not known.

Perceptual Signs and Symptoms

Perceptual signs and symptoms include some dysphonia and the possibility of submucosal vocal fold lesions (Sataloff, Spiegeal, & Rosen, 1996).

Features of Visual Assessment

Visual assessment can reveal an inflammation of the vocal fold mucosa and significantly decreased mucosal wave due to the presence of submucosal nodules (Sataloff et al., 1996).

Management

Microphonosurgical procedures are performed to resect the submucosal lesions if present.

Sarcoidosis

Description and Etiology

Sarcoidosis is a multisystemic, chronic disease of unknown cause that is characterized by the formation of immune granulomas in involved organs .It most commonly presents in African American women in the third through fifth decades of life. Some believe it is triggered by unidentified virus. The lungs and the lymphatic system are predominantly affected. The larynx is involved in 3 to 5% of cases, but more commonly in the supraglottic region. See Mrowka-Kata et al., 2010 for a thorough review.

Perceptual Signs and Symptoms

Perceptual signs and symptoms include evidence of dyspnea and dry cough with or without hoarseness. Sarcoidosis is rarely painful and may present with symptoms of airway obstruction.

Features of Visual Assessment

If present the supraglottal structures may appear swollen (epiglottis, aryepiglottic folds and ventricular folds). Laryngeal involvement is present in 0.5 to 1.4% of sarcoid cases. In very rare cases an isolated true vocal fold paralysis may occur. If present, symptoms invlude hoarseness, stridor, dysphagia, globus sensation, and cough.

Management

The clinical course of sarcoidosis varies from spontaneous resolution within 12 to 36 months to relentless progression and death. Systemic steroid therapy may be recommended. Tracheotomy may be performed to restore patent airway function.

Summary

Structural vocal fold pathologies vary in size and severity, creating various forms of dysphonia. Accurate identification of a structural voice disorders comes primarily from vocal fold imaging and examination. Some pathologic conditions require biopsy. Comprehensive evaluation of voice requires a sophisticated clinical skill set that is composed of intuitive and objective procedures. The accuracy of the clinical voice evaluation is critical in guiding the management decisions and the ultimate care of the patient's voice.

It is apparent that the impact of vocal fold pathology varies in severity creating management challenges for the voice care team. The next chapter describes vocal disorder/pathology stemming from neurologic causes,

followed by vocal rehabilitation strategies used to treat the dysphonia associated with these conditions.

References

Abramson, A. L., Shikowitz, V. M., Mullooly, B. M., Steinberg, C., Amell, A., & Rothstein, H. R. (2006). Clinical effects of photodynamic therapy on recurrent laryngeal papillomas. *Archives of Otolaryngology-Head and Neck Surgery, 118*(1), 1925–1931.

Adler, R. (2006). Transgender/transsexual: An understanding. In R. K. Adler, S. Hirsch, & M. Mordaunt (Eds.), *Voice and communication therapy for the transgender/transsexual client: A comprehensive clinical guide.* San Diego, CA: Plural.

Akif Kilic, M., Okur, E., Yildireim, I., & Guzelsoy, S. (2004). The prevalence of vocal fold nodules in school-age children. *International Journal of Pediatric Otorhinolaryngology, 68*(4), 409–412.

Altman, K. W., Atkinson, C., & Lazarus, C. (2005). Current and emerging concepts in muscle tension dysphonia: A 30-month review. *Journal of Voice, 19*(2), 261–267.

Andrianopoulos, M. V., Gallivan, G. J., & Gallivan, K. H. (1999). PVCM, PVCD, EPL, and irritable larynx syndrome: What are we talking about and how do we treat it? *Journal of Voice, 14,* 607–618.

Andrus, J. G., & Shapshay, S. M. (2006). Contemporary management of laryngeal papilloma in adults and children. *Otolaryngology Clinics of North America, 39*(1), 135–158.

Aronson, A. E. (1990). *Clinical voice disorders.* New York, NY: Thieme.

Avidano, M. A., & Singleton, G. T. (1995). Adjuvant drug strategies in the treatment of recurrent respiratory papillomatosis. *Otolaryngology-Head and Neck Surgery, 112*(2), 197–202.

Baker, S., Kelchner, L., Weinrich B., Lee L., Willging, P., Cotton, R., & Zur, K. (2006). Pediatric laryngotracheal stenosis and airway reconstruction: A review of voice outcomes, assessment, and treatment issues. *Journal of Voice, 20*(4), 631–641.

Ballenger, J. J., & Snow, J. B., Jr. (1996). *Otorhinolaryngology-Head and neck surgery* (15th ed.). Baltimore, MD: Williams & Wilkins.

Bath, A. P., Panarese, A., Thevasagayam, M., & Bull, P. D. (1999). Paediatric subglottic stenosis. *Clinical Otolaryngology and Allied Sciences, 24*(2), 117–121.

Behrman, A., Rutledge, J., Hembree, A., & Sheridan, S. (2008). Vocal hygiene education, voice production therapy, and the role of patient adherence: A treatment effectiveness study in women with phonotrauma. *Journal of Speech, Language, and Hearing Research, 51*(2), 350–366.

Belfasky, P. C., & Postma, G. N. (2003). The laryngeal and esophageal manifestations of Sjogren's syndrome. *Current Rheumotology Reports, 5*(4), 297–303.

Belafsky, P. C., & Postma, G. N. (2004). Vocal fold augmentation with calcium hydrolapatite. *Otolaryngology-Head and Neck Surgery, 131*(4), 351–354.

Belfasky, P. C., Postma, G. N., & Koufman, J. A. (2002). The association between laryngeal pseudosulcus and laryngopharyngeal ref lux. *Otolaryngology-Head and Neck Surgery, 126*(6), 649–652.

Benjamin, B. (1998). *Endolaryngeal surgery.* St. Louis, MO: Mosby.

Benjamin, B., & Inglis, A. (1989). Minor congenital laryngeal clefts. Diagnosis and classification. *Annals of Otology, Rhinology, and Laryngology, 98*(6), 417–420.

Berg, E. E., Hapner, E., Klein, A., & Johns, M. M. (2006). Voice therapy improves quality of life in age-related dysphonia: A case-control study. *Journal of Voice, 22*(1), 70–74.

Bergler, W., & Gotte, K. (2000). Current advances in the basic research and clinical management of juvenile—onset recurrent respiratory papillomatosis. *European Archives of Otorhinolaryngology, 257*, 263–269.

Bhatia, M. S., & Vaid, L. (2000). Hysterical aphonia—an analysis of 25 cases. *Indian Journal of Medical Sciences, 54*(8), 335–338.

Blager, F. B. (1995). Treatment of paradoxical vocal cord dysfunction. *Voice and Voice Disorders, SID3 Newsletter, 5*, 8–11.

Bloch, I., & Behrman, A., (2001). Quantitative analysis of videostroboscopic images in presbylarynges. *Laryngoscope, 111*(11, Pt. 1), 2022–2027.

Bluestone, C. D., & Stool, S. E. (1983). *Pediatric otolaryngology* (Vol. 2). Philadephia, PA: W. B. Saunders & Co.

Boone, D. R., McFarlane, S. C., & Von Berg, S. L. (2005). *Voice and voice therapy* (7th ed.). Boston, MA: Allyn and Bacon.

Bouchayer, M., Cornut, G., Witzig, E., Loire, R., Roch, J. B., & Bastian, R. W. (1985). Epidermoid cysts, sulci, and mucosal bridges of the true vocal cord: A report of 157 cases. *Laryngoscope, 95*(9), 1087–1094.

Butcher, P. (1995). Psychological processes in psychogenic voice disorder. *European Journal of Disordered Communication, 30*(4), 467–474.

Chiang, M. J., Fang, T. J., Li, H. Y., Chen, I. H., & Lee, K. F. (2004). Malignant granular cell tumor in larynx mimicking laryngeal carcinoma. *American Journal of Otlaryngology, 25*(4), 270–273.

Cho, K. J., Nam, I .C., Hwang, Y. S., Shim, M. R., Park, J. O., Cho, J. H., . . . Sun, D. I. (2011). Analysis of factors influencing voice quality and therapeutic approaches in vocal polyp patients. *European Archives of Otorhinolaryngology, 268*(9), 1321–1327

Coll, D. A., Rosen, C. A., Auborn, K., Potsic, W. P., & Bradlow, H. L. (1997). Treatment of recurrent respiratory papillomatosis with indole-3-carbinol. *American Journal of Otolaryngology, 18*(4), 283–285.

Colton, R. H., Casper, J. K., & Leonard, R. (2006). *Understanding voice problems: A physiological perspective for diagnosis and treatment* (3rd ed.). Baltimore, MD: Lippincott, Williams & Wilkins.

Corbitt, G., Zarod, A. P., Arrand, J. R., Longson, M., & Farrington, W. T. (1988). Human papillomavirus (HPV) genotypes associated with laryngeal papilloma. *Journal of Clinical Pathology, 41*(3), 284–288.

Cotran, R., Kumar, V., & Collins, T. (1999) *Robbins pathologic basis of disease* (6th ed.). London, UK: W. B. Saunders.

Cotter, C., Avidano, M., Crary, M., Cassisi, N., & Gorham, M. (1995). Laryngeal complications after type 1 thyroplasty. *Otolaryngology-Head and Neck Surgery, 113*(6), 671–673.

Coyle, S. M., Weinrich, B. D., & Stemple, J. C. (2001). Shifts in the prevalence of laryngeal pathology in a treatment seeking population. *Journal of Voice, 15*(3), 424–440.

Dietrich, M., Verdolini, Abbott, K., Gartner-Schmidt, J., & Rosen, C. A. (2006). The frequency of perceived stress, anxiety, and depression in patients with common pathologies affecting voice. *Journal of Voice, 22*(4), 472–488.

Dubeau, C. E. (2006). The aging lower urinary tract. *Journal of Urology, 175*(3 Pt. 2), S11–S15.

Duffy, J. R. (1995). *Motor speech disorders: Substrates, differential diagnosis, and management.* St. Louis, MO: Mosby.

Farrokhi, F., & Vaezi, M. F. (2007). Laryngeal disorders in patients with gastroesophageal reflux disease. *Minerva Gastroenterologica e Dietologica, 53*(2), 181–187.

Ford, C., Inagi, K., Khidr, A., Bless, D., & Gilchris, K. (1996) Sulcus vocalis: A rational analytical approach to diagnosis and management. *Annals of Otology, Rhinology, and Laryngology, 105*(3), 189–200.

Ford, C., Staskowski, P., & Bless, D. (1995). Autologous collagen vocal fold injection: A preliminary clinical study. *Laryngoscope, 105*(9 Pt. 1), 944–948.

Franco, R., & Andrus, J. (2007). Common diagnoses and treatments in professional voice users. *Otolaryngologic Clinics of North America, 40*(5), 1025–1061.

Gallivan, G. J., Hoffman, L., & Gallivan, K. H. (1996). Episodic paroxysmal laryngospasm: Voice and pulmonary assessment and management. *Journal of Voice, 10*, 93–105.

Gaynor, E. B. (1991). Otolaryngologic manifestations of gastroesophageal reflux. *American Journal of Gastroenterology, 86*(7), 801–808.

Giovanni, A., Chanteret, C., & Lagier, A. (2007). Sulcus vocalis: A review. *European Archives of Oto-rhino-laryngology, 264*(4), 337–344.

Gissmann, L., Diehl, V., Schultz-Coulon, H. J., & zur Hausen, H. (1982). Molecular cloning and characterization of human papilloma virus DNA derived from a laryngeal papilloma. *Journal of Virology, 44*(1), 393–400.

Golub, J. S., Chen, P. H., Otto, K. J., Hapner, E., & Johns, M. M. 3rd. (2006). Prevalence of perceived dysphonia in a geriatric population. *Journal of American Geriatric Society, 54*(11), 1736–1739.

Hamdan, A. L., Sibai, A. M., Srour, Z. M., Sabra, O. A., & Deeb, R. A. (2007). Voice disorders in teachers. The role of family physicians. *Saudi Medical Journal, 28*(3), 422–428.

Harari, P. M., Blatchford, S. J., Coulthard, S. W., & Cassady, J. R. (1991). Intubation granuloma of the larynx: Successful eradication with low-dose radiotherapy. *Head and Neck, 13*(3), 230–233.

Hernando, M., Cobeta, I., Lara, A., García, F., & Gamboa, F. J. (2007). Vocal pathologies of difficult diagnosis. *Journal of Voice, 23* [Epub ahead of print].

Herrington-Hall, B., Lee, L., Stemple, J., Neimi, K., & McHone, M. (1988). Description of laryngeal pathologies by age, sex, and occupation in a treatment-seeking sample. *Journal of Speech and Hearing Disorders, 53*(1), 57–64.

Hirano, M. (1981). *Clinical examination of voice.* New York, NY: Springer-Verlag.

Hirano, M., & Bless, D. M. (1993). *Videostroboscopic examination of the larynx.* San Diego, CA: Singular.

Hochman, I., Sataloff, R. T., Hillman, R. E., & Zeitels, S. M. (1999). Ectasias and varices of the vocal fold: Clearing the striking zone. *Annals of Otology, Rhinology, and Laryngology, 108*(1), 10–16.

Isshiki, N., Shoji, K., Kojima, H., & Hirano, S. (1996). Vocal fold atrophy and its surgical treatment. *Annals of Otology, Rhinology, and Laryngology, 105*(3), 182–188.

Issing, W., Struck, R., & Naumann, A. (1996). Long-term follow-up of larynx leukoplakia under treatment with retinyl palmitate. *Head and Neck, 18*(6), 560–565.

Jackson, C., & Jackson, C. L. (1935). Dysphonia plicae ventricularis: Phonation with ventricular bands. *Archives of Otolaryngology, 21*, 157–167.

Johns, M. (2003) Update on the etiology, diagnosis, and treatment of vocal fold nodules, polyps, and cysts. *Current Opinion in Otolaryngology and Head and Neck Surgery, 11*(6), 456–461.

Johnston, A., De Lisio, M., & Parise, G. (2008). Resistance training, sarcopenia, and the mitochondrial theory of aging. *Applied Physiology, Nutrition, and Metabolism, 33*(1), 191–199.

Jung, A., Schramm, J., Lehnerdt, K., & Herberhold, C. (2005). Recurrent laryngeal nerve palsy during anterior cervical spine surgery: A prospective study. *Journal of Neurosurgery and Spine, 2*(2), 123–127.

Kandogan, T. (2007). The role of thyroplasty in the management of sulcus vocalis. *Kulak Burun Bo az Ihtisas Dergisi, 17*(1), 13–17.

Kashima, H., Mounts, P., Levinthal, B., & Hruban, R. (1993). Sites of predilection in recurrent respiratory papillomatosis. *Annals of Otology, Rhinology, and Laryngology, 102*(8, Pt. 1), 580–583.

Kay, D. J., & Goldsmith, A. J. (2006). Laryngomalacia: A classification system and surgical treatment strategy. *Ear, Nose and Throat Journal, 85*(5), 328–331.

Kleinsasser, O. (1990). *Microlaryngoscopy and endolaryngeal microsurgery: Technique and typical findings.* Philadelphia, PA: Hanley & Belfus.

Kleinsasser, O., & Olieveira e Cruz, G. (1973). "Juvenile" and "adult" papillomas of the larynx. *HNO, 21*(4), 97–106.

Kuruvilla, S., Saldanha, R., & Joseph, L. D. (2008). Recurrent respiratory papillomatosis complicated by aspergillosis: A case report with review of literature. *Journal Postgraduate Medicine, 54*(1), 32–34.

Lee, E. K., & Son, Y. I. (2005). Muscle tension dysphonia in children: Voice characteristics and outcome of voice therapy. *International Journal of Pediatric Otorhinolaryngology, 69*(7), 911–917.

Lemos, E. M., Sennes, L. U., Imamura, R., & Tsuji, D. H. (2005). Vocal process granuloma: Clinical characterization, treatment and evolution. *Revista Brasileira de Otorrinolaringologia (Engl. ed.), 71*(4), 494–498.

Lin, D. S., Cheng, S. C., & Su, W. F. (2008, March 4). Potassium titanyl phosphate laser treatment of intubation vocal granuloma. *European Archives of Otorhinolaryngology* [Epub ahead of print].

Linville, S. E. (1996). The sound of senescence. *Journal of Voice, 10*(2), 190–200.

Marcotullio, D., Magliulo, G., & Pezone, T. (2002). Reinke's edema and risk factors: Clinical and histopathologic aspects. *American Journal of Otolaryngology, 23*(2), 81–84.

Maryn, Y., De Bodt, M. S., & Cauwenberge, P. V. (2003). Ventricular dysphonia: Clinical aspects and therapeutic options. *Laryngoscope, 113*, 859–866.

Mater, N., Amoussa, K., Verduvckt, I., Nolleveaux, M.C., Jamart, J., Lawson, G., & Remacle, M. (2010). C02 laser-assisted microsurgery for intracordal cysts: Technique and results of 49 patients. *European Archives of Otorhinolaryngology, 267*(12), 1905–1909.

Monnier, P., Lang, F., & Savary, M. (2003). Partial cricotracheal resection for pediatric subglottic stenosis: A single institution's experience in 60 cases. *European Archives of Otorhinolaryngology, 260*(6), 295–297.

Morris, M. J., Deal, L. E., Bean, D. R., Grbach, V. X., & Morgan, J. A. (1999). Vocal cord dysfunction in patients with exertional dyspnea. *Chest, 116*, 1676–1682.

Mortenson, M., & Woo, P. (2006). Office steroid injections of the larynx. *Laryngoscope, 116*(10), 1735–1739.

Mounts, P., Shah, K. V., & Kashima, H. (1982). Viral etiology of juvenile- and adult-onset squamous papilloma of the larynx. *Proceedings of the National Academy of Science, 79*, 5425–5429.

Mrowka-Kata, K., Kata, D., Lange, D., Namystowski, G., Czecioir, E., & Banert, K. (2010). Sarcoidosis and its otolaryngological implications. *European Archives of Otorhinolaryngologica, 267*, 1507-1514.

Murry, T., & Rosen, C. (2000). Phonotrauma associated with crying. *Journal of Voice, 14*(4), 575–580.

Murry, T., Tabaee, A., & Aviv, J. E. (2004). Respiratory retraining of refractory cough and laryngopharyngeal reflux in patients with paradoxical vocal fold movement disorder. *Laryngoscope, 114*, 1341–1345.

Myer, C. M., & Hartley, B. E. (2000). Pediatric laryngotracheal surgery. *Laryngoscope, 110*(11), 1875–1883.

Myer, C. M., O'Connor, D. M., & Cotton, R. T (1994). Proposed grading system for subglottic stenosis based on endotracheal tube sizes. *Annals of Otology, Rhinology, and Laryngology, 103*(4, Pt. 1), 319–323.

Neely, J. L., & Rosen, C. (2000). Vocal fold hemorrhage associated with coumadin therapy in an opera singer. *Journal of Voice, 14*(2), 272–277.

Olney, D. R., Greinwald, J. H., Richard, J. H., & Bauman, N. M. (1999). Laryngomalacia and its treatment. *Laryngoscope, 109*(11), 1770–1775.

O'Mara, W., & Hebert, A. F. (2000). External laryngeal trauma. *Journal of the Louisiana Medical State Society, 1152*(5), 218–222.

Orihata, M., & Sarna, S. K. (1994). Contractile mechanism of action of gastroprokinetic agents: Cisapride, metoclopramide, and domperidone. *American Journal of Physiology, 266,* G665–G676.

Otto, K. J., & Johns, M. M. III, (2005). Dysphagia following cervical fusion. *Ear, Nose, and Throat Journal, 84*(6), 344.

Paganelli, R., Di Iorio, A., Cherubini, A., Lauretani, F., Mussi, C., Volpato, S., . . . Ferrucci, L. (2006). Frailty of older age: the role of the endocrine-immune interaction. *Current Pharmaceutical Design, 12*(24), 3147–3159.

Painter, C. (1990). The incidence of voice disorders. *European Archives of Otolaryngology, 247*(3), 197–198.

Paluska, S. A., & Lansford, C. D. (2008). Laryngeal trauma in sport. *Current Sports Medicine Rehabilitation, 7*(1), 16–21.

Pau, H., & Murty, G. E. (2001). First case of surgically corrected puberphonia. *Journal of Laryngology and Otology, 115,* 60–61.

Pinto. J. A., da Silva Freitasm, M. L., Carpes, A. F., Zimath, P., Marquis, V., & Godoy, L. (2007). Autologous grafts for treatment of vocal sulcus and atrophy. *Otolaryngology-Head and Neck Surgery, 137*(5), 785–791.

Pitchenik, A. E. (1991). Functional laryngeal obstruction relieved by panting. *Chest, 100,* 1465–1467

Postma, G., Courey, M., & Ossoff, R. (1998). Microvascular lesions of the true vocal fold. *Annals of Otology, Rhinology, and Laryngology, 107*(6), 472–476.

Prater, R. J., & Swift, R. W. (1984). *Manual of voice therapy.* Boston, MA: Little Brown & Company.

Preciado-Lopez, J., Perez-Fernandez, C., Calzada-Uriondo, M., & Preciado-Ruiz, P. (2007). Epidemilogical study of voice disorders among teaching professional of La Rioja, Spain. *Journal of Voice, 22*(4), 489–508.

Preuss, S. F., Klussmann, J. P., Jungehulsing, M., Eckel, H. E., Guntinas- Lichius, O., & Damm, M. (2007). Long-term results of surgical treatment for recurrent respiratory papillomatosis. *Acta Oto-Laryngology, 127*(11), 1196–1201.

Rahbar, R., Rouillon, I., Roger, G., Lin, A., Nuss, R. C., Denoyelle, F., . . . Garabedian, E. N. (2006). The presentation and management of laryngeal cleft: A 10-year experience. *Archives of Otolaryngology-Head Neck Surgery, 132,* 1335–1341.

Ramig, L. O., Gray, S., Baker, K., Corbin-Lewis, K., Buder, E., Luschei, E., . . . Smith, M. (2001). The aging voice: A review, treatment data and familial and genetic perspectives. *Folia Phoniatriaca et Logopaedia, 53*(5), 252–265.

Ritz, P. (2000). Physiology of aging with respect to gastrointestinal, circulatory, and immune system changes and their significance for energy and protein metabolism. *European Journal of Clinical Nutrition, 54*(Suppl. 3), S21–S25.

Rosen, C. A., Lombard, L. E., & Murry, T. A. (2000). Acoustic, aerodynamic, and videostroboscopic features of bilateral vocal fold lesions. *Annals of Otology, Rhinology, and Laryngology, 109*(9), 823–828.

Rosen, D. C., & Sataloff, R. T. (1997). *Psychology of voice disorders.* San Diego, CA: Singular.

Roy, N., Ford, C. N., & Bless, D. M. (1996). Muscle tension dysphonia and spasmodic dysphonia: The role of manual laryngeal tension reduction in diagnosis and management. *Annals of Otology, Rhinology, and Laryngology, 105*(11), 851–856.

Roy, N., Holt, K. I., Redmond, S., & Muntz, H. (2007). Behavioral characteristics of children with vocal fold nodules. *Journal of Voice, 21*(2), 157–168.

Roy, N., & Leeper, H. (1993). Effects of the manual laryngeal musculoskeletal tension reduction technique as a treatment for functional voice disorders: Perceptual and acoustic measures. *Journal of Voice, 7*(3), 242–243.

Roy, N., Merrill, R. N., Gray, S. D., & Smith, E. M. (2005). Voice disorders in the general population: Prevalence, risk factors, and occupational impact. *Laryngoscope, 115*(11), 1988–1995.

Roy, N., Nissen, S.L., Dromey, C., & Sapir, S. (2009). Articulatory changes in muscle tension dysphonia. Evidence of vowel space expansion following manual circularynggeal therapy.

Journal of Communication Disorders, 42(2), 124–135.

Rutter, M. J., Hartley, B. E., & Cotton, R. T. (2001). Cricotracheal resection in children. *Archives of Otolaryngolgoy-Head and Neck Surgery, 127*(3), 289–292.

Sapienza, C. M., & Stathopoulos, E. T. (1994). Respiratory and laryngeal measures of children and women with bilateral vocal fold nodules. *Journal of Speech and Hearing Research, 37*(6), 1229–1243.

Sataloff, R. T. (1997). *Professional voice: The science and art of clinical care.* San Diego, CA: Singular.

Sataloff, R., Hawkshaw, M., Spiegel, J., & Rosen, D. C. (1996). Vocal fold hemorrhage. *Ear Nose and Throat Journal, 75*(12), 784–789.

Sataloff, R., Spiegel, J., Hawkshaw, M., Rosen, D., & Heuer, R. (1997). Autologous fat implantation for vocal fold scar: A preliminary report. *Journal of Voice, 11*(2), 238–246.

Sataloff, R., Spiegel, J. R., & Rosen, D. C. (1996). Vocal fold consequencys of scleroderma. *Ear, Nose, & Throat Journal, 75*(1), 12-13.

Schweinfurth, J. (2006). *Vascular lesions of the vocal fold.* Retrieved from http://www.emedicine.com/ent/TOPIC608.HTM

Sharma, G., & Goodwin, J. (2006). Effect of aging on respiratory system physiology and immunology. *Clinical Interventions in Aging, 1*(3), 253–260.

Sharma, N., Gill, P., Kauer, J., & Hans, J. M. (2001). Solitary juvenile laryngeal papilloma. *Indian Journal of Otolaryngology and Head and Neck Surgery, 53*(1), 1–3.

Smith, L. J., Praneetvatakul, V., & Sataloff, R. T. (2005). Acute vocal fold hemorrhage. *Ear, Nose, and Throat Journal, 84*(6), 334–335.

Smith, O. D., Callanan, V., Harcourt, J., & Albert, D. M. (2000). Intracordal cyst in a neonate. *International Journal of Perdiatric Otorhinolaryngology, 52*(3), 277–281.

Smith, R. R., & Ferguson, G. B., (1976). Systemic lupus erythematosus causing subglottic stenosis. *Laryngoscope, 86*, 734–738.

Snoeck, R., Wellens, W., Desloovere, C., Van Ranst, M., Naesens, L., De Clercq, E., & Feenstra, L. (1998). Treatment of severe laryngeal papillomatosis with intralesional injections of cidofovir [(s)-1-(3-hydroxy-2-phosphonyl-methoxypropyl) cytosine]. *Journal of Medical Virology, 54*(3), 219–225.

Sontag, S. J. (1990). The medical management of reflux esophagitis: Role of antacids and acid inhibition. *Gastroenterology Clinics of North America, 19*, 683–712.

Spaulding, C. A., Hahn, S. S., & Constable, W. C. (1987). The effectiveness of treatment of lymph nodes in cancers of the pyriform sinus and supraglottis. *International Journal of Radiation, Oncology, Biology, and Physics, 13*(7), 963–968.

Sperfeld, A. D. ,Hanemann, C. O., Ludolph, A. C., & Kassubek, J. (2005). Laryngospasm: An underdiagnosed symptom of X-linked spinobulbar muscular atrophy. *Neurology, 64*, 753–754.

Stathopoulos, E. T., & Sapienza, C. M. (1997). Developmental changes in laryngeal and respiratory function with variations in sound pressure leel. *Journal of Speech, Language, and Hearing Research, 40*(3), 595–614.

Stemple, J., Glaze, L. E., & Klaben, B. G. (2000). *Clinical voice pathology: Theory and management.* San Diego, CA: Singular Thomson Learning.

Sulica, L. (2005). Laryngeal thrush. *Annals of Otolaryngology, Rhinology, and Laryngology, 114*(5), 369–375.

Sulica, L., & Behrman, A. (2003). Management of benign vocal fold lesions: A survey of current opinion and practice. *Annals of Otology, Rhinology, and Laryngology, 112*(10), 2191–2198.

Szkielkowska, A., Miaskiewicz, B., Remacle, M., & Skarzynriski, H. (2011), Quality of voice after implantation of hyaluronic acid to the vocal folds — preliminary report. *Otolaryngologia Polska, 65*(6), 436–442.

Tao, C., & Jiang, J. J. (2007). Mechanical stress during phonation in a self oscillating finate-element vocal fold model. *Journal of Biomechanics, 40*(10), 2191–2198.

Teitel, A. D., MacKenzie, R., & Stern, S. A. (1992) Laryngeal involvement in systemic lupus erythematosus. *Seminars in Arthritis and Rheumotology, 22*(3), 203–214.

Tewfik, T. (2006). *Congenital malformations: Larynx.* Retrieved from http://www.emedicine.com/ent/topic324.htm

Theander, E., & Jacobsson, L.T. (2008). Relationship of Sjogren's syndrome to other connective tissue and autoimmune disorders. *Rheumatic Disease Clinics of North America, 34*(4), 935–947.

Titze, I. R. (1984). Parameterization of the glottal area, glottal flow, and vocal fold contact area. *Journal of the Acoustical Society of America, 75*(2), 570–580.

Tsunoda, K., Ishimoto, S., Suzuki, M., Hara, M., Yamaguchi, H., Sugimoto, M., . . . Tayama, N. (2007). An effective management regimen for laryngeal granuloma caused by gastroesophageal reflux: Combination therapy with suggestions for lifestyle modifications. *Acta Otolaryngologica, 127*(1), 88–92.

Vertigan, A. E., Theodoros, D. G., Winkworth, A. L., & Gibson, P. G. (2007). Chronic cough: A tutorial for speech-language pathologists. *Journal of Medical Speech-Language Pathology, 15*(3), 189–206.

White, J. B., Glade, R., Rossi, C. T., & Bielamowicz, S. (2007). Granular cell tumors of the larynx: Diagnosis and management. *Journal of Voice, 23*(4), 516–517.

Willinger, U., Volkl-Kernstock, S., & Aschauer, H. N. (2005). Marked depression and anxiety in patients with functional dysphonia. *Psychiatry Research, 134*(1), 85–91.

Zeitels, S., Akst, L., Burns, J., Hillman, R., Broadhurst, M., & Anderson, R. (2006). Pulsed angiolytic laser treatment of ectasias and varices in singers. *Annals of Otology, Rhinology, and Laryngology, 115*(8), 571–580.

Chapter 6

Neurologically Based Voice Disorders

Neurologic Voice Disorders

Acting as the command center, the nervous system provides the neural connections for communication within the body. A neurologically based voice disorder occurs when some form of damage affects the normal function of either the central or peripheral nervous system. The central nervous system includes the brain, brainstem, cerebellum, and the spinal cord. The peripheral nervous system includes the peripheral nerves (spinal and cranial) which innervate or control the muscles involved in voice production. The cause of these voice disorders is varied and there are some diseases that are quite rare. The more common etiologies and disorders are covered in this chapter.

Some of the voice disorders stemming from neurologic involvement occur in isolation whereas others are a symptom of a larger disease process (i.e., Parkinson's disease). With diseases that result in alterations to the motor system in general, the voice symptoms are often classified within a dysarthria. A dysarthria is a group of speech disorders attributed to a weakness, slowness, or incoordination affecting the multiple systems involved in communication such as the respiratory, laryngeal, or supralaryngeal systems (Darley, Aronson, & Brown, 1975). The dysarthrias are classified by localization of the neuroanatomic damage including the lower motor neuron system, the upper motor neuron system, the cerebellum, the extrapyramidal system, or combinations of these locations. Therefore, a patient may be classified as having a flaccid dysarthria, spastic dysarthria, ataxic dysarthria, hypokinetic/hyperkinetic dysarthria, or mixed dysarthria depending on the site of lesion. See Table 6–1.

After reading this chapter, you will:

■ Understand which vocal fold pathologies/disorders are classified as neurologic voice disorders
■ Understand the contributing causes and/or factors associated with neurologic voice disorders
■ Understand how to describe the visual, laryngostroboscopic, and perceptual features associated with neurologic voice disorders
■ Understand the management strategies used to treat neurologic voice disorders

By using the DVD accompanying this textbook, it is anticipated that your familiarity will be enhanced in identifying neurologic voice disorders.

Table 6–1. Summary of the Types of Dysarthrias, the Area of Neurologic Damage, Possible Etiologies or Causes, Resulting Voice Quality, and Expected Laryngeal Function

Types of Dysarthrias	Localization Area Affected in Motor System	Etiology	Voice Quality	Laryngeal Function
Flaccid	Damage to the motor neurons of the PNS will disrupt the neural impulses along the LMN (or FCP). Producing a malfunction in one or more of the cranial or spinal nerves	Any process that damages the motor unit, such as: brainstem stroke, tumor, viral or bacterial infection, physical trauma, surgical accidents, neuromuscular junction disease (myasthenia gravis), vascular disorders, infectious processes (polio), demyelinating disease (Guillain-Barré syndrome) and muscle disease (muscular dystrophy or progressive bulbar palsy)	▪ Phonatory Incompetence: *breathy voice, audible inspiration* and short phrases ▪ Resonatory Incompetence: *hypernasality, nasal emission,* imprecise consonants, and short phrases ▪ Phonatory-prosodic insufficiency: harsh voice, monopitch, monoloudness	▪ Muscle weakness ▪ Hypotonia ▪ Diminished reflexes: automatic and voluntary movements ▪ Effects speed, range, and accuracy of speech movements ▪ Atrophy ▪ Fasciculations ▪ Fibrillations
Spastic	Bilateral damage to the UMN system: pyramidal tract (corticobulbar and corticospinal tract) and extrapyramidal tract (indirect activation pathway)	Any process that damages the direct/indirect activation pathways, such as: vascular disease, inflammatory disease (leukoencephalitis), degenerative disease (lateral sclerosis), TBI, and can arise from multiple infarcts	▪ Prosodic excess: excess and equal stress, slow rate of speech ▪ Articulatory- resonatory incompetence: imprecise consonants, distorted vowels, hypernasality	▪ Impaired movement patterns ▪ Loss/reduction in fine, discrete movements ▪ Hyperadduction of the VF—limits length and tense ▪ Excessive muscle tone ▪ Hyperactive reflexes ▪ Reduced range of movement

continues

Types of Dysarthrias	Localization *Area Affected in Motor System*	Etiology	Voice Quality	Laryngeal Function
Spastic *continued*			• Prosodic insufficiency: monopitch, monoloudness, reduced stress, short phrases • Phonatory stenosis: low pitch, harshness strained-strangled voice, pitch breaks, short phrases, slow rate	• Slowness of movement • At rest normal appearing vocal folds
Ataxic	Damage to the cerebellum or to the neural pathways (cerebellar control circuits) that connect the cerebellum to the other parts of the CNS	Any process that damages the cerebellum or cerebellar control circuit, such as: degenerative, demyelinating, vascular, neoplastic, inflammatory, traumatic, and toxic (alcohol abuse)	• Articulatory inaccuracy: imprecise consonants, irregular articulatory breakdowns, vowel distortions • Prosodic excess: excess and equal stress, prolonged phonemes, prolonged intervals, slow rate • Phonatory-prosodic insufficiency— harshness, monopitch, monoloudness • Slurred speech	• Inaccurate movements • Irregular repetitive movements • Slow movements • Reduced muscle tone • Poor coordination • Difficulty initiating purposeful movement

Table 6-1. *continued*

Types of Dysarthrias	Localization *Area Affected in Motor System*	Etiology	Voice Quality	Laryngeal Function
Hypokinetic	Damage is associated with the basal ganglia control circuits, and caused by depletion of the neurotransmitter dopamine	Any damage to the basal ganglia control circuit, such as: degenerative disease (Parkinson's), vascular, toxic, trauma, and infectious (viral encephalitis)	▪ Reduced vocal intensity ▪ Breathy voice quality ▪ Inability to vary vocal pitch ▪ Reduced phonation duration ▪ Reduced intelligibility ▪ Reduced range of motion ▪ Imprecise consonant productions ▪ Slowed movement and incoordination of speech muscles ▪ Tremor or unsteadiness in the voice	▪ Excessive saliva accumulation from infrequent swallowing ▪ Rigidity: slow movement, stiffness or tightness ▪ Bradykinesia: delays or false starts at beginning of movement and slowness of movement; intermittent freezing ▪ Range is reduced ▪ Vocal fold bowing during phonation ▪ Slowness of movement
Hyperkinetic	Damage to the basal ganglia control circuit due to lack in cortical neuronal firing; that effects involuntary movements in speech	Any damage to the basal ganglia control circuit or portions of the cerebellar control circuit, such as: degenerative (Huntington's disease), infections (Sydenham's chorea), vascular (not common), traumatic, toxic, neurogenic (spasmodic dysphonia), and metabolic disease	▪ Abnormal, rhythmic or irregular and unpredictable, rapid or slow involuntary movements ▪ Speech effects result differently to different abnormal movement patterns	Dyskinesias: abnormal involuntary movements Myoclonus: involuntary single or repetitive brief jerks; it can be rhythmic or nonrhythmic Tics: rapid, stereotyped, coordinated or patterned movements that are under partial voluntary control

Types of Dysarthrias	Localization *Area Affected in Motor System*	Etiology	Voice Quality	Laryngeal Function
Hyperkinetic *continued*			• Chorea (Huntington's disease): sudden forced inspiratory/ expiratory, excess loudness, variability in rate and stress; strained-strangled voice; voice stoppages; transient breathiness; grunts; intermittent hypernasality and weak pressure; distortion/ irregular breakdowns	Chorea: involuntary rapid, non-stereotypic, random, purposeless movements; may be present at rest and during sustained postures and voluntary movements. Ballismus: gross, abrupt contractions of axial and proximal muscles of the extremities that can produce wild flailing movements Athetosis: slow, writhing, purposeless movements that tend to flow into one another Dystonia: relatively slow, due to excessive contractions from antagonistic muscles Spasm: various muscular contractions; they can be prolonged, continuous, repetitive, rapid in onset, or brief in duration Tremor: rhythmic (periodic) movement; it can occur during rest, postural, action, or terminal

continues

Table 6–1. *continued*

Types of Dysarthrias	Localization *Area Affected in Motor System*	Etiology	Voice Quality	Laryngeal Function
Unilateral Upper Motor Neuron	Damage to the UMN unilaterally: • Right UMN: problems with lower left side of the face and tongue weakness • Function of the velum, pharynx, and larynx	Any damage to one side of the UMN, such as: stroke, tumors, (TBI), and trauma.	• Harsh voice quality • Slurred speech/ difficulty with pronunciation • Decreased loudness • Slow rate • Irregular articulatory breakdowns • Imprecise articulations	• Reduced range of motion • Mild vocal fold weakness or spasticity
Mixed	Any combination of two or more single dysarthria type Most common: • Flaccid-Spastic • Ataxic-Spastic • Hypokinetic-Spastic • Ataxic-Flaccid-Spastic • Hyperkinetic-Hypokinetic	Can result from combined events, more than one portion of an area is affected or the co-occurrence of two or more diseases, such as: degenerative diseases (Amyotrophic lateral sclerosis and Multiple sclerosis), toxic, vascular, trauma, tumor or infectious/autoimmune disease	Multiple sclerosis: impaired loudness control, harsh voice quality, imprecise articulation, impaired emphasis, decreased vital capacity, hypernasality, inappropriate pitch level, breathiness, increased breathing rate, sudden articulatory breakdowns Amyotrophic lateral sclerosis: imprecise consonants, hypernasality, harsh voice quality, slow rate, monopitch, short phrases, distorted vowels, low pitch, monoloudness, and excess and equal stress	

PNS = peripheral nervous system, LMN = lower motor neuron, UMN = upper motor neuron.

Unilateral True Vocal Fold Paralysis

Description and Etiology

Ninety percent of vocal fold paralysis that occurs is unilateral and caused by damage to the peripheral nervous system. As well, the majority of cases resulting in unilateral vocal fold paralysis are of the adductor type, that is the paralyzed vocal fold cannot adduct or help with closing the glottal space. Unilateral true vocal fold paralysis is the complete immobility (paralysis) in one vocal fold. The term *paralysis* can be contrasted with the term *paresis*, wherein paresis refers to a weakening, and not complete absence of movement in the affected vocal fold. The continuum from paresis to paralysis can lead to a high degree of variability in function when assessing the impaired vocal fold movement with visual examination. This is due to the variable extent to which the recurrent laryngeal nerve or RLN regenerates following injury (Woodson, 2008). The RLN is the nerve primarily responsible for vocal fold ab- and adduction. The RLN is a branch of cranial nerve X, the vagus nerve (see Chapter 2). Because the vagus nerve has a fairly long and "wandering" (the literal translation of the term "vagus") path, there are many points where destruction or disruption of nerve conduction can bring about a potential paralysis of the vocal fold on the same (ipsilateral) side of the body. The resulting voice disorder is classified as a flaccid dysphonia.

When vocal fold paralysis occurs it is typically considered a symptom of an underlying disease process or neurologic disruption which, in one recent study, resulted from surgical trauma (especially thyroidectomy; (40.2%), tumors/neoplasms (especially lung cancer; (29.9%), unknown/idiopathic factors (10.7%), trauma (8%), central nervous system dysfunction (3.8%), radiation (3.4%), inflammatory (2%), cardiovascular (1.7%), and other (0.3%) causes (Chen, Jen, Wang,

Lee, & Lin, 2007). Systemic diseases such as systemic lupus erythematosus, sarcoidosis, and tuberculosis can cause unilateral adductor vocal fold paralysis and it can occur with other more rare systemic diseases. Idiopathic diseases like Lyme disease, herpes simplex virus Type 1, and Epstein-Barr virus have also been implicated in the cause of adductor paralysis.

Perceptual Signs and Symptoms

An individual with an adductor unilateral true vocal fold paralysis may exhibit some aphonia (absence of voice), completely normal voicing, or anything in between these two extremes. The highly variable presentation of unilateral vocal fold paralysis is due to a number of factors including location of the paralyzed fold relative to the nonparalyzed fold as well as ability of the individual to compensate for the paralysis through use of the nonparalyzed fold and/or other compensatory strategies to help close off the glottal space.

For example, a vocal fold that is paralyzed at or just lateral to midline is still likely to form adequate glottal closure with the non-paralyzed fold. In this case, full phonatory capacities are preserved and there may be no audible dysphonia. In other cases, such as when the affected fold is paralyzed in a highly open or *abducted* position the individual may produce a voice that is excessively breathy and weak because the two vocal folds cannot close off the glottis adequately. This breathiness typically corresponds with high rates of airflow through the glottis. Many times, individuals with this type of unilateral adductor paralysis will "fight" against the inability to close the glottis, producing phonation that is perceived as hoarse or strained. Often times the ventricular folds medialize as the person is straining to close off the glottal space.

Dysphagia, particularly for liquid consistencies, is a common side effect of unilateral adductor vocal fold paralysis due to difficulty closing the glottis (Sasaki, Hundal, & Kim, 2005). In extreme instances, this dysphagia can result in recurrent respiratory infections or even death from aspiration pneumonia.

Features of Visual Assessment

Upon laryngostroboscopic assessment, the paralyzed vocal fold may appear weakened or bowed. Saliva or mucous secretions may pool along the piriform sinus as well as the tissue just lateral to the vocal fold. See the DVD for example of unilateral vocal fold paralysis (Appendix 6–1).

> The piriform sinus is a paired mucosal cul-de-sac lying lateral to each side of the larynx.

Although passive vibrations of the paralyzed fold may be evident during phonation due to the flow of exhaled air up and around the paralyzed fold, the arytenoid cartilage on the affected side will not ab- or adduct according to normal phonatory and respiratory patterns. The vibratory pattern of the affected fold will typically not match that of the "normal" fold. This asymmetry is characterized by slower initiation of the mucosal wave on the affected side along with a slower period and reduced amplitude of vibration (Sercarz, Berke, Ming, Garrett, & Natividad, 1992).

Observations of vocal fold immobility can be further confirmed through simultaneous use of needle laryngeal electromyography (EMG) within the thyroarytenoid (TA) or posterior cricoarytenoid (PCA) muscles. EMG activity allows the intrinsic muscle activity of the TA and PCA to be recorded providing information about the extent of neural innervation to those muscle groups.

Management

In cases where direct trauma to the RLN is suspected as the cause of the unilateral adductor paralysis, a "wait and see" approach is often preferred. Here, major surgical or other interventions are postponed for a period of time, typically 6 to 9 months, in order to allow for functional recovery which may occur as a result of nerve regeneration. The overall goal of any treatment for unilateral adductor paralysis is to improve voice and prevent aspiration.

When behavioral voice therapy is initiated for unilateral adductor true vocal fold paralysis guided instruction on techniques to facilitate vocal fold closure or *adduction occur*. Examples of relevant techniques can include (see Chapter 7 for more details):

- Pushing Techniques that take advantage of vocal fold adduction which occurs naturally while pushing or bearing down;
- Vocal Function Exercises (e.g., Stemple, Lee, D'Amico, & Pickup, 1994) that center around a series of exercises performed with *barely adducted* vocal folds;
- Resonant Voice Therapy (e.g., Verdolini, Druker, Palmer, & Samawi, 1998) which emphasizes use of barely adducted vocal fold posture along with use of forward focus;
- Lee Silverman Voice Therapy (LSVT), (e.g., Ramig, Bonitati, Lemke, & Horii, 1994) which focuses on the production of LOUD voice through effortful phonation.

Research evidence suggests that early voice therapy, (between 2 and 6 weeks post-diagnosis of adductor vocal fold paralysis,) can significantly improve acoustic and perceptual measures of phonatory stability after as little as

6 months of treatment, and in the absence of surgical interventions (D'Alatri et al., 2007). Behavioral voice therapy may also enhance the effectiveness of surgical interventions for true unilateral adductor vocal fold paralysis (Heuer et al., 1997).

Surgical interventions for unilateral true adductor vocal fold paralysis primarily consist of medialization (Ishhiki Type I thyroplasty) procedures that attempt to "push" the affected vocal fold to a more medial position. When the vocal fold is in that position it is better able to make contact with the non-paralyzed fold. Thyroplasty procedures are particularly useful when the affected fold is paralyzed in an extremely abducted position relative to the nonparalyzed fold. In instances where the affected fold is paralyzed at a location just lateral to midline, vocal fold augmentation procedures may be the effective and less drastic approach. Arytenoid adduction is another surgical procedure that has often been recommended if there is a large posterior glottic gap or the vocal folds are at different levels. When this occurs, voice improvement can be greater (Li et al., 2011)

Vocal fold augmentation procedures use a variety of injectable substances in order to "plump" the affected vocal fold, allowing for improved contact with the nonparalyzed vocal fold. These injectables are placed lateral to the vocal ligament and have lasting effects from as short as a few months up to 2 years. Teflon (FDA approved) is the only injectable that is permanent. Examples of other injectables include polymethylsiloxane gel, fat, calcium hydroxylapatite (FDA approved), Gelfoam, and collagen (Cymetra, FDA approved), among others (Durson, Boynukalin, Bagis, Ozgursoy, & Coruh, 2008; Randhawa, Ramsey, & Rubin, 2008; Remacle & Lawson, 2007; Rontal & Rontal, 2003). As indicated, vocal fold augmentation procedures frequently need to be repeated as the bulking agent (particularly fat) has a tendency to be reabsorbed by the body. The need for repeat surgical intervention is relatively less common with medialization (thyroplasty) procedures.

Reinnervation surgical procedures can be used to establish new patterns of innervations to the RLN on the affected paralyzed side. One such procedure reinnervates the RLN with branches of the ansa cervicalis, a collection of nerves that arise from cervical nerves I through III. One recent study found this procedure effective at restoring tone to the affected fold while enhancing vocal fold closure and improving perceptual voice variables such as overall severity, roughness, breathiness, and strain (Lorenz et al., 2008; Su, Hsu, Chen, & Sheng, 2007).

In addition to the above studies, there is research exploring the potential application of gene therapy for RLN regeneration (Shiotani, Saito, Araki, Moro, & Watabe, 2007).

Bilateral Abductor True Vocal Fold Paralysis

Description and Etiology

Bilateral abductor vocal fold paralysis most commonly results from surgical trauma (44%), malignancies (17%), endotracheal intubation (15%), neurologic disease (12%), or idiopathic causes (12%) (Benninger, Gillen, & Altman, 1998). It is a potentially life threatening condition when the folds are fixed in the paramedian position (nearly closed). Although phonation may be preserved due to the ability of the vocal folds to vibrate effectively on exhalation, the paralysis produces an airway obstruction with the vocal folds unable to move apart or *abduct*. Bilateral abductor vocal fold paralysis can sometimes be confused with bilateral arytenoid cartilage fixation.

Perceptual Signs and Symptoms

As with unilateral RLN paralysis, the voice associated with bilateral RLN paralysis is highly variable, ranging anywhere from completely normal phonation (in cases where the vocal folds are fixed in the paramedian position and therefore able to establish some semblance of normal vibration on exhalation) to complete aphonia (as when the vocal folds are paralyzed in the abducted position or if the vocal folds are fixed in a more adducted position, inspiratory stridor may be evident In these cases the stridor may signal a more serious problem in the form of airway obstruction. This is because fixing of the true vocal folds in the paramedian position effectively narrows the airway, increasing respiratory effort and potentially contributing to respiratory failure.

Features of Visual Assessment

Endoscopy reveals an appearance of floppy vocal folds or bowed vocal folds. Visual focus on the arytenoid cartilages will indicate no discernible movement in either vocal folds' ab- or adduction during respiration and phonation. This immobility carries over to non-voice functions such as sniffing or whistling. Observations of vocal fold immobility can be further confirmed through simultaneous use of laryngeal EMG within the thryoarytenoid or posterior cricoarytenoid muscles.

Management

If there is no emergent need (e.g., patient's airway is not obstructed by the bilateral abductor vocal fold paralysis) a "wait and see" approach is first recommended wherein major medical or surgical interventions are deferred for a period of 6 to 9 months. In cases where the overriding concern is for airway patency (unobstructed), more drastic and emergency measures may need to be taken on the diagnosis of a bilateral abductor paralysis. An example of such a measure would be tracheotomy, which establishes a direct airway opening through an incision in the neck below the level of the vocal folds (Figure 6–1) (see Arai, Endo, Oshima & Yagi, 2011 in a case of amyotrophic lateral sclerosis).

In some cases of bilateral abductor RLN paralysis (Dennis & Kashima, 1989; Farrior & Bagby, 1950; Helmus, 1972) removal of the arytenoids cartilage or arytenoidectomy and removal of all or a portion of the membranous vocal fold, called a cordectomy, are the necessary surgical procedures for airway restoration. As an alternative to surgical removal of the vocal fold, surgical vocal fold lateralization or cordopexy is an additional treatment option available to permanently widen the glottis. Surgical abduction of the arytenoid cartilages is a procedure used to widen the glottis in cases where the true vocal folds are paralyzed

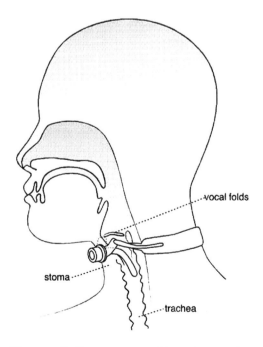

Figure 6–1. Depiction of breathing valve inserted into stoma to aid ventilation.

in a paramedian position. Here, a suture is placed in the muscular process of the arytenoid cartilage which is then rotated to increase the glottal opening. In one recent study, arytenoid adduction was successful at reducing stridor and, in some patients, eliminating the need for tracheostomy. Potential adverse side effects of the procedure included breathiness (Woodson & Weiss, 2007). Arytenoid adduction is most effective in patients with bilateral abductor paralysis of less than 1 year's duration who do not have unfavorable laryngeal adductor activity (Woodson, 2010).

Pacing strategies refer to a class of interventions that use implantable electrical stimulators to trigger vocal fold abduction for respiration. Pacing strategies are considered rather experimental but have been used alone, or in combination with secondary adductor muscle block (with botulinum toxin type A) in order to achieve and maintain sufficient glottal opening (Zealear, Billante, Courey, Sant'Anna, & Netterville, 2002). Reinnervation procedures, such as those used with unilateral RLN paralysis, are highly experimental and largely untested as a treatment approach for bilateral vocal fold paralysis.

Superior Laryngeal Nerve Paralysis

Description and Etiology

The superior laryngeal nerve (SLN) is a branch of the vagus nerve which serves to bilaterally innervate the cricothyroid laryngeal muscles. Recall, from Chapter 2, that the cricothyroid muscle serves a dual role in both laryngeal adduction (contractions in the cricothyroid brings the vocal folds closer together) as well as creating a change in pitch (cricothyroid muscles contract creating a rise in pitch).

As with RLN paralysis, paralysis of the SLN can be brought about via a variety of traumatic, neoplastic, or infectious conditions with viral infections being most commonly implicated (Dursun et al., 1996). The SLN may be damaged during surgery of the thyroid gland. One recent study singled out neuritis (inflammation of the SLN; 69.7%), iatrogenic (10.2%), unknown (10.2%), and trauma (8.9%) as the most frequently observed causes of SLN paralysis (Eckley, Sataloff, Hawkshaw, Spiegel, & Mandel, 1998).

Perceptual Signs and Symptoms

As with RLN paralysis, the perceptual voice characteristics of SLN paralysis exist as an extension of the disruption in vocal fold ability to: (1) adduct and (2) elongate to increase pitch. Common perceptual characteristics of voices of individuals with SLN dysfunction can include a weak, breathy voice. Hoarseness and disruptions to the vocal frequency range are also frequently evident (Eckley et al., 1998).

Features of Visual Assessment

Paralysis or paresis of the SLN can be difficult to diagnose via laryngostroboscopy because of the highly variable manner of presentation. To this end, laryngeal electromyography is often useful for reaching a definitive diagnosis. The visual examination of the larynx reveals the most common findings as ipsilateral (same side as the paralysis) vocal fold bowing and shortening, height asymmetry of the vocal processes (with the affected side higher than the nonaffected side), and ipsilateral hyperadduction of the false vocal fold. These phenomena are frequently visualized only during phonation, with no abnormalities evident at rest (Tsai, Celmer, Bereke, & Chhetri, 2007). Other times at rest the larynx will appear "rotated" toward the weakened side (Newman & Becker, 1981). Additionally, individuals with a unilateral paralysis of the SLN may exhibit true vocal fold movement described clinically as *Gegenschlagen* ("dashing against each other") in which the right and left true vocal folds are observed vibrating 90 degrees out of phase (Mendelsohn, Sung, Bereke, & Chhetri, 2007).

Management

As with RLN dysfunction, a "wait and see" approach deferring major surgical or other medical management of the disorder is a popular preliminary approach. Surgical interventions for SLN paralysis include fusion of the thyroid and cricoid cartilages (Thompson, Ward, & Schwartz, 1984) while other surgical procedures/options for SLN paralysis are being tested in the animal model.

Spasmodic Dysphonia

Description and Etiology

Spasmodic dysphonia (SD) is a focal laryngeal dystonia of relatively unknown origin, resulting in a neurogenic voice disorder. The dystonia affects the laryngeal adductory and/or abductory muscles during voice production.

> A dystonia is a movement disorder often characterized by abnormal muscle tone that results in jerking movements of a body part.

Two varieties of SD exist. The first, known as abductor SD (ABSD), makes up only around 15% of cases and involves uncontrollable opening or abduction of the vocal folds during voicing tasks (Merson & Ginsberg, 1979). These uncontrollable vocal abductions typically produce an excessively breathy and irregular voice. The second, more common subtype is known as adductor SD (ADSD), and features frequent and irregular closure of the vocal folds, producing a characteristic "strain and strangle" type voicing (Miller &

Woodson, 1991; Van Pelt, Ludlow, & Smith, 1994). A small subset of patients demonstrate a "mixed" spasmodic dysphonia characterized by a combination of adductor and abductor symptoms. Patients diagnosed with SD are predominately (nearly 80%) female (Adler, Edwards, & Bansberg, 1997), with onset typically occurring during the fourth decade of life (Schweinfurth, Billante, & Courey, 2002).

Although the etiology remains relatively unknown, evidence is mounting that the basis is neurologic in origin. One study in the early 1990s indicated that of 100 patients with ADSD, 71 had underlying essential tremor, 25 had Meige syndrome, 12 were hypothyroid, and 27 had either a functional disturbance or focal dystonia (Rosenfield et al., 1990).

Diagnosis of SD has also been associated with presence of writer's cramp, essential tremor, and a remote diagnosis of mumps or measles with onset frequently following an upper respiratory illness or major life stress (Schweinfurth et al., 2002). Previously, considered a psychological disorder, primarily affecting anxious individuals, possibly brought about by the "pressures and losses of middle age" (Henschen & Burton, 1978), the current theory holds that psycho emotional correlates of SD are likely symptoms of the primary voice disorder (Aronson, Brown, Litin, & Pearson, 1968; Baylor, Yorkston, Eadie, & Maronian, 2007), rather than the cause of the disorder itself. Other investigations have focused on structural abnormalities involving the RLN but have failed to identify consistent RLN abnormalities in individuals with SD versus healthy controls (Bocchino & Tucker, 1978, Dedo, 1976; Kosaki, Iwamura, & Yamazaki, 1999; Ravits, Aronson, DeSanto, & Dyck, 1979). As stated previously, theory classifies SD as a focal dystonia alongside such disorders as torticollis, blepharospasm, oral mandibular dystonia, and writer's cramp (Ludlow & Connor, 1987). Other research has focused on the role of sensorimotor pathways in the inhibition of laryngeal response to sensory inputs, and potential dysfunction of these pathways (Deleyiannis, Gillespie, Bielamowicz, Yamashita, & Ludlow, 1999; Ludlow, Schultz, Yamashita, & Deleyiannis, 1995). First described by Traube (1871) as a "nervous hoarseness" and, over time, known as "spastic" and later "spasmodic dysphonia," the most recent research has merged neuroimaging technologies with post mortem histopathologic examination to isolate areas of the brain that appear to be different in individuals with SD. The etiology of SD is now possibly moving toward the determination of a definitive neurogenic locus of dysfunction for the disorder. Here, Diffusion Tensor Imaging (DTI; a form of magnetic resonance imaging) identified breakdowns in white matter organization in the right genu of the internal capsule and impaired nerve conduction in the white matter along both sides of the corticobulbar/corticospinal tract in 20 spasmodic dysphonia patients compared to 20 healthy subjects (Simonyan et al., 2008).

Perceptual Signs and Symptoms

The voice quality associated with ABSD is weak and breathy. Voice quality associated with ADSD is strained. Within each condition, abductor and adductor spasms, perceived as stoppages in voice, are heard during both sustained vowel production and connected speech (Braden & Hapner, 2008; Edgar, Sapienza, Bidus, & Ludlow, 2001). Delayed onset of voicing is also common at the initiation of sound production (Edgar et al., 2001). Each of these disorders adversely effects speech intelligibility, impairing communication effectiveness.

ADSD is often confused with muscle tension dysphonia (MTD), where voice symptoms are brought about through excessive muscular tension and maladaptive patterns of voicing. The two disorders can be differentiated acoustically (e.g., Sapienza, Walton,

& Murry, 2000) and, unlike MTD, ADSD appears to be task specific in that voice symptoms manifest as more severe during connected speech (as opposed to sustained vowel) and voiced (as opposed to voiceless) phonemes. In contrast, individuals with MTD typically maintain consistent levels of severity across connected speech, sustained vowel, and during both voiced and voiceless productions (Erickson, 2003; Roy, Gouse, Mauszycki, Merrill, & Smith, 2005; Roy, Mauszycki, Merrill, Gouse, & Smith, 2007).

Features of Visual Assessment

The laryngeal spasms associated with ABSD move the vocal folds in an open position when they should be closing. Likewise, the spasms associated with ADSD move the vocal folds in a closed position when they otherwise should be open. These spasms do not occur at rest or typically during other nonphonatory tasks such as whispering. Interestingly, they do not occur in singing or laughter.

Task production of sustained vowels will reveal the spasmodic nature of the intrinsic laryngeal muscles, primarily the adductory muscles (thyroarytenoid, lateral cricoarytenoid, interarytenoids) and abductory muscle (posterior cricoarytenoid) during laryngotroboscopy. Notably, it is the thyroarytenoid muscle that is significantly more likely than the lateral cricoarytenoid muscle to be the predominant muscle involved in ADSD (Klotz et al., 2004). Connected speech tasks like "Pay Paul a penny" can show ABSD as the transitions from voiceless to voice sound segments occur. Sentences produced like, "We eat apples every day" or "You should use new blue shoes" reveal the adductory movements of the vocal folds as the spasms occur on voicing (Roehm & Rosen, 2004). Some compensatory movements of the false vocal folds and other vocal tract structures may occur as the patient struggles to produce voice.

Management

Botulinum Toxin. For the symptom management of spasmodic dysphonia, injection of botulinum toxin (Botox™ or Myobloc™) into the intrinsic laryngeal muscles has emerged as the preferred approach due to its high rate of success and low risk of side effects (Blitzer, Brin, & Stewart, 1998). For ADSD, Botox™, is injected either unilaterally or bilaterally, into the TA muscle, the muscle primarily implicated in adductory voice spasming. A review on the use of Botox™ injections for ADSD (Boutsen, Cannito, Taylor, & Bender, 2002) concluded that neither the unilateral or bilateral injection technique is consistently associated with better outcomes in terms of symptom relief and overall vocal function. In spite of this, the unilateral technique may minimize adverse side effects such as persistent breathiness and hoarseness and produce better functional results in women (Koriwchak, Netterville, Snowden, Courey, & Ossoff, 1996; Ludlow, Bagley Yin, & Koda, 1992; Maloney & Morrison, 1994).

The technique first used for Botox™ injection into the larynx involved a percutaneous injection, guided into location by EMG signals obtained through use of a Teflon-coated hollow needle. The needle, inserted into the space between the thyroid and cricoid cartilages (located through external palpation) was directed upward toward the TA muscle. Having the patient phonate and observing the resultant EMG signal visually verifies contact with the TA. Injection techniques that allow for other means of locating the injection site have been developed in an effort to increase the accuracy with which the toxin could be administered while eliminating the need for EMG monitoring of injection. These techniques include transoral and transnasal laryngoscopic injections, as well as transcartilaginous "point touch" injections (Ford, Bless, & Lowery, 1990; Green, Berke, Ward, & Gerratt, 1992; Rhew, Fiedler, & Ludlow, 1994) (Figure 6–2).

When injected into a muscle, Botox™ effectively denervates the muscle by temporarily blocking the release of acetylcholine at the

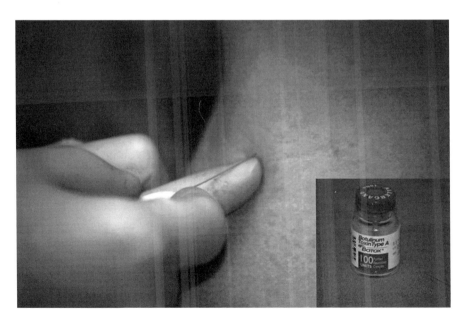

Figure 6–2. Depiction of needle placement, prior to Botox™ injection of the thyroarytenoid muscles.

neuromuscular junction (Ludlow & Mann, 2000). Over a period of time (typically three months) the affected nerve endings recover, and spasmodic symptoms gradually return. In the case of ADSD, partial denervation of the TA temporarily eliminates the uncontrollable spasmodic bursts responsible for the observed voice symptoms.

> Denervation means that the nerve supply is blocked.

Although the popularity and use of Botox™ injections for ADSD continues to grow, the published research to date is not easily characterized or summarized. Two fairly recent publications have made efforts to this end. The first of these found that the "average patient" treated for ADSD with Botox™ treatment experienced a 97% improvement in voice, although no outcome variables demonstrated statistically significant improvement (Whurr, Nye, & Lorch, 1998). In terms of quantitative acoustic measures, Botox™ injections have proved efficacious in reducing the number of phonatory breaks and variation in fundamental frequency while demonstrating less effect on measures associated with vocal breathiness and roughness including speech or harmonic to noise ratio measures, jitter, and shimmer (Boutsen et al., 2002).

Voice Therapy. In many cases, behaviorally driven voice therapy approaches have been discredited and discarded out of frustration as conventional means of vocal rehabilitation fail to offer long-lasting relief to the seemingly impossible to treat patient with spasmodic dysphonia. In spite of this history, during recent years, behavioral therapies have found a niche within the overall picture of clinical management, emerging as a low-risk and (comparatively), low-cost means of assuring optimal treatment outcomes. Existing, as well as new information, suggests that behavioral

therapies may play a role in the management of ADSD. Behavioral treatment approaches for ADSD grew out of frequently observed and well-documented improvement in vocal symptoms achieved through use of specific, volitional voicing behaviors such as whispered or breathy voice, noncommunicative vocalizations (coughing or throat clearing), singing, humming, or pitch alterations (Bloch, Hirano, & Gould, 1985). See Chapter 7 for detailed description of voice therapy strategies for spasmodic dysphonia.

Essential Voice Tremor

Description and Etiology

Often classified as a common hyperkinetic movement disorder, essential tremor is the most common movement disorder (http://www.mayoclinic.com/health/essential-tremor/DS00367). The more frequently occurring essential tremor affects the extremities; the hands and limbs. More common in those of advancing age, essential tremor of the larynx has a varying etiology but is centrally driven. Symptomatically tremor in patients is worsened by anxiety, fatigue, and excitement with symptomatic relief with alcohol intake.

Perceptual Signs and Symptoms

Essential tremor is easy to identify perceptually during vowel prolongation. Audible and rhythmic cycles of the tremor occur every 4 to 6 Hz. Essential tremor may also be characterized by pitch breaks and voice breaks associated with large amplitude tremors of the larynx. These perceptual characteristics sometimes lead to difficulty differentiating essential voice tremor from ADSD. Needle laryngeal electromyography can help differentiate between the two disorders by defining the rhythmic nature of essential tremor (Kimaid et al., 2004). Finnegan, Luschei,

Barkmeier, and Hoffman (2003) found that essential tremor did not appear to occur from one single central oscillating source as their tests of laryngeal muscle activity resulted in distinct timing events for different laryngeal muscles. The same holds true for acoustic analysis which shows differentiation between essential tremor and ADSD based on the presence of cyclic tremor, the degree of voice breaks and other aberrant episodes identified with ADSD that are not identified with essential tremor (Sapienza et al., 2002).

Features of Visual Assessment

Laryngeal examination reveals bilateral tremor of the true vocal folds. Accompanying tremor can also be in the soft palate, tongue, pharyngeal wall, and false vocal folds (Lundy et al., 1996). The larynx moves both at rest and the tremor increases during phonation. To assist in differentially diagnosing essential tremor from ADSD it should be noted that with ADSD, spasms are not seen when the larynx is at rest.

Management

Generally, pharmacologic management controls essential tremor including the use of beta-blockers and propranolol and metoprolol (LoPressor, Toprol XL). These are considered first-line choices, particularly propanolol and the beta-blockers which seem to be best tolerated by younger patients. Other drug treatments include the use of anticonvulsants, benzodiazepines, calcium channel blockers, and Botox (Pahwa & Lyons, 2003; Roehm & Rosen, 2004). Deep brain stimulation results for one patient, reported by Yoon, Munz, Satalof, Spiegel, and Heuer (1999), illustrated substantial effects with about a three-fold drop in tremor rate when the deep brain stimulator was on. This finding was similar in a study by Moringlane, Putzer, and Barry (2004) in another case study of a patient suffering from

not only vocal tremor but other tremor of the head and upper extremities. Finally, Botox has been tried with 13 patients with vocal tremor and shown to improve following bilateral injection (Adler et al., 2004).

Myasthenia Gravis

Description and Etiology

Myasthenia gravis is caused by reductions in the peripheral nervous system neurotransmitter, acetylcholine, via an autoimmune mechanism, resulting in a severe decline in a muscle's ability to contract. The hallmark symptom of myasthenia gravis is muscle weakness. Receptors in the peripheral nervous system receive the neurotransmitter acetylcholine and its action can be either excitatory or inhibitory depending on the type of tissue and the nature of the receptor with which it interacts. In the case of myasthenia gravis the excitatory response is diminished causing the muscles to contract with less force. The typical onset of myasthenia gravis is between the third and sixth decade of life for females and males respectively (http://www.ninds.nih.gov/disorders/myasthenia_gravis/detail_myasthenia_gravis.htm).

Perceptual Signs and Symptoms

A telling sign that a patient may have myasthenia gravis is that as activity increases; for example, sound prolongation, muscle weakness exhibits. As a result of the disease, weakness in the supralaryngeal and laryngeal structures results causing a dysarthria that is characterized as flaccid and a dysphonia characterized as weak and breathy. When muscle force production returns to normal with a period of rest, myasthenia gravis, is the likely diagnosis. Other voice and speech symptoms associated with myasthenia gravis include inspiratory stridor, reduced vocal loudness, monotone voice, hypernasality, hoarseness, and tremor

(Toth, Pap, Diozaeghy, & Sziklai, 1999). Persons with myasthenia gravis may also have an associated dysphagia. Other primary muscles involved in myasthenia gravis include the eye and eyelids, facial muscles, respiratory muscles, and sometimes limb muscles.

Features of Visual Assessment

Stroboscopy results gained from the most comprehensive study of persons with myasthenia gravis reveal fluctuating impairment of vocal fold mobility (Mao et al., 2001) either unilaterally or bilaterally with reductions in phase closure and vibratory amplitude.

Management

According to the National Institute for Neurological Disorders and Stroke (http://www .ninds.nih.gov/disorders/myasthenia_gravis/ detail_myasthenia_gravis.htm) several management strategies exist for the treatment of myasthenia gravis. These include pharmacologic treatments that act as anticholinesterase agents. These drugs help to maintain acetylcholine at the receptor site improving the neuromuscular transmission and therefore the muscle's contractile ability. Specifically, the drug blocks the active site of acetylcholinesterase, the enzyme that breaks down acetycholine. By diminishing the amount of acetylcholine broken down it gives acetylcholine a chance to complete its action. These drugs are neostigmine and pyridostigmine. Other drug classes include immunosuppressive drugs such as prednisone, cyclosporine, and azathioprine. These medications improve muscle strength by suppressing the production of abnormal antibodies.

A surgical option for myasthenia gravis includes a procedure called a thymectomy. A thymectomy removes the thymus gland and is done because the thymus gland is often abnormal in persons with myasthenia gravis.

> The main function of the thymus gland is in the processing and maturation of special lymphocytes called T-cells. T-cells help destroy invading bacteria and viruses.

Thymectomy can reduce symptoms in more than 70% of patients with myasthenia gravis by rebalancing the immune system. Other therapies used to treat myasthenia gravis include plasmapheresis, a procedure in which abnormal antibodies are removed from the blood, and high-dose intravenous immune globulin are given, which temporarily modifies the immune system and provides the body with normal antibodies from donated blood (http://www.ninds.nih.gov/disorders/myas thenia_gravis/detail_myasthenia_gravis.htm).

Hypophonia Associated with Parkinson's Disease

Description and Etiology

The etiology of Parkinson's disease (PD), thought to be a neurodegenerative disease of the extrapyramidal system, is unknown. There is evidence of both genetic and environmental triggers (Moore, West, Dawson, & Dawson, 2005; Tansey, McCoy, & Frank-Cannon, 2007; Zhang et al., 2005).

> The extrapyramidal system includes the basal ganglia, the red nucleus, the substantia nigra, the reticular formation, and the cerebellum.

Perceptual Signs and Symptoms

Parkinson's disease and the associated changes to the central nervous system cause an alteration in speech and voice. The classification of these changes to the speech and voice production system is termed hypokinetic dysarthria. Most patients with PD present vocal symptoms of decreased vocal pitch and loudness range, because of impaired intrinsic laryngeal muscle movement. Other voice characteristics include breathiness, roughness, hoarseness, and vocal tremor. The speech of person's with PD is altered in its timing with slower than normal speech rate. But, there is also evidence that PD can also result in an abnormally fast rate of speech. Most recently in a study of 121 persons with PD, acoustic evidence emerged indicating a stronger acceleration of articulatory rate and a significant reduction in the total number of pauses (Skodda & Schlegel, 2008).

Features of the Visual Assessment

Vocal fold structure and movement associated with the hypokinetic dysarthria varies as a function of the patient's age and the duration and severity of the PD. That said, sometimes upon visual laryngeal examination the vocal folds appear normal during phonation and other times they appear bowed, related most likely to the presence of muscle atrophy. In characterizing the laryngeal abnormalities of patients with PD, Perez, Ramig, Smith, and Dromey (1996) completed visual-perceptual ratings of endoscopic and laryngostroboscopic examinations of 22 persons diagnosed with PD. Of the 22 patients, 55% were rated as presenting with primarily vertical laryngeal tremor and abnormal phase closure and phase asymmetry. Vibratory amplitude and mucosal wave were judged to be normal.

Management

Parkinson's disease and the hypokinetic dysarthria associated with them, can be difficult to treat. The reason for this is that persons with PD present with a set of heterogeneous symptoms, meaning that the symptoms vary with time of day, medication state, mood, age, sex, disease severity, and so forth, and of course, patient motivation with regard to treatment interest (Denny & Behari, 1999; Jankovic, 2005).

One popular and widely used treatment for the dysphonia associated with PD is LSVT (see Chapter 7). Although there is no long-term efficacy of LSVT beyond two years and little data supporting its generalization in conversational speech, to date there are no other treatments that have been experimentally tested to the degree of LSVT. And although summary findings from several reviews on the efficacy of speech therapy indicate that there remains insufficient evidence to support speech therapy as a sole treatment in any indication of PD, this should not deter the future examination of these important multisystem treatments (Ramig, Fox, & Sapir, 2008).

Sapienza and colleagues have been using a therapy technique called expiratory muscle strength training (EMST) to study whether expiratory muscle strengthening can improve functions like breathing, cough and voice/speech in persons with PD (see Chapter 7). See also Troche et al., 2010.

Effects of dual task on the outcomes of talking and mobility are most recent suggesting that degree of cognitive loading will affect outcomes of motoric abilities (e.g. Dromey, Jarvis, Sondrup, Nissen, Foreman, & Dibble, 2010; Lapointe, Stierwalt & Maitland, 2010).

Multiple Sclerosis

Description and Etiology

Multiple sclerosis (MS) is an autoimmune and inflammatory disease of neurogenic origin within the white and gray matter of the central nervous system (Svejgaard, 2008). Demyelination and axonal damage that present from the earliest stage of the disease, account for the progressive disability. Primary progressive MS is the chronic demyelinating degenerative disorder whereas relapsing remitting MS is characterized as a gradual symptomatic deterioration. In the United States, there are approximately 400,000 people with MS, with more females diagnosed than men. Caucasians of northern European ancestry are more likely than other ethnic groups to get MS. There are identifiable patterns in the distribution of MS that may be related to genetics and demographics, such as the geographic location in which the person with MS was raised. MS is more widespread in areas that are farther from the equator and less widespread in areas closer to the equator, which may relate to the exposure to sunlight. Triggering factors that have been examined in the cause of MS for those with genetic susceptibility include exposure to environmental toxins, trace metal exposure, and climate (as described above) (Alonso, Hernan, & Ascherio, 2008; Ebers, 2008; Johansson, Ytterber, Hillert, Widen Homqvist & von Koch, 2008; Poser & Brinar, 2007).

Physical findings and symptoms reported by the patient through a case history interview help determine a diagnosis of MS. Symptoms often reported include fatigue, numbness, difficulty with walking or balance, bowel and bladder dysfunction, vision problems, depression, and other cognitive/emotional changes. Speech, voice, and swallow disorders occur less frequently and typically are demonstrated later in the disease process. As the disease progresses, symptom severity worsens (e.g., Poser & Brinar, 2004).

In order to diagnose the condition of MS there must be evidence of damage to at least two separate areas of the central nervous system and evidence that damage occurred at different points in time, at least one month apart. Imaging techniques like magnetic resonance imaging and analysis of cerebrospinal fluid are tests used to examine central nervous system damage. Visual evoked potentials are another test used to record the nervous system's electrical response to stimulation. If demyelination is present the response time of the nervous system will be reduced. Each of these tests, in combination, and not in isolation, serves to help with the diagnosis of MS (e.g., Chowdhury, Lin, & Sadiq, 2008).

Perceptual Signs and Symptoms

Ataxic, or mixed dysarthria characterize the speech production impairments in those with MS. The earliest description of speech impairments associated with MS was that of scanning speech (Hartelius, Buder, & Strand, 1997; Hartelius & Svensson, 1994). The symptoms of the speech production disorder can include abnormally long pauses between words or individual syllables of words and/or words are slurred or a hypernasal sound quality. Additionally, impaired communication, particularly difficulty raising the vocal loudness may occur due to the inability to generate sufficient expiratory muscle force. Weak phonation, characterized by harshness, and disturbances of the respiratory cycle are two of five major characteristics of the speech impairment associated with MS, resulting from weakened expiratory and /or laryngeal muscles (Darley, Brown, & Goldstein, 1972; Dogan et al., 2007; Espir, Watkin, & Smith, 1966).

Features of Visual Assessment

Individuals with MS demonstrate reduced vocal fold closure upon laryngeal examination (Hartelius, Buder, & Strand, 1997). Dogan et al (2007) reported that 16 of 27 patients with MS who were examined stroboscopically had a posterior glottal chink/opening. Aside from the voice effects associated with laryngeal muscle weakness, reduced laryngeal muscle strength impairs sufficient vocal fold closure required for cough and other functions like swallowing.

Management

Currently, there are no management therapies that directly modify the course of MS but there are a broad range of available symptomatic treatments. The details of each of the treatments are beyond the scope of this text; however, they include the use of pharmacologic therapies that are immune modulating drugs administered as injectable treatments or infusion treatments. These include Interferon beta 1a and 1b, chemotherapeutic agents such as mitoxantrone administered by IV, as well as others. Corticosteroids such as prednisone either IV or taken orally may be used, as well as pain medications and antidepressants, if symptomatic. Diet and lifestyle modifications, exercise therapies, and alternative and complementary therapies are also highly advocated and most typically a combination of all or most of these are prescribed or tried by the patient with MS (Baumhackl, 2008; Ciccone et al., 2008).

Amyotrophic Lateral Sclerosis

Description and Etiology

Amyotrophic lateral sclerosis (ALS), commonly called Lou Gehrig's disease is one of the most devastating neurologic disease processes. Considered a motor neuron disease, it fatally attacks the neurons responsible for controlling voluntary muscle contraction (movement) http://www.ninds.nih.gov/disorders/amyotrophiclateralsclerosis/detail_ALS.htm. Although a small percentage of the individuals stricken with ALS have genetically inherited the disease, the disease process affects most individuals randomly and they present with no associated risk factors with its onset.

Perceptual Signs and Symptoms

Initially, the motor symptoms associated with ALS are not so obvious. A person may at first experience weakness or cramping in their muscle(s) and eventually muscle(s) twitching. The first motor symptoms tend to be in the leg. In about one-quarter of the cases of ALS, the symptoms may start off in the corticobulbar system affecting the muscle movements involved in voice, speech, and swallowing via the cranial nerves.

> Muscle twitching is referred to as fasciculations.

When respiratory muscles become involved, particularly the diaphragm, the patient with ALS will likely be placed on a ventilator to aid breathing. With regard to the voice and speech production deterioration, the mixed dysarthria is characterized by weak voice, hoarseness, roughness, and strained voice and some hypernasality with decreased speech intelligibility and slow rate of speech.

Features of Visual Assessment

Chen and Garrett (2005), through a retrospective review, diagnosed 1,759 patients with voice disturbance that came to both a voice center and neurology clinic with ALS. Incomplete vocal fold closure was the commonly presenting laryngoscopic finding of these patients. Chen and Garret cautioned that neuromuscular disease was missed in 8 of 19 ALS patients seen by the otolaryngologists and that patients presenting with a combination of dysarthria, dysphonia, and dysphagia should be referred to Neurology with a diagnosis of

ALS considered. A case report by Watts and Vanryckeghem (2001) discussed similar laryngoscopic features for patients with ALS.

Management

There is no cure for ALS. With regard to treatment of the dysarthria (dysphonia included), augmentative communication devices may best serve the patient because of the rapid neurodegeneration of muscle function (Brownlee & Palovcak, 2007) and critical need to functionally communicate. Augmentative devices can include computer-based communication systems and/or speech synthesizers. The swallow difficulties become life threatening and ultimately feeding tubes are required when the patient can no longer feed him/herself. The use of a feeding tube reduces the risk of choking and pneumonia that can result from inhaling liquids into the lungs.

Most recently, the Food and Drug Administration has approved the first drug for treatment of ALS called riluzole (Rilutek). Clinical trials with ALS patients showed that riluzole prolongs survival by several months, mainly in those with difficulty swallowing by reducing the motor neuron damage.

Huntington's Disease/Chorea

Diagnosis and Etiology

Huntington's disease (HD) is an inherited autosomal dominant disorder with complete penetrance resulting from a mutation on chromosome 4. Neuronal destruction with HD is differentially targeted to the basal ganglia and cerebral cortex but it is not understood why.

> Penetrance is the chance that a clinical state will occur when a particular genotype is present.

Perceptual Signs and Symptoms

Considered a hyperkinetic neurologic disorder because of its effect on the basal ganglia, HD produces abnormal and jerky movements of the body called chorea. In 1986, Ramig reported on one of the first preliminary study outcomes of HD voice. Although the research article discussed the findings from an acoustic analysis of HD voice, the examination also yielded information about the voice quality. The voice of those with HD was characterized by adductory and abductory stoppages, a hoarse and rough voice quality, and variability in the pitch and loudness of the voice. The dysarthria associated with HD is also characterized by slowness of articulatory movements and difficulty coordinating breathing with speech (see Duffy, 2005 for further details of the hyperkinetic dysarthria related with HD).

The voice symptoms associated with HD may seem similar to other neurologic/neurodegenerative diseases, as described earlier, that is why other signs and symptoms like dysphagia and choreic movements of the limbs and/or oral structures will help differentiate the disorder, but the ultimate diagnostic test for HD comes from genetic testing.

Features of Visual Assessment

Of the few reported studies on the laryngoscopic and/laryngostroboscopic characteristics with HD, laryngeal movement is characterized by adductor spasm.

Management

Today, drug treatments for neurologic diseases are developed to try to protect the central nervous system from further breakdown or in the case of inherited disease process, potentially to slow or negate the onset of the condition. This drug feature is referred to as neuroprotective. In the case of HD, there is no drug to date that is effective in providing a neuroprotective therapy. Several different types of drugs have been tried to treat the symptoms of HD including dopamine depleters for motor dysfunction, antidepressants for mood disorders, antiglutamatergic drugs (drugs designed to prevent cell damage), GABA agonists (drugs used to relax the body, antispasmodic effect), antiepileptic medications, and acetylcholinesterase inhibitors (to diminish the activity of the enzyme that breaks down acetylcholine, see explanation under Myasthenia Gravis and Botox). See review of drug treatments clinically investigated for HD by Venuto et al., 2012. Recently, surgical approaches including pallidotomy, deep brain stimulation, and fetal cell transplants have also been tried with patients having HD (Adam & Jankovic, 2008; Bonelli & Hofman, 2004). In these cases, the individual outcomes were very reliant on the patient profile of the disease and its symptoms. As such the results of these surgical approaches, whether good or poor, should not be over generalized to all patients with HD.

> Pallidotomy is a surgical procedure where cells are killed in a region of the brain called the globus pallidus with the intent to reduce the symptoms of rigidity, tremor and slowness of movement.

> The globus pallidus is a small part of the basal ganglia.

Progressive Supranuclear Palsy

Description and Etiology

Progressive supranuclear palsy (PSP) is another neurodegenerative disorder with unknown etiology, yet symptoms reflect an abnormal accumulation of the tau protein in the basal ganglia, brainstem, prefrontal cortex, and cerebellum resulting in neurofibrillary tangles. "The diagnosis of PSP is exclusively clinical. Use of laboratory tests and imaging exams cannot detect the disease, but rather help rule out other pathologies" (Zampieri & Di Fabio, 2006, p. 872).

> A neurofibrous tangle is a twisted fiber of the protein tau. The protein tau is important for maintaining the internal structure of a cell.

Perceptual Signs and Symptoms

See Table 6–2.

Features of Visual Assessment

The laryngeal function is not well defined for the population diagnosed with PSP, although some case reports reveal adductor laryngeal spasm during inspiration and/or bilateral vocal fold abductor paralysis (Yokoji, Nakamura, & Ideda, 1997).

Management

To date, there are no effective medications or surgical treatments to cure or delay the progression of the symptoms in PSP. Although palliative interventions (treatments to alleviate symptoms without curing the disease) may be used to alleviate major symptoms, no drug efficiently treats the origin of the problem.

Voice Therapy. Clinically, the use of therapies like the LSVT, delayed auditory feedback, and alternative augmentative communication have been used therapeutically for PSP (i.e., Hanson & Metter, 1980); given the complex relationship between visual, cognitive, language, and speech functioning in these patients, outcomes are usually less than optimal with little generalization or maintenance of treatment effects. This experience can be frustrating and tire-

Table 6–2. Progressive Supranuclear Palsy Impairments

Memory impairment	*Learning*	*Executive Function*
Mild to moderate impaired recall and access to stored information, but no deficits in recognition	Deficit in generating implicit procedural rules, but explicit learning deficits partially compensated by using semantic cues	Severe, early planning deficit; deficits in problem-solving; concept-formation; abstract reasoning
Frontal Signs	*Other Cognitive Factors*	*Visuospatial Impairments*
Utilization, prehension, and imitation behavior	Severe slowness in thought processes	Visual grasping; vertical plane inattention; spatial perception
Aphasia	*Apraxia*	*Dysarthria* (Kluin et al., 2001)
Decreased letter fluency; transcortical motor or dynamic aphasia	Mild ideomotor apraxia; no ideatory apraxia	1. Hypokinetic dysarthria, specifically loudness. 2. Spastic dysarthria. 3. Ataxic dysarthria

Source: Adapted from Magherini and Litvan, 2005.

some for the patient, the therapist and the caregiver, as success in therapy does not transfer to daily interactions. Therefore, it is essential to determine how cognitive and language factors affect speech production in an empirical manner based on a theoretical framework in order to identify appropriate therapeutic targets (e.g. Helfer, Chevalier, & Freyman, 2010).

Multiple System Atrophy (MSA)

Description and Etiology

Occurring about half as frequently as PSP, MSA is a rapidly progressive neurodegenerative disease process that appears related to glial changes and glial-neuronal interactions (Castellani, 1998) and relatively widespread degeneration of myelin formed by the glial cell, the oligodendrocyte (Matsuo et al., 1998). There are several subtypes of MSA

and Castellani provides a very good review of these subtypes and the pathophysiologic signs associated with each type. The disorder can be further subdivided into predominant cerebellar ataxia (MSA-C) and predominant parkinsonism (MSA-P) with cognitive dysfunction observed more frequently with the parkinsonism type (Kawai et al., 2008). MSA is frequently misdiagnosed as idiopathic Parkinson's disease (PD) , but can be conclusively distinguished from PD through a variety of biochemical markers (Goldstein et al., 2008).

Perceptual Signs and Symptoms

Voice quality associated with MSA is breathy and strained with episodes of reduced vocal loudness, monopitch, and monoloudness and could be associated with a bilateral vocal fold paresis (Blumin & Berke, 2002). The speech production disorder is a flaccid dysarthria typified by imprecise consonants, reduced speech intelligibility, variations in rate, and rate-slowing, suggesting a flaccid type of dysarthria (Hanson, Ludlow, & Bassich, 1992).

Features of Visual Assessment

Large samples of laryngostroboscopic findings do not exist for patients with MSA, but some case reports indicate the presence of bilateral vocal fold paresis with the potential for airway obstruction (Blumin & Berke, 2002). Interestingly, in some cases inspiratory stridor and narrowing of the glottal airway are more apparent during sleep than wake. Seven patients with MSA who had nocturnal stridor were studied with laryngoscopy during both sleep and wake. When awake, about half of the patients with MSA demonstrated normal vocal fold movement, half demonstrated mild glottal restriction with abduction, and one demonstrated paradoxic movement. When asleep, all showed paradoxic movement accompanied by high pitched inspiratory stridor (Isozaki et al., 1996). This comparison points out very well how different tasks, conditions, and environment can influence laryngeal behavior and as such should be considered in the assessment plan particularly for complex neurologic cases. Though frequently observed in early stages of the disorder, this laryngeal dysfunction is observed with increasing frequency as the disease progresses and is associated with earlier mortality compared with individuals with MSA but no laryngeal dysfunction (Yamaguchi, Arai, Asahina, & Hattori, 2003).

Management

There is no cure for MSA. The time from diagnosis to death is typically 5 to 10 years. A number of drugs are used to treat the many symptoms of MSA but the progression does not seem to be slowed by their use. These drugs include treatment for limb motor disturbances, orthostatic hypertension and depression as well as others (http://www.shydrager.org).

Other Neurologic Cases

Cerebral vascular accident (CVA) and traumatic brain injury are complex conditions with different symptomotology depending on the extent of the brain damage. The laryngeal examination will reveal a central laryngeal dysmotility disorder with the representation of movement being either hypo- or hypertonic depending on the location of the CVA or traumatic event. With traumatic brain injury, rather than an isolated voice disorder the patient may demonstrate reductions in speech intelligibility, aprosodia and potentially post-traumatic mutism. McHenry (2000) found the most frequently occurring abnormal voice quality to be breathiness.

Management of Voice in CVA

Recently, the effectiveness of a 4-week LSVT program was reported for the treatment of 10 individuals with dysarthria following CVA. Perceptual and acoustic measures and everyday communication outcome measures were made before, immediately following and 6 months post LSVT treatment. Following treatment, patients demonstrated increased vocal loudness in sustained phonation and connected speech, increased vocal frequency range, and improved word and sentence intelligibility (Wenke, Theodoros, & Cornwell, 2008).

Summary

Neurologic voice disorders can originate from either peripheral and/ or central nervous system disorders. The etiology of these disorders is often difficult to define. Therefore, treatment is often focused on symptomatic management of the condition. These include surgical, pharmacologic, and behavioral options. Chapter 7 covers behavioral management of voice disorders including those of neurologic origin.

References

Adam, O. R., & Jankovic, J. (2008). Symptomatic treatment of Huntington's disease. *Neurotherapeutics*, 5(2), 181–197.

Adler, C. H., Bansberg, S. F., Hentz, J. G., Ramig, L. O., Buder, E. H., Witt, K., . . . , Caviness, J. N. (2004). Botulinum toxin type A for treating voice tremor. *Archives of Neurology*, 61(9), 1416–1420.

Adler, C. H., Edwards, B.W., & Bansberg, S. F. (1997). Female predominance in spasmodic dysphonia. *Journal of Neurology, Neurosurgery and Psychiatry*, 63(5), 688.

Alonso, A., Hernan, M. A., & Ascherio, A. (2008). Allergy, family history of autoimmune diseases, and the risk of multiple sclerosis. *Acta Neurologica Scandanavica*, 117(1), 15–20.

Arai, M., Endo, S., Oshima, G., & Yagi, Y. (2011). A case of amyotrphic lateral sclerosi with bilateral vocal cord paralysis necessitating tracheotomy. *Rinsho Shinkeigaku*, 51(10), 765–769.

Aronson, A. E., Brown, J. R., Litin, E. M., & Pearson, J. S. (1968). Spastic dysphonia. I. Voice, neurologic, and psychiatric aspects. *Journal of Speech and Hearing Disorders*, 33(3), 203–218.

Baumhackl, U. (2008). The search for a balance between short and long-term treatment outcomes in multiple sclerosis. *Journal of Neurology*, 255(1), 75–83.

Baylor, C. R., Yorkston, K. M., Eadie, T. L. & Maronian, N. C. (2007). The psychosocial consequences of Botox injections for spasmodic dysphonia: A qualitative study of patients' experiences. *Journal of Voice*, 21(2), 231–247.

Benninger, M. S., Gillen, J. B. & Altman, J. S. (1998). Changing etiology of vocal fold immobility. *Laryngoscope*, 108(9), 1346–1350.

Blitzer, A., Brin, M. F., & Stewart, C. F. (1988). Botulinum toxin management of spasmodic dysphonia (laryngeal dystonia): A 12-year experience on more than 900 patients, *Laryngoscope*, 108(10), 1435–1441.

Bloch, C. S., Hirano, M., & Gould, W. J. (1985). Symptom improvement of spastic dysphonia in response to phonatory tasks. *Annals of Otology, Rhinology, and Laryngology*, 94(Pt. 1), 51–54.

Blumin, J. H., & Berke, G. S. (2002). Bilateral vocal fold paresis and multiple system atrophy. *Archives of Otolaryngology-Head and Neck Surgery*, 128(12), 1404–1407.

Bocchino, J. V., & Tucker, H. M. (1978). Recurrent laryngeal nerve pathology in spasmodic dysphonia. *Laryngoscope*, 88(8, Pt. 1), 1274–1278.

Bonelli, R. M., & Hofmann, P. (2004). A review of the treatment options for Huntington's disease. *Expert Opinions on Pharmacotherapy*, 5(4), 767–776.

Boutsen, F., Cannito, M. P., Taylor, M., & Bender, B. (2002). Botox treatment in adductor spasmodic dysphonia: A meta-analysis. *Journal of Speech, Language, and Hearing Research*, 45(3), 469–481.

Braden, M. N., & Hapner, E. R. (2008). Listening: The key to diagnosing spasmodic dysphonia. *Society of Otorhinolaryngology and Head-Neck Nurses*, 26(1), 8–12.

Brownlee, A., & Palvocak, M. (2007). The role of augmentative communication devices in the medical management of ALS. *Neurorehabilitation*, 22(6), 445–450.

Castellani, R. (1998). Multiple system atrophy: Clues from inclusion. *American Journal of Pathology*, 153(3), 671–676.

Chen, A., & Garrett, C. G. (2005). Otolaryngologic presentations of amyotrophic lateral sclerosis. *Otolaryngology-Head and Neck Surgery*, 132(3), 500–504.

Chen, H. C., Jen, Y. M., Wang, C. H., Lee, J. C., & Lin, Y. S. (2007). Etiology of vocal cord paralysis. *Journal of Otorhinolaryngology and Its Related Specialties*, 69(3), 167–171.

Chowdhury, S. A., Lin, J., & Sadiq, S. A. (2008). Specificity and correlation with disease activity of cerebrospinal fluid osteopontin levels in patients with multiple sclerosis. *Archives of Neurology*, 65(2), 232–235.

Ciccone, A., Berretta, S., Brusaferri, F., Galea, I., Prottic, A., & Spreafico, C. (2008). Corticosteroids for the long-term treatment in multiple sclerosis. *Cochrane Database System Review*, 23(1), CD006264. Review.

D'Alatri, L., Galla, S., Rigante, M., Antonelli, O., Buldrini, S., & Marchese, M. R. (2007). Role of early voice therapy in patients affected by unilateral vocal fold paralysis. *Journal of Laryngology and Otology, 24,* 1–6.

Darley, F. L., Aronson, A. E., & Brown, J. R. (1975). *Motor speech disorders.* Philadephia, PA: W. B. Saunders.

Darley, F. L., Brown, J. R., & Goldstein, N. P. (1972). Dysarthria in multiple sclerosis. *Journal of Speech and Hearing Research, 15,* 229–245.

Dedo, H. H. (1976). Recurrent laryngeal nerve section for spastic dysphonia. *Annals of Otology, Rhinology, and Laryngology, 85,* 451–459.

Deleyiannis, F. W., Gillespie, M., Bielamowicz, S., Yamashita, T., & Ludlow, C. L. (1999). Laryngeal long latency response conditioning in abductor spasmodic dysphonia. *Annals of Otology, Rhinology, and Laryngology, 108*(6), 612–619.

Dennis, D. P. & Kashima, H. (1989). Carbon dioxide laser cordectomy for treatment of bilateral vocal cord paralysis. *Annals of Otology, Rhinology, and Laryngology, 98*(12 Pt. 1), 930–934.

Denny, A. P., & Behari, M. (1999). Motor fluctuations in Parkinson's disease. *Journal of Neurological Sciences, 165*(1), 18–23.

Dogan, M., Midi, I., Yazici, M. A., Kocak, I., Gunal, D., & Sehitoglu, M. A (2007). Objective and subjective evaluation of voice quality in multiple sclerosis. *Journal of Voice, 21*(6), 735–740.

Dromey, C., Jarvis, E., Sondrup, S., Nissen, S., Foreman, K. B., & Dibble. L. E., (2010). Bidirectional interference between speech and postural stability in individuals with Parkinson's disease. *International Journal of Speech-Language Pathology, 12*(5), 446–454.

Duffy, J. (2005). *Motor speech disorders: Substrates, differential diagnosis, and management.* Amsterdam, Netherlands: Elsevier.

Dursun, G., Boynukalin, S., Bagis Ozgursoy, O., & Coruh, I. (2008). Long-term results of different treatment modalities for glottic insufficiency. *American Journal of Otolaryngology, 29*(1), 7–12.

Dursun, G., Sataloff, R. T., Spiegel, J. R., Mandel, S., Heuer, R. J., & Rosen, D. C. (1996). Superior laryngeal nerve paresis and paralysis. *Journal of Voice, 10*(2), 206–211.

Ebers, G. C. (2008). Environmental factors and multiple sclerosis [Review]. *Lancet Neurology, 7*(3), 268–277.

Eckley, C. A., Sataloff, R. T., Hawkshaw, M., Spiegel, J. R., & Mandel, S. (1998). Voice range in superior laryngeal nerve paresis and paralysis. *Journal of Voice, 12*(3), 340–348.

Edgar, J. D., Sapienza, C. M., Bidus, K., & Ludlow, C. L. (2001). Acoustic measures of symptoms in abductor spasmodic dysphonia, *Journal of Voice, 15*(3), 362–372.

Erickson, M. L. (2003). Effects of voicing and syntactic complexity on sign expression in adductor spasmodic dysphonia. *American Journal of Speech-Language Pathology, 12*(4), 416–424.

Espir, M. L., Watkins, S. M., Smith, H. V. (1966). Paroxysmal dysarthria and other transient neurological disturbances in disseminated sclerosis. *Journal of Neurology, Neurosurgery and Psychiatry, 29*(4), 323–330.

Essential tremor. (n.d.). Retrieved from http://www.mayoclinic.com/health/essential-tremor/DS00367

Farrior, J. B., & Bagby, R. A. (1950). Bilateral laryngeal paralysis: Relief of respiratory obstruction by arytenoidectomy. *Journal of the Florida Medical Association, 36*(11), 692.

Finnegan, E. M., Luschei, E. S., Barkmeier, J. M., & Hoffman, H. T. (2003). Synchrony of laryngeal muscle activity in persons with vocal tremor. *Archives of Otolaryngology-Head and Neck Surgery, 129*(3), 313–318.

Ford, C. N., Bless, D. M. & Lowery, J. D. (1990). Indirect laryngoscopic approach for injection of botulinum toxin in spasmodic dysphonia. *Otolaryngology-Head and Neck Surgery, 103,* 752–758.

Goldstein, D. S., Holmes, C., Bentho, O., Sato, T., Moak, J., Sharabi, Y., Imrich, R., Conant, S., & Eldadah, B. A (2008). Biomarkers to detect central dopamine deficiency and distinguish Parkinson disease from multiple system atrophy. *Parkinsonism and Related Disorders,14*(8), 600–607.

Green, D. C., Berke, G. S., Ward, P. H., & Gerratt, B. R. (1992). Point-touch technique of botulinum toxin injection for the treatment of spasmodic dysphonia. *Annals of Otology, Rhinology, and Laryngology, 101,* 883–887.

Hanson, D. G., Ludlow, C. L., & Bassich, C. (1992). Vocal fold paresis in Shy-Drager syndrome. *Annals of Otology, Rhinology, and Laryngology, 92*(1), 85–90.

Hanson, W. R., & Metter, E. J. (1980). DAF as instrumental treatment for dysarthria in progressive supranuclear palsy: A case report. *Journal of Speech and Hearing Disorders, 45*(2), 268–276.

Hartelius, L., Buder, E. H., & Strand, E. A. (1997). Long-term phonatory instability in individuals with multiple sclerosis. *Journal of Speech, Language, and Hearing Research, 40*(5), 1056–1072.

Hartelius L., & Svensson, P. (1994). Speech and swallowing symptoms associated with Parkinson's disease and multiple sclerosis: A survey. *Folia Phoniatrica Logopaedia, 46*(1), 9–17.

Helfer, K. S., Chevalier, J. & Freyman, R. L. 2010). Aging, spatial cues, and single-versus dual task performance in competing speech perception. *Journal of the Acoustical Society of America, 128*(6), 3625–3633.

Helmus, C. (1972). Microsurgical thyrotomy and arytenoidectomy for bilateral recurrent laryngeal nerve paralysis. *Laryngoscope, 82*(3), 491–503.

Henschen, T. L., & Burton, N. G. (1978). Treatment of spastic dysphonia by EMG biofeedback. *Biofeedback and Self-Regulation, 3*(1), 91–96.

Heuer, R. J., Sataloff, R. T., Emerick, K., Rulnick, R., Baroody, M., Spiegel, J. R., Durson, G., & Butler, J. (1997). Unilateral recurrent laryngeal nerve paralysis: The importance of "preoperative" voice therapy. *Journal of Voice, 11*(1), 88–94. http://www.ninds.nih.gov/disorders/amyotrophiclateralsclerosis/detail_ALS.html. Accessed March 2012.

Isozaki, E., Naito, A., Horiguchi, S., Kawamura, R., Hayashida, T., & Tanabe, H. (2005). Early diagnosis and stage classification of vocal cord abductor paralysis in patients with multiple system atrophy. *Journal of Neurology, Neurosurgery, and Psychiatry, 60*(4), 399–402.

Jankovic, J. (2005). Motor fluctuations and dyskinesias in Parkinson's disease: Clinical manifestations [Review]. *Movement Disorders, 20*(11), S11–S16.

Johansson, S., Ytterber, C., Hillert, J., Widen Homqvist, L., & von Koch, L. (2008). A longitudinal study of variations in and predictors of fatigue in multiple sclerosis. *Journal of Neurosurgery and Psychiatry, 79*(4), 454–457.

Kawai, Y., Suenaga, M., Takeda, A., Ito, M., Watanabe, H., Tanaka, F., . . . Sobue, G. (2008). Cognitive impairments in multiple system atrophy: MSA-C vs. MSA-P. *Neurology, 15*(70, Pt. 2), 1390–1396.

Kimaid, P. A., Quagliato, E. M., Crespo, A. N., Wolf, A., Viana, M. A., & Resende, L. A. (2004). Laryngeal electromyography in movement disorders: Preliminary data. *Arquivos de Neuro-Psiquiatria, 62*(3A), 741–744.

Klotz, D. A., Maronian, N. C., Waugh, P. F., Shahinfar, A., Robinson, L., & Hillel, A. (2004). Findings of multiple muscle involvement in a study of 214 patients with laryngeal dystonia using fine-wire electromyography. *Annals of Otology, Rhinology, and Laryngology, 113*(8), 602–612.

Koriwchak, M., Netterville, J. L., Snowden, T., Courey, M., & Ossoff, R. (1996). Alternating unilateral botulinum toxin type A injections for spasmodic dysphonia. *Laryngoscope, 106,* 1476–1481.

Kosaki, H., Iwamura, S., & Yamazaki, I. (1999). Histologic study of the recurrent laryngeal nerve in spasmodic dysphonia. *Otolaryngology-Head and Neck Surgery, 120*(1), 129–133.

Lapointe, L. L., Stierwalt, J. A., & Maitland, C. G. (2010). Talking while walking: Cognitive loading and injurious falls in Parkinson's disease. *International Journal of Speech Language Pathology, 12*(5), 455–459.

Li, A. J., John, M. M., Jackson-Menaldi, C., Dailey, S. Heman-Ackah, Y., Meratia, A., & Rubin, A. D. (2011). Glottic closure patterns: type 1 thyroplasty versus type 1 thyroplasty with arytenoids adduction. *Journal of Voice, 25*(3), 259–264.

Lorenz, R. R., Esclamado, R. M., Teker, A. M., Strome, M., Scharpf, J., Hicks, D., Milstein, C., & Lee, W. T. (2008). Ansa cervicalis to recurrent laryngeal nerve anastomosis for unilateral vocal fold paralysis: Experience of a single institution. *Annals of Otology, Rhinology, and Laryngology, 117*(1), 40–45.

Ludlow, C. L., Bagley, J., Yin, S. G., & Koda, J. (1992). A comparison of injection techniques using botulinum toxin injection for the treatment of the spasmodic dysphonias. *Journal of Voice, 6,* 380–386.

Ludlow, C. L., & Connor, N. (1987). Dynamic aspects of phonatory control in spasmodic dysphonia, J*ournal of Speech and Hearing Research, 30*(2), 197–206.

Ludlow, C. L. & Mann, E. A. (2000). Management of spasmodic dysphonia. In J. Rubin, R. Sataloff, & G. Korovin, (Eds.), *Diagnosis and treatment of voice disorders* (2nd ed.). San Diego, CA: Singular.

Ludlow, C. L., Schultz, G. M., Yamashita, T., & Deleyiannis, F. W. (1995). Abnormalities in long latency responses to superior laryngeal nerve stimulation in adductor spasmodic dysphonia. *Annals of Otology, Rhinology, and Laryngology, 104*(12), 928–935.

Lundy, D. S., Casiano, R. R., Lu, F. L., & Xue, J. W. (1996). Abnormal soft palate posturing in patients with laryngeal movement disorders. *Journal of Voice,* 10(*4*), *348–353.*

Magherini, A., & Litvan, I. (2005). Cognitive and behavioral aspects of PSP since Steele, Richardson, and Olszewski's description of PSP 40 years ago and Albert's delineation of the subcortical dementia 30 years ago. *Neurocase, 11,* 250–262.

Maloney, A. P., & Morrison, M. D. (1994). A comparison of the efficacy of unilateral versus bilateral botulinum toxin injections in the treatment of adductor spasmodic dysphonia. *Journal of Otolaryngology, 23*(3), 160–164.

Mao, V., Abaza, M., Spiegel, J. R., Mandel, S., Hawkshaw, R., Heuer, R. J., & Sataloff, R. T. (2001). Laryngeal myasthenia gravis: Report of 40 cases. *Journal of Voice, 15*(1), 122–130.

Matsuo, A., Akiguchi, I., Lee. G. C., McGeer, E. G., McGeer, P. L., & Kimura, J. (1998). Myelin degeneration in multiple system atrophy detected by unique. *American Journal of Pathology, 153,* 735–744.

McHenry, M. (2000). Acoustic characteristics of voice after severe traumatic brain injury. *Laryngoscope, 110*(7), 1157–1161.

Mendelsohn, A. H., Sung, M. W., Berke, G. S., & Chhetri, D. K. (2007). Strobokymographic and videostroboscopic analysis of vocal fold motion in unilateral superior laryngeal nerve paralysis. *Annals of Otology, Rhinology, and Laryngology, 116*(2), 85–91.

Merson, R. M., & Ginsberg, A. P. (1979). Spasmodic dysphonia:abductor type A. A clinical report of acoustic, aerodynamic and perceptual characteristics, *Laryngoscope, 89*(1), 129–138.

Miller, R. H., & Woodson, G. E. (1991). Treatment options in spasmodic dysphonia, *Otolaryngologic Clinics of North America, 24*(5), 1227–1237.

Morgan, J. E., Zraick, R. I., Griffin, A. W., Bowen, T. L., & Johnson, F. L. (2007). Injection versus medialization laryngoplasty for the treatment of unilateral vocal fold paralysis. *Laryngoscope, 117*(11), 2068–2074.

Moringlane, J. R., Putzer, M., & Barry, W. J. (2004). Bilateral high-frequency electrical impulses to the thalamus reduce voice tremor: Acoustic and electroglottographic analysis: A case report. *European Archives of Otorhinolaryngology, 261*(6), 334–336.

Moore, D. J., West, A. B., Dawson, V. L., & Dawson, T. M. (2005). Molecular pathophysiology of Parkinson's disease. *Annual Review of Neuroscience, 28,* 57–87.

Myasthenia gravis fact page. Retrieved from http://www.ninds.nih.gov/disorders/myasthenia_gravis/detail_myasthenia_gravis.htm

National Institute of Neurological Disease and Stroke. *Amyotrophic lateral sclerosis fact sheet.* Retrieved from http://www.ninds.nih.gov/disorders/amyotrophiclateralsclerosis/detail_amyotrophic lateralsclerosis.htm

National Institute of Neurological Disease and Stroke. *Myasthenia gravis fact sheet.* Retrieved from http://www.ninds.nih.gov/disorders/myasthenia_gravis/detail_myasthenia_gravis.htm

Newman, A. N., & Becker, S. P. (1981). Superior laryngeal nerve paralysis and benign thyroid disease. *Archives of Otolaryngology, 107*(2), 117–119.

Pahwa, R., & Lyons, K. E. (2003). Essential tremor: Differential diagnosis and current therapy. *American Journal of Medicine, 115*(2), 34–42.

Perez, K. S., Ramig, L. O., Smith, M. F., & Dromey, C. (1996). The Parkinson larynx:

Tremor and videostroboscopic findings. *Journal of Voice*, *10*(4), 354–361.

Poser, C. M., & Brinar, V. V. (2004). The nature of multiple sclerosis. *Clinical Neurology and Neurosurgery*, *106*(3), 159–171.

Poser, C. M., & Brinar, V. V. (2007). The accuracy of prevalence rates of multiple sclerosis: A critical review. *Neuroepidemiology*, *29*(3–4), 150–155.

Ramig, L. O. (1986). Acoustic analysis of phonation in patients with Huntington's disease. *Annals of Otology, Rhinology, and Laryngology*, *3*, 288–293.

Ramig, L., Bonitati, C., Lemke, J., & Horii, Y. (1994). Voice treatment for patients with Parkinson disease: Development of an approach and preliminary efficacy data. *Journal of Medical Speech Language Pathology*, *2*, 191–209.

Ramig, L. O., Fox, C., & Sapir, S. (2008). Speech treatment for Parkinson's disease. *Expert Review of Neurotherapeutics*, *8*(2), 299–311.

Randhawa, P. S., Ramsey, A. D., & Rubin, J. S. (2008). Foreign body reaction to polymethylsiloxane gel (Bioplastique trademark) after vocal fold augmentation. *Journal of Laryngology and Otology*, *122*(7), 750–753.

Ravits, J. M., Aronson, A. E., DeSanto, L. W., & Dyck, P. J. (1979). No morphometric abnormality recurrent laryngeal nerve in spastic dysphonia. *Neurology*, *29*(10) 1376–1382.

Remacle, M., & Lawson, G. (2007). Results with collagen injection into the vocal folds for medialization. *Current Opinion in Otolaryngology and Head and Neck Surgery*, *15*(3), 148–152.

Rhew, K., Fiedler, D. A., & Ludlow, C. L. (1994). Technique for injection of botulinum toxin through the flexible nasolaryngoscope. *Otolaryngology-Head and Neck Surgery*, *111*(6), 787–794.

Roehm, P., & Rosen, C. (2004). Dynamic voice assessment using flexible laryngoscopy—how I do it: A targeted problem and its solution. *American Journal of Otolaryngology*, *25*(2), 138–141.

Rontal, E., & Rontal, M. (2003). Permanent medialization of the paralyzed vocal fold utilizing botulinum toxin and Gelfoam. *Journal of Voice*, *17*(3), 434–441.

Rosenfield, D. B., Donovan, D. T, Sulek, M., Viswanath, N. S., Inbody, G. P., & Nudelman, H. B. (1991). Neurologic aspects of spasmodic dysphonia. *Journal of Otolaryngology*, *19*(4), 231–236.

Roy, N., Gouse, M., Mauszycki, S. C., Merrill, R. M., & Smith, M. E. (2005). Task specificity in adductor spasmodic dysphonia versus muscle tension dysphonia. *Laryngoscope*, *115*(2), 311–316.

Roy, N., Mauszycki, S. C., Merrill, R.M., Gouse, M., & Smith, M. E. (2007). Toward improved differential diagnosis of adductor spasmodic dysphonia and muscle tension dysphonia. *Folia Phoniatrica*, *59*(2), 83–90.

Sapienza, C. M., Cannito, M. P., Murry, T., Branski, R., & Woodson, G. (2002). Acoustic variations in reading produced by speakers with spasmodic dysphonia pre-Botox injection and within early stages of post-Botox injection. *Journal of Speech Language and Hearing Research*, *45*(5), 830–843.

Sapienza, C. M., Walton, S., & Murry, T. (1999). Acoustic variations in adductor spasmodic dysphonia as a function of speech task. *Journal of Speech and Hearing Research*, *42*(1), 127–140.

Sasaki, C. T., Hundal, J. S., & Kim, Y. H. (2005). Protective glottic closure: Biomechanical effects of selective laryngeal denervation. *Annals of Otology, Rhinology, and Laryngology*, *114*(4), 271–275.

Schweinfurth, J. M., Billante, M., & Courey, M. S. (2002). Risk factors and demographics in patients with spasmodic dysphonia. *Laryngoscope*, *112*(2), 220–223.

Sercarz, J. A., Berke, G. S., Ming, Y., Gerratt, B. R., & Natividad, M. (1992).Videostroboscopy of human vocal fold paralysis. *Annals of Otology, Rhinology, and Laryngology*, *101*(7), 567–577.

Shiotani, A., Saito, K., Araki, K., Moro, K., & Watabe, K. (2007). Gene therapy for laryngeal paralysis. *Annals of Otology, Rhinology, and Laryngology*, *116*(2), 115–122.

Simonyan, K., Tovar-Moll, F., Ostuni, J., Hallett, M., Kalasinsky, V. F., Lewin- Smith, M. R., . . . Ludlow, C. L. (2008). Focal white matter changes in spasmodic dysphonia: A combined diffusion tensor imaging and neuropathological study. *Brain*, *131*,(Pt. 2), 447–459.

Skodda, S., & Schlegel U. (2008). Speech rate and rhythm in Parkinson's disease. *Movement Disorders, 23*(7), 985–992.

Stemple, J. C., Lee, L., D'Amico, B., & Pickup, B. (1994). Efficacy of vocal function exercises as a method of improving voice production. *Journal of Voice, 8*, 271–278.

Su, W. F., Hsu, Y. D., Chen, H. C. & Sheng, H. (2007). Laryngeal reinnervation by ansa cervicalis nerve implantation for unilateral vocal cord paralysis in humans. *Journal of the American College of Surgery, 204*(1), 64–72.

Svejgaard, A. (2008). The immunogenetics of multiple sclerosis. *Immunogenetics, 60*(6), 275–286.

Tansey, M. G., McCoy, M. K., & Frank-Cannon, T. C. (2007). Neuroinflammatory mechanisms in Parkinson's disease: Potential environmental triggers, pathways, and targets for early therapeutic intervention. *Experimental Neurology, 208*(1), 1–25.

Thompson, J. W., Ward, P. H., & Schwartz, I. R. (1984). Experimental studies for correction of superior laryngeal nerve paralysis by fusion of the thyroid to cricoid cartilages. *Otolaryngology-Head and Neck Surgery, 92*(5), 498–508.

Toth, L., Pap, U., Diozaeghy, P., & Sziklai, I. (1999). Phoniatric studies in myasthenia gravis patients. *HNO, 47*(11), 981–985.

Traube, L. (1871). Spastische Form der Nervosen Heiserkeit. *Ges Beitr Pathology and Physiology, 2*, 677.

Troche,M. S., Okun, M. S., Rosenbek, J. C., Musson, M., Fernandex, H. H. Rodriguez, R., . . . Sapienza, C. M. (2010). *Neurolgoy, 75*(21), 1923–1919.

Tsai, V., Celmer, A., Berke, G. S., & Chhetri, D. K. (2007). Videostroboscopic findings in unilateral superior laryngeal nerve paralysis and paresis. *Otolaryngology-Head and Neck Surgery, 136*(4), 660–662.

Van Pelt, F., Ludlow, C. L., & Smith, P. J. (1994). Comparison of muscle activation patterns in adductor and abductor spasmodic dysphonia. *Annals of Otology, Rhinology, and Laryngology, 103*(3), 192–200.

Venuto, C.S., McGarry, A., Ma, Q., & Kieburtz, K. (2012). Pharmacologic approaches to the treatment of Huntingon's disease. *Movement Disorders, 27*(1), 31–41.

Verdolini, K., Druker, D. G., Palmer, P. M., & Samawi, H. (1998). Laryngeal adduction in resonant voice. *Journal of Voice, 12*, 315–327.

Watts, C. R., & Vanryckeghem, M. (2001). Laryngeal dysfunction in amyotrophic lateral sclerosis: A review and case report. *BMC Ear, Nose and Throat Disorders, 1*(1), 1.

Wenke, R. J., Theodoros, D., & Cornwell, P. (2008). The short- and long- term effectiveness of the LSVT(R) for dysarthria following TBI and stroke. *Brain Injury, 22*(4), 339–352.

Whurr, R., Nye, C., & Lorch, M (1998). Meta-analysis of botulinum toxin treatment of spasmodic dysphonia: A review of 22 studies. *International Journal of Language and Communication Disorders, 33*(3), 327–329.

Woodson, G. (2008). Evolving concepts of laryngeal paralysis. *Journal of Laryngology and Otology, 122*(5), 437–441.

Woodson, G., (2010). Arytenoid abduction: indications and limitations. *Annals of Otology, Rhinology and Laryngology, 119*(11), 742–748.

Woodson, G., & Weiss, T. (2007). Arytenoid abduction for dynamic rehabilitation of bilateral laryngeal paralysis. *Annals of Otology, Rhinology, and Laryngology, 116*(7), 483–490.

Yamaguchi, M., Arai, K., Asahina, M., & Hattori, T. (2003). Laryngeal stridor in multiple system atrophy. *European Neurology, 49*(3), 154–159.

Yokoji, I., Nakamura, S., & Ideda, T. (1997). A case of progressive supranuclear palsy associated with bilateral vocal cord abductor paralysis. *Rinsho Shinkeigaku, 37*, 523–525.

Yoon, M. S., Munz, M., Sataloff, R. T., Spiegel, J. R., & Heuer, R. J. (1999). Vocal tremor reduction with deep brain stimulation. *Stereotactic and Functional Neurosurgery, 72*, (2–4), 241–244.

Zampieri, C., & Di Fabio, R. (2006). Progressive supranuclear palsy: Disease profile and rehabilitation strategies. *Physical Therapy, 86*(6), 870–880.

Zealear, D. L., Billante, C. R., Courey, M. S., Sant'Anna, G. D., & Netterville, J. L. (2002). Electrically stimulated glottal opening combined with adductor muscle Botox blockade restores both ventilation and voice in a patient with bilateral laryngeal paralysis. *Annals of Otology, Rhinology, and Laryngology, 111*(6), 500–506.

Zhang, L., Shimoji, M., Thomas, B., Moore, D. J., Yu, S. W., Marupudi, N. I., . . . Dawson, V. L. (2005). Mitochondrial localization of the Parkinson's disease related protein dj-1: Implications for pathogenesis. *Human Molecular Genetics, 14*(14), 2063–2073.

Appendix 6–1
DVD Table of Contents: Images

Case 1: Bilateral Abductor Vocal Fold Paralysis

Case 2: Bowing and Hypofunction in Parkinson's Disease, Laryngopharyngeal Reflux

Case 3: Bowing Small Pinpoint Vocal Fold Polyp and Ectasia

Case 4: Bowing and Anteroposterior, Lateral Compression

Case 5: Hypofunction due to Parkinson's Disease and Laryngopharyngeal Reflux

Case 6: Left True Vocal Fold Bowing and Paresis

Case 7: Post Thyroplasty, Left True Vocal Fold

Case 8: Left True Vocal Fold Adductor Paralysis

Case 9: Unilateral Vocal Fold Paralysis

Chapter 7

Vocal Rehabilitation

Voice Therapy

Interventions are programs specifically designed to help particular disorders and diseases. They can take the form of behavioral, surgical, and medical therapies. The success of a particular intervention is based on its process for achieving remediation of symptoms associated with a disease/disorder. Other factors that define the success of an intervention are how much it costs in terms of money and time with regard to its implementation. Health care today requires the use of cost-effective techniques based on empirical evidence for their use.

After reading this chapter, you will:

- Understand the importance of vocal rehabilitation in the remediation of voice disorders
- Understand the categories of voice therapy regimens
- Understand the rationale and basis of physiologically based voice rehabilitation programs including: Vocal Function Exercises, Lessac-Madsen Resonant Voice, and Lee Silverman Voice Treatment Program
- Understand the basis of other rehabilitation techniques for treating voice disorders

- Understand the role of biofeedback techniques in the treatment of voice disorders

Voice therapy is provided by a licensed voice pathologist, for patients determined to be candidates for voice remediation that was established by the results of the comprehensive diagnostic evaluation completed by a voice care team. Selecting voice therapy as the treatment option suggests that this is the best option to modify the voice (e.g., Aronson, 1990; Boone & McFarlane, 1988; Colton & Casper, 1996; Stemple, Glaze, & Klaben, 2000). A therapy technique should not be chosen because of its popularity but because of its known effectiveness and efficacy (Pannebacker, 1998). A technical report written by an ASHA committee and a committee from the American Academy of Otolaryngology Head and Neck Surgery (AAO-HNS) in 2005 detailed the use of voice therapy in the treatment of dysphonia (http:www.asha .org/docs/html/TR2005-00158.html). This report summarized studies and provided evidence for behavioral voice therapy with a variety of patient populations. It should be used as a reference source for providing evidence for both independent treatment and within a combined modality paradigm, particularly in combination with phonosurgical techniques.

For each treatment program discussed in this chapter, the target population is identified, the protocol is outlined, the treatment outcomes are defined and the evidence for treatment effectiveness and efficacy are included, if they exist. Where no empirical studies exist of a particular treatment, it is stated. *Note:* single case studies and small-scale intervention studies are not satisfactory for defining a treatment's effect.

As a highly individualized process each patient brings to the therapeutic setting their own etiologic factors that contribute to the voice disorder, a history characterized by a certain amount of voice use demands, medical complexities, occupational and social issues, and degree of patient motivation. Consequently, there is no set regimen for voice therapy. Chapter 4 described the steps and procedures to a thorough diagnostic evaluation. If followed, a comprehensive dataset is collected that informs the voice pathologist about etiology, patient symptoms, and the physiologic consequence of the disorder.

The successful diagnostic session dictates the success or failure of the rehabilitation process, serving to motivate the patient toward the therapeutic course. The information gained in the diagnostic session(s) provides the clinician with a collection in which to educate the patient about the disorder/disease. The clinician's role is to describe to the patient the normal anatomy and physiology of voice production versus the current condition. The cause and effect relationships between etiologic factors and current symptoms require explanation to the patient. For example, by explaining the negative effects of a long history of cigarette smoking and daily symptoms of reflux on the cause of their vocal fold edema and leukoplakia, the patient will better understand why cessation of smoking is imperative to optimizing vocal fold function. The clinician's explanation that leukoplakia is a precancerous condition may be the only

stimulus that is needed to motivate the patient to quit smoking or the patient may be more motivated to comply with a smoking cessation program.

Another example is the case of a second-grade schoolteacher who is diagnosed with vocal fold nodules and is in a situation where voice use cannot be modified easily. The behavior that led to the development of the nodules is not the primary problem. Rather, the compensatory vocal behaviors that currently affect her condition and serve to help her meet her occupational voice demand (given the existence of vocal nodules) requires clarification. Although it seems to be common sense, this patient needs to be educated about the nature of her voice disorder, why compensatory strategies arise, and what the implications of continued phonotraumatic behaviors will have, not only on her current condition, but on the progression of a worsening condition. This type of case is observed commonly in the clinical setting. There are other cases where the larynx simply is not physically able to meet the demands of phonation. In these cases, a treatment program must provide a mechanism to structurally aid vocal fold function, which can then be enhanced by behavioral modifications.

The Evolving Process of Voice Therapy

The management of voice disorders began in the 1930s with introductory texts by West, Kennedy, and Carr (1937) and Van Riper (1939). During this time frame, there was an appreciation defining the underlying to the voice condition and to make it clear how symptoms can be traced back to an underlying reason. These texts strongly advocated a thorough assessment including laryngeal imaging and examination of pitch, loudness, and quality in order to guide a sensible rehabilitation. Over the years, many of the introductory methods have been modified but the underlying principles are the same.

Today, clinicians use numerous therapy approaches to modify a patient's voice production. But, the approaches evolved from the techniques introduced by Van Riper, as well as Brodnitz (1954) and Brodnitz and Froeschels (1954). This chapter discusses the various orientations to voice therapy, and explains in more detail the steps for some specific therapy techniques. It is by no means an exhaustive presentation of all voice therapy techniques available to the clinician, nor does it advocate one technique over the other. In fact, the clinician with a good skill set will select the best voice therapy strategy based on individual patient presentation. We do not advocate a "one size fits all" approach. Most of the time, the clinician will need to sample a variety of approaches before settling on the best therapeutic strategy for their patient or select a combined modality approach that is better suited to meet the patient's functional outcome goals.

Goals of Voice Therapy

Voice therapy goals are specific for each patient given the etiologic factors contributing to the voice disorder. However, a general goal of voice therapy is to restore the best voice possible, one that will be functional for purposes of employment opportunities, social interactions, and activities of daily living (Colton, Casper, & Leonard, 2006). Setting realistic expectations with the patient at the onset of voice therapy and during the therapy process is critical. This is particularly important in cases when "normal" voice is not physiologically possible even in the hands of the "most skilled" voice clinician. This realization can be devastating and distressing for persons who

have relied heavily on their voice use for their livelihood, as is the case of singers, actors, public speakers, realtors, sales personnel, teachers, and so forth. Ultimately, regardless of the form of treatment, the rehabilitation goal is to develop a program that reeducates the patient on how to most effectively and efficiently use the voice and eliminate the reformation of the voice disorder/pathology.

Initial Steps in the Therapy Process

- Gauge patient motivation for making changes to (vocal) lifestyle
- Empower the patient to take responsibility for their voice care
- Provide patient with a timeline of the therapeutic process (even though this may change over time)
- Develop home practice materials so the patient takes responsibility in voice care

Definition of Treatment Efficacy

Treatment efficacy is how well a treatment affects the symptoms of a disorder in comparison to other standard treatments (Carding, 2000; Robey, 2004).

In general, there are few behavioral treatments, currently used to rehabilitate voice disorders, that are sufficiently operationalized to permit rigorous study of their outcomes and, therefore, defining treatment efficacy has been left incomplete.

Who Is the Target Population of Voice Therapy?

Any person who complains of a disturbance to the voice that results in an impairment, disability, or handicap regardless of age, sex, race, and culture.

Accurate Diagnosis Guides Treatment Planning

The voice pathologist does not provide the diagnostic label for a voice condition, their role is integral in the evaluation, development, and implementation of the treatment plan. There will be situations where an otolaryngologist may provide a diagnostic label after completing an indirect laryngoscopy. However, following the videolaryngostroboscopic examination, conducted by (most) voice pathologists, the diagnosis may be modified based on the more sophisticated view of the vocal fold structure and its function (Bless, Hirano, & Feder, 1987). The change in diagnosis, ultimately made by the otolaryngologist, typically results from team discussion. In cases where no diagnostic label is provided, voice therapy can still be initiated following the same goals and guidelines stated above. Although it is rarer that a diagnostic label is not provided, there are certain circumstances where this can occur. For example:

- Biopsy of pathology has not been made and a diagnostic label cannot be given
- Medically complex conditions require further evaluation (such as neurologic, endocrine, pulmonary, CT/MRI images are needed, allergy testing, etc.)
- An idiopathic condition occurs where a diagnostic label cannot be made
- Malingering—is present when a person pretends to be ill for secondary gain (escape work, garnish attention, and/or make a financial claim)

Contributing to Successful Therapy Outcome

Patient responsibility:

- Taking responsibility for their condition
- Making a time commitment to the treatment process
- Completing their home practice
- Incorporating suggested vocal lifestyle changes. Examples include:
  - Vocal health education
  - Using amplification
  - Modifying voice usage in social or work settings
- Acceptance of disability
- Compliance with prescriptive management
- Compliant with postphonosurgical care

Clinician responsibility (Colton, Casper, & Leonard, 2006):

- Knowledge and skill of normal and disordered voice production
- Knowledge and skill of therapeutic process
- Compassion, understanding, and empathy
- Superb listening skills
- Counseling skills
- Motivation skills: the ability to inspire action for change

Factors Related to Therapy Outcomes: Prognostic Indicators

Many factors can influence prognosis for therapy and require consideration, exploration, and discussion with the person. First and foremost, in any therapeutic process the person must recognize that a problem exists.

A person has an internal reference for what they feel is a "normal" voice and has opinions about what they should sound like. Although a person may agree that their voice is not "normal," they may not agree that it is as impaired as the clinician does and may not be agreeable to the clinician's rehabilitation goals (Colton, Casper, & Leonard, 2006). Other factors affecting prognosis include:

- Agreement of the therapy process: a patient must agree to comply with the therapy process, practice exercises in and outside of the therapy room, and assume responsibility for the development and maintenance of the existing problem. Patients who are seeking a "quick fix" so that they do not have to assume responsibility will likely fail in the therapeutic process or take a much longer time to meet the therapy goals. Although the patient is equally responsible for their therapeutic outcome they often become frustrated with the voice pathologist because they view the voice pathologist as the ultimate endpoint in their care and/or the "change agent" for the current condition
- Willingness to change: the patient must possess a willingness to change traumatic habits, risk factors, alter diet, lifestyle, and so forth, not just in an isolated environment but in their everyday activities. This is one of the most challenging aspects of the therapeutic process and can hinder the generalizability of the treatment program
- Elimination of other medical problems: if present, eliminating other medical and/or psychiatric problems is imperative. These have the potential to hinder therapy

progress. For example, a patient who is a chronic allergy sufferer may experience a plateau effect in their therapy progress when the allergen(s) (potentially causing changes in laryngeal function) have not been fully evaluated and treated
- Development of realistic expectations: developing realistic expectations (whether appropriate or not) needs to be considered from both the patient and clinician perspective. For example, the nature of the disorder may not be amenable to voice improvement due to the extent of damage to laryngeal structure and function. This needs to be shared with the patient
- Consideration of other health problems: other medical/ health conditions may preclude a patient from being able to participate in voice therapy or even attend voice therapy sessions
- Development of a trusting rapport between clinician and patient: The patient must sense the clinician's skill set, confidence, understanding, empathy, and diligence in meeting the therapeutic goals. The clinician's ability to openly communicate with their patient is critical for successful treatment outcomes

Voice Therapy Approaches: What Are They?

Complete Voice Rest Versus Modified Voice Rest

Historically, the care of structural voice pathologies, has called for complete voice rest as a first-order treatment. However, complete voice rest does not aid in the process to reprogram the patient to healthier voice use patterns. Obviously, if one eliminates any and all vocal fold tissue contact the pathologic tissue may heal. Complete voice rest is sensible after a phonosurgical procedure that requires the complete vocal rest for the healing process to occur or in acute conditions such as vocal fold hemorrhage, acute laryngitis, and trauma. There is recent evidence that suggests that extended vocal rest (beyond three to five days) may be more harmful then good (Rousseau et al., 2008). This is because tissue health relies on a certain amount of vocal fold activity, helping to guide cell behavior so that wound healing happens effectively, minimizing the development of scar tissue. One area that is currently being researched in our field is how to reduce the degree of inflammatory response associated with vocal fold injury and define the type of conditions that minimize the inflammatory response (Welham, Lim, Tateya, & Bless, 2008). One such mechanism for minimizing inflammation may be voice therapy by stimulating fibroblasts via stretching as shown recently using a rabbit model (Branski, Verdolini, Sandulache, Rosen, & Hebda, 2006) and assisting with modulating the inflammatory response (Welham et al., 2008). Therefore, rather than counseling a patient to completely rest their voice, vocal fold mobility should be encouraged, though not at too high a level that would be considered stressful to the tissue. Subsequently, a more contemporary pattern of practice in the remediation of structural lesions is to incorporate a modified voice rest program (also referred to as a vocal conservation program). This is where the patient is directed to eliminate excessive voice use, using the voice only when absolutely necessary and in a therapeutic manner. Voice use durations associated with modified vocal rest should be patient specific, taking into account the extent of the pathology, the vibratory characteristics, lifestyle, and personality factors.

Hygienic

Vocal hygiene is a program focused on patient education. The goal is the elimination of behaviors that are considered to be traumatic to the structural health and function of the vocal folds. It is often a first step in voice management and voice prevention programs. These factors were reviewed in Chapter 3. Examples of phonotraumatic behaviors include, shouting, talking too loudly, coughing, throat clearing, making vocal noises (grunts, growl, animal noises, etc.), using an unnatural pitch or tense in voice, persistent use of glottal fry, and poor hydration. And although vocal hygiene education is involved in almost all voice therapy programs as an independent form of treatment, it fails to compete with direct voice therapy methods (Roy et al., 2001) for changing vocal behaviors (Chan, 1994; Timmermans, DeBodt, Wuyts, & Van de Heyning, 2004). Rather, hygiene therapy is best suited as an adjunct to other forms of treatment.

Symptomatic

Symptomatic voice therapy focuses on the modification of aberrant vocal symptoms either observed by the patient or the voice pathologist during the diagnostic session. These aberrant symptoms might include a pitch that is produced too high or too low, a voice that is too breathy or too tense, too soft or too loud, the use of persistent glottal fry, hard glottal attacks, etc. Dr. Daniel Boone (1971) was the first to introduce the symptomatic therapy orientation to our profession and provided a series of techniques for eliciting desired behavioral patterns. In this orientation, the desired behavior is elicited, it is then shaped, stabilized, and habituated using a hierarchical pattern: progressing through therapy that increases in difficulty as therapy progresses. The first step for the patient and clinician is to identify the behaviors that need to be eliminated or modified. The second step is to stimulate the desired target behavior by using a facilitating technique. Facilitating techniques are listed below. *Note*: although readily used in the voice clinic, many of the methods below have little to no supporting published evidence on their outcome.

1. Auditory Feedback: clinician provides a recorded sample of the patient's voice for them to judge correct versus incorrect production.

2. Change of Loudness: clinician educates the patient about how vocal loudness impacts vocal fold vibration and modifies vocal loudness (either elevating or softening), based on the physical condition of the vocal folds.

3. Chant Talk: clinician uses this technique with hyperfunctional voice disorders. The words used as stimuli run continuously together without changes in stress or prosody, like Legato (in singing, (see Glossary, Chapter 10). The chant uses elevated pitches, sustained vowels, no syllable stress, and an elimination of hard glottal attacks. The chant is then modified to progress into conversational speech.

4. Chewing: clinician uses this technique with hyperfunctional voice disorders, particularly for those patients demonstrating minimal mouth movement, thus suppressing oral resonance. The chewing technique is used to facilitate greater oral movements to improve oral resonance, reduce extrinsic laryngeal muscle tension, and reduce vocal strain.

5. Confidential Voice: clinicians use this technique with hyperfunctional voice disorders as first described by Colton and Casper (1990, 1996). The confidential voice treatment uses a soft, easy onset, and relaxed voice.

6. Counseling (Explanation of Problem): clinician helps a patient with conse-

quences of a voice disorder, helping the patient explore the many intrinsic or extrinsic factors that relate to the condition and/or refering the patient for help with psychological issues when those issues go beyond the scope of practice for the voice pathologist.

7. Digital Manipulation: clinicians use physical pressure on the thyroid cartilage to help reduce excessive extrinsic muscle contraction that is minimizing laryngeal movement. See discussion of laryngeal reposturing techniques.

8. Elimination of "Abuses" (Phonotrauma): clinicians help the patient identify the behaviors that are causing harmful effects on laryngeal anatomy and/or function.

9. Establishing a New Pitch: clinicians most clearly understand that there is no such thing as the concept of "optimal pitch." However, slight alterations in vocal pitch may be necessary to ensure that the patient is not straining the vocal folds beyond their normal anatomic range.

10. Focus: clinicians use this technique to help patients generate a voice source that is optimal with regard to resonance. The direction to the patient is to "move" the voice from the back of the throat to the front of the mouth while feeling vibrations in the nasal cavity. Optimal coupling of the supraglottal and glottal cavities is necessary for best possible voice production.

11. Glottal Fry: clinicians strive to reduce glottal fry in cases of hyperfunctional voice disorders. According to Boone, McFarland, and Von Berg (2005) it can be used as a relaxing technique, apparently because the vocal folds are vibrating in a more lax state when a low fundamental frequency is produced.

12. Head Positioning: clinicians advocate a good posture. Most recently, a group of researchers invented a "posturometer" to help maintain elevated chin position

and optimize voice production (Denizoglu & Pehlivan, 2008). Head turning has been used with cases of unilateral vocal fold paralysis by turning the head to the affected side to aid in vocal fold adduction.

13. Hierarchy Analysis: clinicians use this analysis to help the patient identify the most stressful or anxiety provoking events, comparing situations that create a good voice or a worse voice (Wolpes, 1987). Basically, a deconditioning approach is used to help the patient learn relaxation strategies to reduce the stressful or anxious response.

14. Inhalation Phonation: clinicians use voice production on inspiration rather than expiration to help modify ventricular phonation or for those who are unable to resist voice change when using expiration.

15. Laryngeal Massage: clinicians use a modified approach to Aronson's (1990) technique of circumlaryngeal therapy whereby the larynx is gently massaged to reduce extrinsic laryngeal muscle tension and a lower laryngeal position.

16. Masking: clinicians use a source of noise to induce the Lombard effect (Newby, 1972), which is known to elevate vocal loudness when noise is introduced to the patient via headphones. Voice clarity may result.

17. Nasal/Glide Stimulation: clinicians use words predominated by nasals and glides as therapy stimuli for those with hyperfunctional voice production as it relaxes the articulators and optimizes nasal resonance.

18. Open Mouth Approach: clinicians encourage patients to open their mouth to reduce dampening of sound production and increase oral resonance.

19. Pitch Inflections: clinicians use pitch inflections for patients with monotone voice to help activate the cricothryoid muscle.

20. Redirected Phonation: clinicians use this technique for patients who are unable to produce any voice often due to excessive vocal strain. Vegetative tasks or others can be used to help facilitate any sound production.

21. Relaxation: clinicians use this technique to help patients reduce stress via relaxation exercises.

22. Respiration Training: clinicians realize that the support for voice production is subglottal pressure. As such respiration training teaches the patient how to coordinate the inspiratory and expiratory phases of voice production, optimizing lung volumes for speech.

23. Tongue Protrusion /i/: clinicians work to minimize extreme cases of hyperfunction by posturing the tongue in the position for vowel production of /i/. The high tongue position helps to reduce pharyngeal squeezing and is often used in cases of ventricular hyperfunction/phonation.

24. Visual Feedback: clinicians use visual techniques to aid patients in identifying correct from incorrect voice productions, such as that used in the KayPentax Visi-Pitch 3950 for modulating vocal pitch and loudness.

25. Yawn-Sigh: clinicians use this technique in cases of hyperfunctional voice disorders by lowering the position of the larynx, widening the pharynx, moving the tongue forward, and reducing extrinsic laryngeal muscle tension.

Psychogenic

Certain patients presenting with voice disorders often develop vocal habits as a reaction to emotional, occupational, or social stresses. In serious cases, these patients should be referred for a psychiatric evaluation as emotional disturbances such as depression and anxiety can be potentially life threatening or life altering. In more mild situations, the voice pathologist acts with the multidisciplinary team to help the patient cope with excessive muscle tension. In most cases the laryngeal structure is essentially normal upon visual examination. The voice problem is functional, due to difficulty initiating and coordinating phonation (Aronson, 1990). The voice pathologist's role is to discern whether the voice symptoms are due to structural, physiologic or neurophysiologic reasons, and if not, work toward helping the patient remediate the emotional disturbances associated with the onset or maintenance of the condition. For example, a young woman came to our clinic who was due to get married but had recently lost her voice. She reported general anger and anxiety associated with planning her wedding and an extreme amount of sleep deprivation associated with her job as an emergency room nurse.

After speaking to the voice pathologist and otolaryngologist, and intensely expressing her feelings, the otolaryngologist prescribed her general rest and she was given a medical release from work. The voice pathologist met with her twice and facilitated enough voice to allow her to explore the psychodynamics of her voice disorder onset and allow her the freedom to express herself openly. She appeared to greatly appreciate the process, particularly given the calmness and nonjudgmental manner of the voice pathologist. Weeks later she called the office and her voice was not recognizable as it was back to normal. The "cure" was telling her future mother-in-law to allow her to plan the wedding and taking control of her wedding plans. With adequate sleep and sense of control, her voice returned to normal. No further formal voice therapy was needed.

Physiologic

Physiologic voice therapy is likened to a physical therapy approach in that direct exercises are used to facilitate laryngeal muscle activity as well as work with the other subsystems involved in voice production, including the respiratory and supraglottal systems. The techniques described below are highlighted because they are guided by structured principles and protocols and have some experimental testing to their use, although this testing is not homogeneous for all programs. As Pannebacker (1998) pointed out, voice therapy techniques should be selected based on empirical evidence for their use and effectiveness rather than their popularity or promotion (1998). Examples of physiologic therapy techniques include Vocal Function Exercises (Stemple, Lee, D'Amico, & Pickup, 1994), Lessac-Madsen Resonant Voice Therapy (Verdolini, 2000), and the Lee Silverman Voice Treatment technique (Ramig, Countryman, Thompson, & Horii, 1995). There are others such as inspiratory and expiratory muscle strength training that work primarily on respiratory muscle force as well as other types of techniques that rely on physiologic principles and/or manipulations of strength and endurance (Sapienza, 2008).

Eclectic

Eclectic therapy is a relatively new model of voice rehabilitation that involves using multiple behavioral therapy orientations to address patient care. It does not rely only on one technique. For example, the Lee Silverman Voice treatment technique is advocated for all patients with Parkinson's disease and does not exemplify an eclectic voice therapy method. On the other hand, a general group of patients better served by an eclectic approach may be those with hyperfunctional voice disorders. There are some cases of hyperfunction that are related to extreme voice demand and others that are due to psychosocial reasons or poor vocal technique. In these cases, one treatment approach often results in a plateau of recovery requiring the clinician to quickly select another method to facilitate improved voice production. For example, in a patient with an intracordal cyst and generalized edema, the initial step would be to use a hygienic voice therapy program to help minimize the swelling and optimize a postsurgical healing process by reducing inflammation. If phonotraumatic behaviors exist the clinician would work to reduce them. Once the inflammation and swelling were reduced, surgical intervention would occur. Following surgery, the patient is already familiarized with the purpose of voice therapy and ready to engage in a behavioral voice therapy strategy to help minimize the reoccurrence of the condition. The postsurgical approach is more often than not a physiologic therapy approach to help patients meet their voice demands.

In summary, the voice pathologist is encouraged to be well versed in a variety of techniques given the many profiles of patients even though they may have the same condition.

Combined Modality

Many centers have adopted combined modality therapy as the standard treatment approach for patients with voice disorders. That is because voice disorders/diseases can stem from medically complex conditions. As a result, a combination of behavioral, pharmacologic and surgical interventions may be necessary to normalize voice production. Each treatment modality outlined above may be used independently but when symptoms do not resolve in a reasonable time period or when symptoms are known to stem from a physiologic cause (such as gastroesophageal disease or a neurodegenerative disease process), other forms of treatment may be necessary.

Physiologic Therapy Approaches

Semioccluded Vocal Tract

Semioccluded vocal tract is a voice therapy technique with a long history of use. Voice clinicians,

singing voice teachers, and vocal coaches have implemented various forms of semi occluded vocal tract with use of lip trills, tongue trills, bilabial fricatives, humming, and phonation into tubes or straws. According to Titze (2010), the purpose of the semioccluded vocal tract exercise(s) is to improve vocal fold adduction, vocal registration, and epilarynx tube narrowing in order to achieve the best acoustic power transfer from the glottis to the lips.

However, until recently, little has been studied in order to understand the physiological basis for this technique and the various semi-occluded vocal tract shapes. In a computer simulation study by Titze (2006) use of a self-oscillating vocal fold model and a 44 section vocal tract to understand the source–filter interactions for the lip and epilarynx tube found that semiocclusion in the front of the vocal tract (at the lips) heightens source–tract interaction by raising the mean supraglottal and intraglottal pressures. This study also demonstrated that impedance matching by vocal fold adduction and epilarynx tube narrowing results in more efficient and economic vocal use (in terms of tissue collision). A series of YouTube videos have been produced for an introduction to this technique that the reader may find benefit from watching. The video depicts the regimen with demonstrations that students can easily follow. The regimen includes a series of pitch glides, from a low pitch to a high pitch gradually increasing the pitch and loudness followed by vocalizing a song through a straw or other semioccluded vocal tract shape.

Vocal Function Exercises

Vocal function exercises (VFE) were developed and are currently promoted by Dr. Joseph Stemple. VFE exercises are used with all age groups and like the Lessac Resonant Voice Treatment (described next) are well suited to use with patients that have hyper- and hypofunctional voice disorders. A formal certification program is not necessary to implement this technique, although attendance in Dr. Stemple's workshop is worthwhile for learning how to implement the steps of VFE.

VFE outcome has been tested on a randomized group of subjects with normal voice who were placed into experimental, placebo, and control groups. After 4 weeks of VFE, the experimental group improved phonation volumes, phonation times, and frequency range compared to the placebo and control groups (Stemple et al., 1994). In another study, a group of singers were split into experimental and control groups and assessed after 4 weeks of VFE (Sabol, Lee, & Stemple, 1995). Again, those who participated in the VFE treatment produced improved measures of flow rate, phonation volume, maximum phonation time, and increased glottal efficiency. Another study by Roy et al. (2001) examined the functional effects of two voice therapy programs on a group of nearly 40 teachers with voice disorders; one therapy approach was VFE and the other was a vocal hygiene program. An untreated control group of 20 teachers was also included. Findings indicated that the VFE group had an overall greater improvement, and ease and clarity in their voice production. In the future, a comparison with patient groups is definitely needed to determine the efficacy of the VFE program, as this remains untested. For example, contrasting VFE outcome with another physiologic voice treatment approach such as the Lessac-Madsen Resonant Voice Treatment Program would be an excellent clinical trial comparison.

Protocol. The VFE protocol includes the following four steps to the program and each step is completed twice with the entire program completed twice per day by the patient. Stemple presents an analogy to clinicians when he presents information on VFE. He likens the vocal mechanism to other skeletal systems in the body. And, like other skeletal systems in the body, the vocal folds are made up of skeletal muscle and respond to exercise and conditioning based treatments.

Steps to the program are: vocal warm-up, pitch glides, and prolonged phonation of /o/ at selected pitches.

The steps to the program are the following:

1. (Warm-up) Sustain the vowel (ee) for as long as possible on the musical note.

    Goal = _____ seconds.*

    *The ranges for sustaining a vowel maximally will vary depending on the age and sex of the patient as well as the initial lung volume the task is started at.

2. (Stretching) Glide from your lowest note to your highest note on: (the word "knoll") (a tongue trill) (a lip trill) (the word "whoop").

    Goal = No voice breaks.

3. (Contracting) Glide from a comfortable high note to your lowest note on: (the word "knoll") (a tongue trill) (a lip trill) (the word "boom").

    Goal = No voice breaks.

4. (Adductory Power) Sustain the musical notes for as long as possible on the sound "ol."

    Goal = _____ seconds.

These productions should be made with a softly engaged voice with the least amount of effort without any breaks, wavering, or breathiness in voice quality. The patient should pay attention to posture, breathing, tone placement, and onset.

Lessac-Madsen Resonant Voice Therapy (LMRVT)

As an honor to two great mentors and voice teachers, Professor Arthur Lessac and Dr.

Mark Madsen, Dr. Verdolini Abbott (2000) developed the formal, programmatic version of "Lessac-Madsen Resonant Voice Therapy" (Verdolini Abbott, 2000). The LMRVT program augments initial introductory approaches to "resonant voice" training and incorporates a training program that leads to a stronger resonant voice after a few weeks in the program. Conducted during 30 to 45-minute sessions once or twice weekly, for 4 to 8 weeks, LMRVT is appropriate to use with adolescent and adult voice patients with hypo and hyperfunctional voice disorders. A formal certification program is not necessary to implement this technique, although attendance in Dr. Verdolini-Abbott's workshop is highly recommended to learn the detailed steps of the program.

The basic premise of LMRVT is that a target laryngeal configuration produces the strongest voice while using the least amount of respiratory effort and impact stress on the vocal folds, thus reducing laryngeal injury. Another premise of the technique is that outcomes of LMRVT can be enhanced by attention to sensory information relative to gestures rather than verbal, mechanistic explanations.

As a physiologically based treatment approach, LMRVT outcome has not been well tested in experimentally controlled studies. As a relatively new systematic approach, LMRVT outcome studies are needed. Currently, clinical trials are ongoing with the intent to provide evidence like that available for the Lee Silverman Voice Treatment Program. Likewise, a similar program for children is under development.

LMRVT Protocol. During the first therapy session, attention is paid to collecting patient case history data and educating the patient about voice care. The second therapy session starts with the introduction of the "Resonant Voice Basic Training Gesture" (RV BTG).

This gesture is the catalyst for the remainder of therapy. The clinician teaches the patient how to produce voice on very simple sounds, in a way that both sounds good, and feels good. The process continues with further training in the BTG, on words and phrases. Many opportunities for practice on resonant voice are given on a large number of words and sentences, using "variable practice." According to Verdolini-Abbott, variable practice allows resonant voice to be learned very thoroughly, resulting in better generalization. The remaining therapy sessions continue to involve training in resonant voice, always emphasizing sensory processing and variable practice.

Example of Exercises in Session 2 of LMRVT

- Stretches (3 to 10 seconds per stretch)

RV Core Exercises: Basic Training Gesture (BTG)

- "mmmmm" — explore making vibrations wider and narrower
- "mmmmm" — explore making vibrations narrower and narrower, and voice easier and easier
- "mmmmm" — explore what happens to vibrations shifting tongue in mouth
- "mmmmm" — explore what happens to vibrations gliding through pitch range; sustain pitch in range where vibrations are strongest, voice easiest (not about "optimal pitch" but rather awareness)
- "mmmmm" — sustain comfortable pitch and imagine pitch is increasing, but it's not; notice shift in vibrations

RV Core Exercises: Examples of Words

Mention Moon Mundane Man

Mum

Motion

RV Core Exercises: Examples of Phrases

The machine is broken

Morgan likes ice cream

RV Chant

- /mi mi mi mi mi mi/ (one pitch).
- /mi mi pi pi mi mi/ (one pitch; to criterion).
- Meet me Peter, meet me (one pitch; to criterion).
- Meet me Peter, meet me (gradually increasing inflection over several trials, to criterion).

- Hi, my name's Peter. What am I supposed to do this afternoon? (Response, with natural inflection: Meet me, Peter, meet me!)

RV Vocal Communicator (VC)

- Regular conversation, in quiet, at short distance, in the treatment room.

Table 7–1 shows the outline of the tasks as a function of treatment session number as the program continues along a hierarchical approach.

Lee Silverman Voice Treatment (LSVT)

The Lee Silverman Voice Treatment Program was developed and is currently promoted by

Table 7–1. Outline of LMRVT Tasks

Session	Stretches	RV Core	RV Chant	RV "VC"	RV "Mini"	RV Messa de Vocce	Conver-sation	Own Treat-ment
1	X	X						
2		X	X	X			C1	
3		X	X	X	(X)		C2	
4		X		X	(X)	X	C1 + C2	
5		X		X	(X)	X	C3	
6		X			X	X	C4	
7		X				X	C5	
8		X					C6	X

C1 = normal conversation; C2 = quiet conversation on telephone, Dictaphone, or other as relevant patient; C3 = loud voice (over distance) as relevant to patient; C4 = speech in background noise as relevant to patient; C5 = emotional speech as relevant to patient; C6 = "challenge" conversation; VC = Vocal Communicator.

Dr. Lorraine Ramig. In the developer's opinion (Ramig et al., 1995, 1996, 2001), LSVT is a proven, effective speech treatment for patients with Parkinson's disease (PD). Promoting models of exercise-based theories into the model of LSVT, this treatment requires clinicians to be certified via a 1.5-day certification and workshop program.

The LSVT program uses vocal loudness as a "trigger" for stimulating increased effort and coordination during speech production (http://www.lsvt.org/main_site.html). Other symptoms targeted by the program include breathiness, pitch, and reduced articulatory movements and respiration associated with the hypokinetic nature of the dysarthria linked with PD. The LSVT program is considered to be an intensive treatment program. It occurs over a 4-week time frame and includes 16, one-hour sessions of treatment. The program is designed to develop patient awareness such that the individual involved in LSVT is able to cue himself or herself for changing vocal loudness. The training involves memory, learning and reliance on self-cuing and self-regulation (Sapir et al., 2007). One important consideration in using this intervention for patients with PD is the cognitive deficit associated with PD. Cognitive deficits associated with PD include impairment in executive functioning, language, and working memory (for a review see Owen, 2004). Some of these deficits can be masked in less complex tasks, but impede generalization to more complex speech and language. Therefore, the degree of impairment in these domains must be assessed and therapeutic targets selected that challenge the patient sufficiently to maintain speech and voice related gains.

The LSVT program is based on five fundamental concepts: (1) thinking loud, (2) high speech effort, (3) intensive treatment, (4) recalibrating loudness level, and (5) quantifying improvements. The protocol followed within the LSVT program is hierarchical in nature, much like the other physiologic voice therapy techniques. This means that the targets are first worked on within sound production during sustained vowel production, followed by the production of the targets within more complex speech production utterances such as words, phrases, sentences, and conversation. There is now an extended version of the traditional LSVT program called LSVT-X where the program is extended from 4 to 8 weeks and treatments are administered 2 times per week as opposed to 4 times per week for one-hour sessions (Spielman et al., 2007).

LSVT research has resulted in both short and long-term efficacy data (Ramig et al., 1995, 1996, 2001a, 2001b).

Outcomes studies on LSVT indicate the following:

- LSVT increases vocal loudness on average by 8 dB SPL following 4 weeks of its intervention with patients with PD
- The extended LSVT program called LSVT-X increases dB SPL of vocal output consistent with traditional LSVT, on the order of 8 dB SPL, with maintenance of the effects after 6 months
- LSVT has some positive effect on swallow function: completed on a trial of 8 patients with PD (El Sharkawi et al., 2002)
- LSVT may alter facial expression in patients with PD following 4 weeks of treatment (Spielman, Borod, & Ramig, 2003)
- LSVT effects were superior for increasing dB SPL, compared to a low effort respiratory treatment protocol in patients with PD (Baumgartner, Sapir, & Ramig, 2001).

Laryngeal Relaxation with Circumlaryngeal Massage and Reposturing Techniques

Aronson (1990) first described circumlaryngeal massage along with laryngeal reposturing. Its concept has been further studied by Roy and Leeper (1993) and Roy, Ford, and Bless (1996). This technique is most applicable in cases when laryngeal tension is impairing phonation. If the patient experiences laryngeal tension for an extended period of time, the larynx can become positioned high in the neck, restricting laryngeal movement.

To evaluate a patient's level of extrinsic laryngeal muscle tension the clinician directs pressure in three areas of the neck, described below. When palpating the neck the clinician should also be observing if a pain response is elicited from the patient:

1. From the thyroid notch, move superiorly finding the hyoid bone and place direct pressure on the two major cornu of the hyoid bone
2. From the thyroid notch move just superiorly, finding the superior cornu of the thyroid notch and apply pressure
3. From the thyroid notch move laterally to feel along the anterior side of the sternocleidomastoid muscle, then move up to palpate the submandibular muscles
4. Find the thyroid notch and apply "traction," pulling the larynx down during vocalization to determine if there is an improvement in voice quality. If voice quality significantly improves then laryngeal repositioning may be a key factor in remediating the patient's dysphonia

The final step of this procedure is to apply manual tension reduction or the circumlaryngeal massage techniques using the clinician's or the patient's fingers. Pressure is applied in a circular motion with downward pressure to the following locations:

1. Over the two major horns of the hyoid bone,
2. Between the hyoid bone and the thyroid cartilage (thyrohyoid space), and
3. Along the thyroid cartilage (remembering the downward pressure that is also to be applied).

Roy and Leeper (1993) demonstrated a significant return of voice quality with this technique and have shown that it can be used to differentiate muscle tension dysphonia from adductor spasmodic dysphonia (Roy et al., 1996; Roy, Mauszycki, Merrill, Gouse, & Smith, 2007).

Expiratory Muscle Strength Training

Expiratory muscle strength training (EMST) is a technique based on the notion that the strength of skeletal muscles, such as limb muscles, occurs fairly rapidly due to neural mechanisms and eventual muscle hypertrophy as training progresses past a period of approximately 4 weeks (Powers & Howley, 2004). The expiratory muscles involved in voice production, like the abdominal and internal intercostal muscles, are skeletal muscles and have many of the same structural and metabolic properties as limb muscles. Similarities in muscle fiber type distribution between respiratory and limb muscles suggest that the expiratory muscles may be capable of using similar metabolic processes for the creation of energy necessary for muscle contraction.

Capitalizing on this notion, the EMST technique uses an experimental pressure threshold device to accomplish expiratory muscle strength training. The device requires patients to develop an expiratory pressure while blowing forcefully through the device. The EMST device can be calibrated up to a pressure range of 150 cm H_2O allowing for the pressure load to be varied as muscle strength improves. This is similar to increasing a weight being lifted during exercise. Expiratory muscle strength is determined by measuring maximum expiratory pressure. Maximum expiratory pressure has been used historically as an indirect measure of expiratory muscle strength (Clanton & Diaz, 1995) and is sampled with a pressure transducer as the patient maximally blows into a tube. The device is set at 75% of the patient's maximum expiratory pressure and reset as their maximum expiratory pressure improves with training.

When training with the device, patients must overcome the threshold load by generating an expiratory pressure sufficient to open the expiratory spring-loaded valve within the device. The individual must sustain this pressure level throughout the expiration. If the patient does not generate the threshold pressure, the valve remains closed.

A very important distinction exists between pressure threshold devices and traditional resistance training devices. The resistance devices marketed for clinical use (PEEP, incentive spirometry, etc.) allow the rate of airflow produced into the trainer to be varied, thus minimizing the potential gains in muscle strength. It would be analogous to swimming across a pool either fast or slow. The rate of swimming alters the degree of the training effect. With the pressure threshold trainer, the user cannot modify airflow mechanics. That is, a steady airflow must be maintained during the exercise. Therefore, the pressure threshold device offers a specific stimulus to the expiratory muscles as the patient cannot remove the load. It is an activity that is considered a short duration, high intensity exercise.

It is believed that use of the EMST device can help patients develop a greater ability to generate expiratory pressures for voice and speech production while reducing perception of physiologic effort. Other improved functions include improvements in cough, swallow and breathing (Gonzalez-Rothi, Musson, Rosenbek, & Sapienza, 2008; Kim, Davenport, & Sapienza, 2008; Sapienza, 2008). The latest clinical trial work with EMST describes outcomes for airway protection in those with Parkinson's disease (Troche et al., 2010). EMST can be used therapeutically with pediatrics (under close supervision) and adults with hypofunctional, hyperfunction, and neurogenic populations (Jones, Moss, Edwards & Kishnani, 2011; Pinto, Swash & de Carvalho, 2012; Sapienza, Troche, Pitts, & Davenport, 2011).

Special Cases

Management of Paradoxic Vocal Fold Dysfunction

In cases of paradoxic vocal fold dysfunction, medical treatment of asthma and reflux should be optimized first. If these comorbid factors are ignored, then progress with any behavioral treatment may be unlikely. The patient may be prescribed bronchodilators, steroids, reflux medications, anti-allergens, and others. Other factors can trigger paradoxic vocal fold dysfunction like stress, anxiety, food products, environmental factors, air pollutants, perfume products, airborne allergens, airborne chemical agents, and exercise. Exposure to these factors should all be minimized, when possible, when working on treatment.

Behavioral Approaches

Pitchenik (1991) described a panting maneuver as an effective emergency measure for relief. Martin et al. (1987) introduced a multiple-step level program that included:

- Helping the patient acknowledge the sensations and emotion that accompany stridor, fear, and helplessness associated with paradoxic vocal fold dysfunction
- Using behavioral and self-awareness approaches to establish good breathing pattern and to allow voluntary control when airway obstruction occurs
- Teaching inspiratory and expiratory breath coordination and self-awareness of breathing. Patients are also taught how to use proper inspiratory and expiratory breathing techniques to provide the "pressure support" for voice production. Patients are encouraged to develop and maintain an expiratory count, and avoid gasping for air
- Teaching "wide-open throat" breathing, concentrating on having the lips closed, the tongue lying flat on the floor of the mouth behind the lower front teeth, with the buccal (cheek) areas of the mouth relaxed, then releasing the jaw gently and using inhalation/exhalation techniques

Bastian and Nagorsky (1987) introduced laryngeal image biofeedback as did Altman, Mirza, Ruiz, and Sataloff (2000). While conducting voice therapy techniques, patients viewed their laryngeal posture from the videolaryngoscopy display helping them alter, if able, the improper tendencies toward adduction on inspiration. Relaxation maneuvers and breathing control with "sniffing" helped reduce the likelihood of improper vocal fold adduction.

Inspiratory muscle strength training was tried in one case of a rower with exercise-induced paradoxical vocal fold dysfunction.

A substantial improvement was made in both inspiratory muscle strength training and the complete reduction in paradoxical activity during exercise (Hoffman-Ruddy, Sapienza, Lehman, Davenport, & Martin, 2004). This is a single case and more work needs to be done to clearly understand the mechanism of the result. It is thought that the elimination of the paradoxing in this case was related to the principle of neural adaptation and crossover effects that accompany physical training (Powers & Howley, 2004).

Psychotherapy Approach

The initial aim of psychotherapy is to allow patients to retain many of their psychiatric symptoms without needing to use paradoxic vocal fold dysfunction as a coping syndrome. Martin et al. (1987) recommended voice therapy along with short-term psychotherapy as the treatment of choice. The first step is simply informing patients that they have a problem, clearly explaining to them what happens when they have an attack, explaining that treatments do work to remediate the condition, and so forth. Attempts should be made to explain to the patient that this voice disorder is not "all in their head," so they do not actively resist voice therapy or psychotherapy.

Patients' fears concerning their health should be discussed as well as discussion about their family and work dynamics associated with the illness. Associated psychiatric conditions including depression, obsessive-compulsive personality, borderline personality, passive-dependent personality, adjustment reaction, or somatization disorder, and dealing with the common patient factors of difficulty in directly expressing anger, sadness, pleasure, or other emotions are important in psychotherapy over the long term. On the other hand, it may be worthwhile to explain to the patient the role of precipitating psychological factors, muscle tension, and anticipatory anxiety in the production of the disorder. Hypnosis and hypnotic suggestion may be of value.

Management of Abductor Spasmodic Dysphonia

Treatment options for ABSD are limited and primarily involve injection of botulinum toxin (Botox™) into the posterior cricoarytenoid muscles, but even this technique does not appear to offer optimal outcomes (Bielamowicz, Squire, Bidus, & Ludlow, 2001).

Management of Adductor Spasmodic Dysphonia

Initially addressed through behavioral therapy alone, today a number of treatment options exist for individuals with ADSD. These include surgical, chemodenervation, alternative, behavioral, and combined modality approaches.

Surgical Treatments

Surgical treatment of ADSD focus on modifying the mechanics of phonation, reducing vocal fold adduction by altering nervous system control of the larynx. This can be accomplished through resection (Barton, 1979; Dedo, 1976), selective sectioning (Carpenter, Henley-Cohn, & Snyder, 1979), or crushing (Biller, Som, & Lawson, 1979) of the recurrent laryngeal nerve (RLN), the nerve responsible for vocal fold adduction. These procedures create a surgically induced partial or total paralysis of one or both vocal folds, reducing or eliminating the ability of the vocal folds to spasmodically close. Failure rates for this type of surgical procedure appear relatively high with return of symptoms frequently observed anywhere from 4 months to 3 years postsurgery (Aronson & DeSanto, 1981; Fritzell et al.,

1993; Izdebski, Dedo, Shipp, & Flower, 1981; Levine, Wood, Batza, Rusnov, & Tucker, 1979; Wilson, Oldring, & Mueller, Learned compensation in the form of overadduction of the nonparalyzed fold or false vocal fold adduction (Aronson & DeSanto, 1981), and neural regrowth (Fritzell et al., 1993; Ludlow, Naunton, Fujita, & Sedory, 1990; Schiratzki & Fritzell, 1991; Shindo, Herzon, Hanson, Cain, & Sahgal, 1992; Wilson et al., 1980) are frequently implicated as reasons why surgical interventions for ADSD fail. Companion surgical procedures such as vocal fold bulking (Belafsky & Postma, 2004; Hill, Meyers, & Harris, 1991; Izdebski, Dedo, Shipp, & Flower, 1981; Hirano, Tanaka, Tanaka, & Hibi, 1990; Peppas & Benner, 1980; Schramm, May, & Lavorato, 1978) and thinning (Izdebski et al., 1981) can be used to improve an overly breathy or still-spasmodic vocal quality following RLN procedures.

Selective bilateral denervation/reinervation procedures emerged in the early 1990s and were designed to eliminate vocal fold hyperadduction while minimizing the potential undesirable surgical side effects of excessive breathiness, airway compromise, and neural regrowth with symptom return (Allegretto, Morrison, Rammage, & Lau, 2003; Chhetri & Berke, 2006; Sercarz, Berke, Ming, Rothschiller, & Graves, 1992). Here, the RLN is sectioned bilaterally, and then reinnervated by branches of the ansa cervicalis. This preserves the action of vocal fold adduction for voicing and airway protection while permanently eliminating the capacity for overadduction, or vocal fold spasming (Allegretto et al., 2003; Berke et al., 1999). This procedure has been successful in long-term symptom resolution for some patients (Chhetri, Mendelsohn, Blumin, & Berke, 2006). Other less popular surgical procedures used in the treatment of ADSD include midline lateralization type II thyroplasty (Chan, Baxter, Oates, & Yorkston, 2004; Isshiki, 1998; Isshiki, Haji, Yamamoto,

Mahieu, 2001; Isshiki, Tsuji, Yamamoto, & Iizuka, 2000), anterior commissure retrusion (Tucker, 1989), autologous replacement of the vocal fold (Tsunoda, Amagai, Kondou, Baer, Kaga, & Niimi, 2005), thermotherapy of terminal RLN branches (Remacle, Plouin-Gaudon, Lawson, & Abitbol, 2005), thyro-arytenoid muscle myectomy (muscle tissue removal), (Su, Chuang, Tsai, & Chiu, 2007), and implantation of a RLN stimulator (Friedman, Toriumi, Grybauskas, & Applebaum, 1989; Friedman, Wernicke, & Caldarelli, 1994).

Chemodenervation Treatments

Botulinum toxin type A (Botox™), acts as a temporary paralytic, inactivating muscle fibers into which it is injected (Blitzer & Sulica, 2001). Botox™, injected into one or both of the thyroarytenoid muscles, paralyzes the muscle fibers through blockage of acetylcholine release at the neuromuscular junction (Bielamowicz & Ludlow, 2000). When successful, this chemical denervation of the TA eliminates the uncontrollable spasmodic bursts that bring about the primary voice symptoms of ADSD (Bielamowicz & Ludlow, 2000).

Observed physiologic changes following Botox™ chemodenervation include reduced airway impedance and increases in airflow rates and stability during phonation (Adams, Durkin, Irish, Wong, & Hunt, 1996; Cantarella, Berlusconi, Maraschi, Ghio, & Barbieri, 2006; Finnegan, Luschei, Gordon, Barkmeier, & Hoffman, 1999; Fisher, Scherer, Guo, & Owen, 1996; Miller, Woodson, & Jankovic, Wong et al., 1995; Zwirner, Murry, Swenson, & Woodson, Perceptual and acoustic effects of Botox™ injection include improvements in voice quality, reduced presence of voice breaks, reduced aperiodicity, and reductions in shifts in vocal fundamental frequency (F0) with less effect on noise to harmonic ratio, jitter, and shimmer (e.g., Blitzer, Brin, & Stewart,

1998; Boutsen, Cannito, Taylor, & Bender, 2002; Damrose, Goldman, Groessl, & Orloff, 2004; Langeveld et al., 2001; Mehta et al., 2001; Sapienza, Cannito, Murry, Branski, & Woodson, 2002; Whurr, Nye, & Lorch, 1998; Zwirner, Murry, & Woodson, 1997) Botox™ also appears to exert beneficial effects on quality of life (Baylor, Yorkston, Eadie, & Maronian, 2007; Bhattacharyya & Taray, 2001; Courey et al., 2000; Epstein, Stygall, & Newman, 1997; Hogikyan, Wodchis, Spak, & Kileny, 2001; Langeveld et al., 2001; Rubin, Wodchis, Spak, Kileny, & Hogikyan, 2004; Wingate et al., 2005). Over time (typically a matter of months), the toxin is eliminated from the muscle fibers, and symptoms return.

In spite of its widespread clinical use, there are very few studies which have examined the effects of Botox™ within the context of a randomized, clinically controlled trial (e.g., Boutsen et al., 2002; Watts, Nye, & Whurr, 2006; Watts, Whurr, & Nye, 2004). As previously discussed, Botox™ has the potential to exert a wide array of positive effects on both physical and quality of life variables. However, injection failure rates have been documented as high as 29% (Galardi et al., 2001), Also, given that Botox™ injections must be administered repeatedly to achieve lasting symptom relief, the issue of acquired immunoresistence to Botox™ has emerged within the research literature (Park, Simpson, Anderson, & Sataloff, 2003; Smith & Ford, 2000). Future research should continue with clinical trials, examining Botox™ effectiveness in combination with voice therapy.

Alternative Treatments

Acupuncture has been used as an alternative treatment for ADSD and, anecdotally, has been associated with improvements in voice performance (Crevier-Buchman, Laccourreye, Papon, Nurit, & Brasnu, 1997; Lee et al., 2003). These changes do not necessarily translate into improvements in perceptual measures of voice symptom severity and, in fact, continued acupuncture treatment was not desired by a majority of participants in one recent study (Lee et al., 2003).

There also exists a single case study examining the effect of chiropractic manipulation of the first and second cervical vertebrae in an individual with ADSD hypothesizing that manipulations reduce vagus nerve compression restoring normal nerve conduction. Treatment occurred five times during a 2-week period and was reported to display some improvement in phonation after two sessions, with complete symptom resolution by the conclusion of five treatment sessions (Wood, 1991).

Behavioral Treatments

The primary voice symptoms of ADSD are typically reduced during whisper or breathy voice (performed with complete or partial vocal fold abduction), cough, throat clearing, singing, humming, and altered pitch maneuvers (Bloch, Hirano, & Gould, 1985). Observation of these effects has led to the development of various styles of voicing that can be trained therapeutically to help minimize the primary voice symptoms of ADSD. Other behavioral techniques seek to reduce laryngeal tension, a separate and secondary phenomenon that may contribute to reduced vocal quality.

Use of vocal abductor muscles to counteract the adductor spasms associated with ADSD is the rationale behind use of a technique called inverse phonation. Here, individuals with ADSD are taught to phonate on inhalation, rather than exhalation. There are isolated reports of success with this technique; however, difficulty in carryover and habituation of this style of voicing have limited its therapeutic use (Harrison, Davis, Troughear, & Winkworth, 1992; Miller & Woodson,

1991). General body relaxation or muscle tension reduction techniques are ineffective at eliminating ADSD symptoms (Henschen & Burton, 1978). Laryngeal massage targets extrinsic laryngeal musculature to achieve a lowering of the resting position of the larynx. This technique has not been shown to be an effective treatment for ADSD, but can be a useful tool in the differentiation of ADSD from MTD where it can produce substantial and long-term symptom relief (Roy, Ford, & Bless, 1996).

Conventional voice therapy for ADSD seeks to minimize adverse vocal symptoms through use of easy onset voicing while enhancing breath support for speech. These behaviors are first learned in isolation, and then carried over into conversational contexts through guided practice (Miller & Woodson, 1991). Although this approach has been set forth as an independently effective cure for ADSD (Cooper, 1990), it has largely been abandoned as a stand-alone treatment and is more frequently used as an adjunctive therapy to surgery (Dedo & Izdebski, 1983) or Botox™ injection (Miller & Woodson, 1991; Murry & Woodson, 1995).

Combined Modality Treatments

In a review of treatment options for ADSD, Miller and Woodson (1991) stressed the importance of continued research into the role of voice therapy, in combination with Botox™ injections, in the treatment of ADSD. In spite of this, to date there is only one published study, now over a decade old, which addresses the role of voice therapy in a combined modality approach to the treatment of ADSD (Murry & Woodson, 1995). The investigation involved 27 participants with ADSD and no prior history of Botox™ treatment. Participants were injected, and then returned to clinic three weeks later where they were offered a course of voice therapy. Those who declined voice therapy were assigned to the Botox™ only group, and those who accepted were assigned to the combined modality group. Dependent variables examined were durational (time, in weeks, between initial and repeat Botox™ injection, acoustic (standard deviation of F0, jitter, shimmer, and signal to noise ratio — SNR), aerodynamic (mean airflow rates during /a/), and speech (words per minute) variables. Participants in the combined modality group were observed to go longer between injections (M = 27.4 weeks, range = 13 to 54 weeks) than the Botox™ only group (M = 9 weeks, range = 9 to 26 weeks). This between-groups difference in durational effect rose to the level of statistical significance. Within groups, analysis revealed that participants in the combined modality group achieved statistically significant improvements in mean airflow rates, standard deviation of F0, jitter, shimmer, and following voice therapy compared to the Botox™ only group, suggesting this approach should be investigated more thoroughly, along with the inclusion of a placebo group.

Voice Therapy for School-Age Children with Voice Disorders

Traditional models for pediatric voice therapy have largely focused on eliminating vocal behaviors that are not conducive to vocal health (a "don't do" approach). Consequently, scientific literature and anecdotal clinical reports indicate that this is rarely a successful model. Current opinions (Andrews, 2002; Stemple, Glaze, & Gerdeman, 2000) have advocated a combination of hygienic and physiologic models of voice therapy in order to address rehabilitation in pediatric voice disorders. For example, a child will forget that shouting or making truck/animal noises is not vocally healthy. As it is nearly impossible to stop

the child from engaging in phonotraumatic behavior, it may be beneficial to train them to make these sounds more therapeutically.

Voice therapy occurs in the school setting for most children with identified vocal pathology, and as a result, there is a federal guideline know as "The Individuals with Disabilities Education Act (IDEA) Amendments of 1997 (P. L. 105-17)" which outline parameters for services that are provided in an educational setting. The final Part B section of the document states that a child is only eligible for services if the impairment "adversely impacts educational performance." However, students with voice disorders may fail to receive therapeutic services due to the misconception that their disability will not adversely affect academic performance or achievement; a misunderstanding of IDEA (Andrews, 2002; Hoffman-Ruddy & Sapienza, 2004). In an effort to clarify some of the adverse effects a voice impairment can have on a child's educational performance or achievement, Andrews (2002), and Hoffman-Ruddy and Sapienza (2004), suggest that children may have:

- ■ difficulty being heard or communicating in educational environments inside or outside of the classroom setting limited participation in public speaking activities fear of participating in oral reading activities
- ■ limited participation in classroom discussions with peer groups fear of conversing in interpersonal interactions (i.e., raising hand to request to go to the bathroom)
- ■ limited participation in regular physical education routines due to compromised physiologic aspects of the laryngeal anatomy
- ■ limited participation in music education (vocal and instrumental) due to a compromised upper airway

- reluctance to participate in activities, such as school plays, cheerleading, and debate
- limited participation in secondary education co-op activities
- negative attention from peers, teachers, and other school personnel
- hindrance of academic goals of other classroom students (i.e., a child's voice quality may be distracting to other classmates who may focus on the abnormal voice quality instead of the content of the message).

Further readings specific to childhood voice disorders (Andrews, 2002; Lee, Stemple, Glaze, & Kelchner, 2004) should be consulted as this area of management continues to evolve.

Biofeedback Techniques

Biofeedback is the feedback of biological information to gain control of bodily processes that normally cannot be controlled voluntarily. The use of biofeedback with voice patients appears effective and is easily integrated into a treatment program with a variety of patient types. Electromyography is (EMG) is one method used to provide feedback to patients with regard to the degree of muscle activity they are producing during voicing tasks. This can be particularly helpful for patients exhibiting above average muscle tension or hyperfunctional voicing characteristics. By strategically placing surface electrodes over the extrinsic laryngeal muscles, visual feedback can be provided of the muscle's force activities. Higher amplitude of an EMG signal reflects greater muscle activity, and lower amplitude of an EMG waveform reflects lower muscle activity. In the treatment of those with voice disorders,

the clinician has the patient monitor both perceptual and physiologic processes associated with the voice disorder while implementing a particular treatment regime that attempts to reduce the hyperfunctional behaviors. Likewise, real-time visually presented feedback can be useful through oscillographic displays or online computer monitoring systems to help enhance breathing pattern.

Murdoch, Pitt, Theodoro, and Ward (1999) used biofeedback with the inductance plethysmography (or Respitrace) to provide real-time, continuous visual biofeedback of rib cage circumference during breathing in a child with traumatic brain injury. Results showed very good success with the biofeedback technique when compared to traditional instructions for proper speech breathing and Murdoch and colleagues believed that the visual biofeedback techniques brought about far superior outcome when compared to traditional methods.

Defining a Voice Outcome

The value of defining outcomes with therapy should not be underestimated given the increasing demands by patients, insurance companies, and policy writers. The outcomes that are selected for making judgment about improvements in vocal performance or quality of life with intervention need to be selected carefully based on their validity and reliability. Objective measures that have reliability and validity provide the underpinning(s) for accountability (see Chapter 4). And, although those involved in voice have progressed forward in the generation of a database of outcomes, we must continue to design experimental trials that are of excellence in procedural methods so we can best determine the most effective and efficacious practice(s).

Criteria for Termination of Therapy

There are several criteria for terminating therapy including resolution of the vocal pathology, patient satisfaction with the voice outcome, and the unfortunate circumstance when managed care and reimbursement issues limit the patient's ability to continue with services. In these cases, a home-based voice therapy program can be developed with medical reevaluation that is typically covered by third-party pay. Some conditions require ongoing reassessment like those affected by laryngeal cancer.

Definition of Treatment Effectiveness

An applied treatment is deemed effective when it successfully addresses the needs and complaints of the patient is deemed effective (Carding, 2000). There can be varying levels of the "complaint" and these variations led the World Health Organization (WHO) to define terms such as impairment, disability, and handicap. The WHO defined impairment as the loss or abnormality of psychological, physiologic, or anatomic structure or function. Disability is defined as any restriction or lack (resulting from impairment) of ability to perform an activity in the (normal) manner. And, finally, handicap is defined as a disadvantage, resulting from an impairment or disability that limits or prevents fulfillment of a (normal) role (http://www.who.int/medicines/publications/essentialmedicines/en/).

Therefore, with regard to a voice disorder, the impairment might be impairment of pitch or loudness. The disability would be the restriction of ability to produce song production (disability in singing) or talking with a resulting handicap that does not allow the person to engage in regular occupational activities, restricts a career choice, or the engagement in particular social activities.

When faced with a patient presenting a voice disorder, we are called on, and are responsible for, addressing the patient's complaint. But, our treatments may not be effective in addressing all levels of the complaint and may only be able to target the impairment with the hope that the disability and handicap will dissipate as the impairment is resolved.

Summary

Voice therapy strategies are carefully selected based on the pathophysiology of the disease and the patient's presentation of symptoms. There are several distinct treatment modalities to select from and combinations of these modalities may best serve the patient. The clinician must carefully select the interventional tools and ensure that outcomes are being tracked diligently in order to document patient improvement or determine whether a treatment plan should be changed or terminated.

References

Adams, S. G., Durkin, L. C., Irish, J. C., Wong, D. L., & Hunt, E. J. (1996). Effects of botulinum toxin type A injections on aerodynamic measures of spasmodic dysphonia. *Laryngoscope*, *106*(3 Pt. 1), 296–300.

Allegretto, M., Morrison, M., Rammage, L., & Lau, D. P. (2003). Selective denervation: Reinnervation for the control of adductor spasmodic dysphonia. *Journal of Otolaryngology*, *32*(3), 185–189.

Altman, K. W., Mirza, N., Ruiz, C., & Sataloff, R. T. (2000). Paradoxical vocal fold motion: Presentation and treatment options. *Journal of Voice, 14*(1), 99–103.

Andrews, M. (2002). *Voice treatment for children and adolescents*. San Diego, CA: Singular.

Aronson, A. E. (1990). *Clinical voice disorders: An interdisciplinary approach*. New York, NY: Thieme.

Aronson, A. E., & DeSanto, L. W. (1981). Adductor spastic dysphonia: 1 1/2 years after recurrent laryngeal nerve resection. *Annals of Otolology, Rhinology, and Laryngology, 90*(1 Pt. 1), 2–6.

Barton, R. T. (1979). Treatment of spastic dysphonia by recurrent laryngeal nerve section. *Laryngoscope, 89*(2 Pt. 1), 244–249.

Bastian, R. W., & Negorsky, M. J. (1987). Laryngeal image biofeedback. *Laryngoscope, 97*(11), 1346–1349.

Baumgartner, C. A., Sapir, S., & Ramig, L. O. (2001). Voice quality changes following phonatory-respiratory effort treatment (LSVT) versus respiratory effort treatment for individuals with Parkinson's disease. *Journal of Voice, 15*(1), 105–114.

Baylor, C. R., Yorkston, K. M., Eadie, T. L., & Maronian, N. C. (2007). The psychosocial consequences of botox injections for spasmodic dysphonia: A qualitative study of patients' experiences. *Journal of Voice, 21*(2), 231–247.

Belafsky, P. C., & Postma, G. N. (2004). Vocal fold augmentation with calcium hydroxylapatite. *Otolaryngology-Head and Neck Surgery, 131*(4), 351–354.

Berke, G. S., Blackwell, K. E., Gerratt, B. R., Verneil, A., Jackson, K. S., & Sercarz, J. A. (1999). Selective laryngeal adductor denervation-reinnervation: A new surgical treatment for adductor spasmodic dysphonia. *Annals of Otology, Rhinology, and Laryngology, 108*(3), 227–231.

Bhattacharyya, N., & Tarsy, D. (2001). Impact on quality of life of botulinum toxin treatments for spasmodic dysphonia and oromandibular dystonia. *Archives of Otolaryngology-Head and Neck Surgery, 127*(4), 389–392.

Bielamowicz, S., & Ludlow, C. L. (2000). Effects of botulinum toxin on pathophysiology in spasmodic dysphonia. *Annals of Otology, Rhinology, and Laryngology, 109*(2), 194–203.

Bielamowicz, S., Squire, S., Bidus, K., & Ludlow, C. L. (2001). Assessment of posterior cricoarytenoid botulinum toxin injections in patients with abductor spasmodic dysphonia. *Annals of Otology, Rhinology, and Laryngology, 110*(5 Pt. 1), 406–412.

Biller, H. F., Som, M. L., & Lawson, W. (1979). Laryngeal nerve crush for spastic dysphonia. *Annals of Otolaryngology, Rhinology, and Laryngology, 88*(4 Pt. 1), 531–532.

Bless, D. M., Hirano, M., & Feder, R. J. (1987). Videostroboscopic evaluation of the larynx. *Ear, Nose, and Throat Journal, 66*(7), 289–296.

Blitzer, A., Brin, M. F., & Stewart, C. F. (1998). Botulinum toxin management of spasmodic dysphonia (laryngeal dystonia): A 12-year experience in more than 900 patients. *Laryngoscope, 108*(10), 1435–1441.

Blitzer, A., & Sulica, L. (2001). Botulinum toxin: Basic science and clinical uses in otolaryngology [Review]. *Laryngoscope, 111*(2), 218–226.

Bloch, C. S., Hirano, M., & Gould, W. J. (1985). Symptom improvement of spastic dysphonia in response to phonatory tasks. *Annals of Otology, Rhinololgy and Laryngology, 94*(1 Pt. 1), 51–54.

Boone, D. R. (1971). *The voice and voice therapy*. Englewood Cliffs, NJ: Prentice-Hall.

Boone, D. R., & McFarlane, S. C. (1988). *The voice and voice therapy*. Englewood Cliffs, NJ: Prentice-Hall.

Boone, D. R., McFarland, S., & Von Berg, S. (2005). *The voice and voice therapy* (7th ed.) Boston, MA: Allyn and Bacon.

Boutsen, F., Cannito, M. P., Taylor, M., & Bender, B. (2002). Botox treatment in adductor spasmodic dysphonia: A meta-analysis. *Journal of Speech, Language, and Hearing Research, 45*(3), 469–481.

Branski, R. C., Verdolini, K., Sandulache, V., Rosen, C. A., & Hebda, P. A. (2006). Vocal fold wound healing: A review for clinicians. *Journal of Voice, 20*(3), 432–442.

Brodnitz, F. S. (1954). Voice problems of the actor and singer. *Journal of Speech and Hearing Disorders, 19*(3), 322–326.

Brodnitz, F. S., & Froeschels, E. (1954). Treatment of nodules of vocal cords by chewing method. *AMA Archives of Otolaryngology, 59*(5), 560–565.

Cantarella, G., Berlusconi, A., Maraschi, B., Ghio, A., & Barbieri, S. (2006). Botulinum toxin injection and airflow stability in spasmodic dysphonia. *Otolaryngology-Head and Neck Surgery, 134*(3), 419–423.

Carpenter, R. J., 3rd, Henley-Cohn, J. L., & Snyder, G. G., 3rd. (1979). Spastic dysphonia: Treatment by selective section of the recurrent laryngeal nerve. *Laryngoscope, 89*(12), 2000–2003.

Carding, P. (2000). *Evaluating voice therapy: Measuring the effectiveness of treatment.* London, UK: Whurr.

Chan, R. W. (1994). Does the voice improve with vocal hygiene education? A study of some instrumental voice measures in a group of kindergarten teachers. *Journal of Voice, 8*(3), 279–291.

Chan, S. W., Baxter, M., Oates, J., & Yorston, A. (2004). Long-term results of type ii thyroplasty for adductor spasmodic dysphonia. *Laryngoscope, 114*(9), 1604–1608.

Chhetri, D. K., & Berke, G. S. (2006). Treatment of adductor spasmodic dysphonia with selective laryngeal adductor denervation and reinnervation surgery. *Otolaryngologic Clinics of North America, 39*(1), 101–109.

Chhetri, D. K., Mendelsohn, A. H., Blumin, J. H., & Berke, G. S. (2006). Long-term follow-up results of selective laryngeal adductor denervation-reinnervation surgery for adductor spasmodic dysphonia. *Laryngoscope, 116*(4), 635–642.

Clanton, T. L., & Diaz, P.T. (1995). Clinical assessment of the respiratory muscles [Review]. *Physical Therapy, 75*(11), 983–995.

Colton, R., & Casper, J. (1996). *Understanding voice problems: A physiological perspective for diagnosis and treatment* (2nd ed). Baltimore, MD: Lippincott Williams & Wilkins.

Colton, R., Casper, J., & Leonard, R. (2006). *Understanding voice problems: A physiological perspective for diagnosis and treatment* (3rd ed). Baltimore, MD: Lippincott Williams & Wilkins.

Cooper, M. (1990). Spastic dysphonia simplified. *ASHA, 32*(8), 3.

Courey, M. S., Garrett, C. G., Billante, C. R., Stone, R. E., Portell, M. D., Smith, T. L., & Netterville, J. R. (2000). Outcomes assessment following treatment of spasmodic dysphonia with botulinum toxin. *Annals of Otology, Rhinology, and Laryngology, 109*(9), 819–822.

Crevier-Buchman, L., Laccourreye, O., Papon, J. F., Nurit, D., & Brasnu, D. (1997). Adductor spasmodic dysphonia: Case reports with acoustic analysis following botulinum toxin injection and acupuncture. *Journal of Voice, 11*(2), 232–237.

Damrose, J. F., Goldman, S. N., Groessl, E. J., & Orloff, L. A. (2004). The impact of long-term botulinum toxin injections on symptom severity in patients with spasmodic dysphonia. *Journal of Voice, 18*(3), 415–422.

Dedo, H. H. (1976). Recurrent laryngeal nerve section for spastic dysphonia. *Annals of Otology, Rhinology, and Laryngology, 85*(4 Pt. 1), 451–459.

Dedo, H. H., & Izdebski, K. (1983). Intermediate results of 306 recurrent laryngeal nerve sections for spastic dysphonia. *Laryngoscope, 93*(1), 9–16.

Denizoglu, I., & Pehlivan, M. (2008). *Vocal posturometer.* 37th Annual Symposium: Care of the Professional Voice. May 28–June 1; Philadelphia, PA.

El Sharkawi, A., Ramig, L., Logemann, J. A., Pauloski, B. R., Rademaker, A. W., Smith, C. H., . . . Werner, C. (2002). Swallowing and voice effects of Lee Silverman Voice Treatment (LSVT): A pilot study. *Journal of Neurology, Neurosurgery and Psychiatry, 72*(1), 31–36.

Epstein, R., Stygall, J., & Newman, S. (1997). The short-term impact of botox injections on speech disability in adductor spasmodic dysphonia. *Disability and Rehabilitation,19*(1), 20–25.

Finnegan, E. M., Luschei, E. S., Gordon, J. D., Barkmeier, J. M., & Hoffman, H. T. (1999). Increased stability of airflow following botulinum toxin injection. *Laryngoscope, 109*(8), 1300–1306.

Fisher, K. V., Scherer, R. C., Guo, C. G., & Owen, A. S. (1996). Longitudinal phonatory characteristics after botulinum toxin type A injection. *Journal of Speech and Hearing Research, 39*(5), 968–980.

Friedman, M., Toriumi, D. M., Grybauskas, V. T., & Applebaum, E. L. (1989). Implantation of a recurrent laryngeal nerve stimulator for the treatment of spastic dysphonia. *Annals of Otology, Rhinology, and Laryngology*, *98*(2), 130–134.

Friedman, M., Wernicke, J. F., & Caldarelli, D. D. (1994). Safety and tolerability of the implantable recurrent laryngeal nerve stimulator. *Laryngoscope*, *104*(10), 1240–1244.

Fritzell, B., Hammarberg, B., Schiratzki, H., Haglund, S., Knutsson, E., & Martensson, A. (1993). Long-term results of recurrent laryngeal nerve resection for adductor spasmodic dysphonia. *Journal of Voice*, *7*(2), 172–178.

Galardi, G., Guerriero, R., Amadio, S., Leocani, L., Teggi, R., Melloni, G., & Comi, G. (2001). Sporadic failure of botulinum toxin treatment in usually responsive patients with adductor spasmodic dysphonia. *Neurological Sciences*, *22*(4), 303–306.

Gonzalez-Rothi, L. H., Musson, N., Rosenbek, J. C., & Sapienza, C. M. (2008). Neuroplasticity and rehabilitation research for speech, language, and swallowing disorders [Review]. *Journal of Speech-Language and Hearing Research*, *51*(1), S222–S224.

Harrison, G. A., Davis, P. J., Troughear, R. H., & Winkworth, A. L. (1992). Inspiratory speech as a management option for spastic dysphonia. Case study. *Annals of Otology, Rhinology, and Laryngology*, *101*(5), 375–382.

Henschen, T. L., & Burton, N. G. (1978). Treatment of spastic dysphonia by emg biofeedback. *Biofeedback and Self-Regulation*, *3*(1), 91–96.

Hill, D. P., Meyers, A. D., & Harris, J. (1991). Autologous fat injection for vocal cord medialization in the canine larynx. *Laryngoscope*, *101*(4 Pt. 1), 344–348.

Hirano, M., Tanaka, S., Tanaka, Y., & Hibi, S. (1990). Transcutaneous intrafold injection for unilateral vocal fold paralysis: Functional results. *Annals of Otology, Rhinology, and Laryngology*, *99*(8), 598–604.

Hoffman-Ruddy, B., Davenport, P., Baylor, J., Lehman, J. Baker, S., & Sapienza, C. (2004). Inspiratory muscle strength training with behavioral therapy in a case of a rower with presumed exercise-induced paradoxical vocalfold dysfunction. *International Journal of Pediatric Otorhinolaryngolgy*, *68*(10), 1327–1332.

Hoffman-Ruddy, B., & Sapienza, C. M (2004). Treating voice disorders in the school based setting: Working in the framework of IDEA. *Language, Speech and Hearing in Schools*. *35*(4), 327–332.

Hogikyan, N. D., Wodchis, W. P., Spak, C., & Kileny, P. R. (2001). Longitudinal effects of botulinum toxin injections on voice-related quality of life (V-RQOL) for patients with adductory spasmodic dysphonia. *Journal of Voice*, *15*(4), 576–586.

Individuals with Disabilities Education Act Amendments of 1997, PUB.105-17.20 U.S.C., 1400 *et seq.*

Isshiki, N. (1998). Vocal mechanics as the basis for phonosurgery. *Laryngoscope*, *108*(12), 1761–1766.

Isshiki, N., Haji, T., Yamamoto, Y., & Mahieu, H. F. (2001). Thyroplasty for adductor spasmodic dysphonia: Further experiences. *Laryngoscope*, *111*(4 Pt. 1), 615–621.

Isshiki, N., Tsuji, D. H., Yamamoto, Y., & Iizuka, Y. (2000). Midline lateralization thyroplasty for adductor spasmodic dysphonia. *Annals of Otology, Rhinology, and Laryngology*, *109*(2), 187–193.

Izdebski, K., Dedo, H. H., Shipp, T., & Flower, R. M. (1981). Postoperative and follow-up studies of spastic dysphonia patients treated by recurrent laryngeal nerve section. *Otolaryngology-Head and Neck Surgery*, *89*(1), 96–101.

Jones, H. N., Moss, T., Edwards, L., & Kishnani, P. S. (2011). Increased inspiratory and expiratory muscle strength following respiratory muscle strength training (RMST) in two patients with late-onset Pompe disease. *Molecular Genetics and Metabolism*, *104*(3), 417–420.

Kim, J., Davenport, P. D., & Sapienza, C. M. (2008). Effect of expiratory muscle strength training on elderly cough function. *Archives of Gerontology and Geriatrics* [Epub ahead of print].

Langeveld, T. P., Luteijn, F., van Rossum, M., Drost, H. A., & Baatenburg de Jong, R. J. (2001). Adductor spasmodic dysphonia and botulinum toxin treatment: The effect on well-being. *Annals of Otology, Rhinology, and Laryngology*, *110*(10), 941–945.

Lee, L., Daughton, S., Scheer, S., Stemple, J. C., Weinrich, B., Miller-Seiler, T., Goeller, S., & Levin, L. (2003). Use of acupuncture for the treatment of adductor spasmodic dysphonia: A preliminary investigation. *Journal of Voice*, *17*(3), 411–424.

Lee, L., Stemple, J. C., Glaze, L., & Kelchner, L. (2004). Quick screen for voice and supplementary documents for identifying pediatric voice disorders. *Language Speech and Hearing Services in Schools*, *35*, 305–319.

Levine, H. L., Wood, B. G., Batza, E., Rusnov, M., & Tucker, H. M. (1979). Recurrent laryngeal nerve section for spasmodic dysphonia. *Otolaryngology-Head and Neck Surgery*, *88*(4 Pt. 1), 527–530.

Ludlow, C. L., Naunton, R. F., Fujita, M., & Sedory, S. E. (1990). Spasmodic dysphonia: Botulinum toxin injection after recurrent nerve surgery. *Otolaryngology-Head and Neck Surgery*, *102*(2), 122–131.

Martin, R. J., Blager, F. B., Gay, M. L., & Wood, R. P. II. (1987). Paradoxic vocal cord motion in presumed asthmatics. *Seminars in Respiratory Medicine*, *8*(4), 332–337.

Mehta, R. P., Goldman, S. N., & Orloff, L. A. (2001). Long-term therapy for spasmodic dysphonia: Acoustic and aerodynamic outcomes. *Archives of Otolaryngology-Head and Neck Surgery*, *127*(4), 393–399.

Miller, R. H., & Woodson, G. E. (1991). Treatment options in spasmodic dysphonia. *Otolaryngology Clinics of North America*, *24*(5), 1227–1237.

Miller, R. H., Woodson, G. E., & Jankovic, J. (1987). Botulinum toxin injection of the vocal fold for spasmodic dysphonia. A preliminary report. *Archives of Otolaryngology-Head and Neck Surgery*, *113*(6), 603–605.

Murdoch, B. E., Pitt, G., Theodoros, D. G., & Ward, E. C. (1999). Real-time continuous visual biofeedback in the treatment of speech breathing disorders following childhood traumatic brain injury: Report of one case. *Pediatric Rehabilitation*, *3*(1), 5–20.

Murry, T., & Woodson, G. E. (1995). Combined-modality treatment of adductor spasmodic dysphonia with botulinum toxin and voice therapy. *Journal of Voice*, *9*(4), 460–465.

Newby, H. A. (1972). *Audiology*. New York, NY: Appleton-Century-Crofts.

Owen, A. M. (2004). Working memory: Imaging the magic number four. *Current Biology*, *14*(14), R573–R574.

Pannebacker, M. (1998). Voice treatment techniques: A review and recommendations for outcome studies. *American Journal of Speech-Language Pathology*, *7*(3), 49–64.

Park, J. B., Simpson, L. L., Anderson, T. D., & Sataloff, R. (2003). Immunologic characterization of spasmodic dysphonia patients who develop resistance to botulinum toxin. *Journal of Voice*, *17*(2), 255–264.

Peppas, N. A., & Benner, R. E., Jr. (1980). Proposed method of intracordal injection and gelation of poly (vinyl alcohol) solution in vocal cords: Polymer considerations. *Biomaterials*, *1*(3), 158–162.

Pinto, Swash, M., & de Carvalho, M. (2012). Respiratory exercise in amyotrophic lateral sclerosis. *Amoyotrphoic Lateral Sclerosis*, *13*(1), 33–43.

Pitchenik, A. E. (1991). Functional laryngeal obstruction relieved by panting. *Chest*, *100*, 1465–1467.

Powers, S. K., & Howley, E. T. (2004). *Exercise physiology: Theory and applications to fitness and performance* (5th ed.). Boston, MA; Toronto, Canada: McGraw-Hill.

Ramig, L., Countryman, S., O'Brien, C., Hoehn, M., & Thompson, L. (1996). Intensive speech treatment for patients with Parkinson disease: Short and long-term comparison of two techniques. *Neurology*, *47*, 1496–1504.

Ramig, L. O., Countryman, S., Thompson, L. L., & Horii, Y. (1995). Comparison of two forms of intensive speech treatment for Parkinson's disease. *Journal of Speech and Hearing Research*, *38*(6), 1323–1351.

Ramig, L. O., Sapir, S., Countryman, S., Oaywlas, A. A., O'Brien, C., Hoehn, M., & Thompson, L. L. (2001). Intensive voice treatment (LSVT) for patients with Parkinson's disease: A 2-year follow-up. *Journal of Neurology, Neurosurgery, and Psychiatry*, *71*(4), 493–498.

Ramig, L., Sapir, S., Fox, C., & Countryman, S. (2001). Changes in vocal intensity following intensive voice treatment (LSVT®) in individuals with Parkinson disease: A comparison with untreated patients and normal age-matched controls. *Movement Disorders, 16,* 79–83.

Remacle, M., Plouin-Gaudon, I., Lawson, G., & Abitbol, J. (2005). Bipolar radiofrequency-induced thermotherapy (RFITT) for the treatment of spasmodic dysphonia. A report of three cases. *European Archives of Otorhinolaryngology, 262*(10), 871–874.

Robey, R. R. (2004). A five-phase model for clinical-outcome research. *Journal of Communication Disorders, 37*(5), 401–411.

Rousseau, B., Ge, P., Ohno, T., French, L. C., Thibeault, S. L., & Ossoff, R. H. (2008). *Investigation of experimental induced phonation on gene expression of the vocal fold 48 hours after injury.* 37th Annual Symposium: Care of the Professional Voice, Philadelphia, PA.

Roy, N., Ford, C. N., & Bless, D. M. (1996). Muscle tension dysphonia and spasmodic dysphonia: The role of manual laryngeal tension reduction in diagnosis and management. *Annals of Otology, Rhinology, and Laryngology, 105*(11), 851–856.

Roy, N., Gray, S. D., Simon, M., Dove, H., Corbin-Lewis, K., & Stemple, J. C. (2001). An evaluation of the effects of two treatment approaches for teachers with voice disorders: A prospective randomized clinical trial. *Journal of Speech Language and Hearing Research, 44*(2), 286–296.

Roy, N., & Leeper, H. A. (1993). Effects of the manual laryngeal musculoskeletal tension reduction technique as a treatment for functional voice disorders: Perceptual and acoustic measures. *Journal of Voice, 7*(3), 242–249.

Roy, N., Mauszycki, Merrill, R. M., Gouse, M., & Smith, M. E. (2007). Toward improved differential diagnosis of adductor spasmodic dysphonia and muscle tension dysphonia. *Folia Phoniatrica et Logopaedia, 59*(2), 83–90.

Rubin, A. D., Wodchis, W. P., Spak, C., Kileny, P. R., & Hogikyan, N. D. (2004). Longitudinal effects of botox injections on voice-related quality of life (V-RQOL) for patients with adductory spasmodic dysphonia: Part II. *Archives of Otolaryngology-Head and Neck Surgery, 130*(4), 415–420.

Sabol, J. W., Lee, L., & Stemple, J. C. (1995). Efficacy of vocal function exercises in the practice regimen of singers. *Journal of Voice, 9*(1), 27–36.

Sapienza, C. M. (2008). Respiratory muscle strength training application. *Current Opinions of Otolaryngology-Head and Neck Surgery, 16*(3), 216–220.

Sapienza, C. M., Cannito, M. P., Murry, T., Branski, R., & Woodson, G. (2002). Acoustic variations in reading produced by speakers with spasmodic dysphonia pre-Botox injection and within early stages of post-Botox injection. *Journal of Speech Language and Hearing Research, 45*(5), 830–843.

Sapienza, C., Troche, M., Pitts, T., & Davenport, P. (2011). Respiratory strength training: concept and intervention outcomes. *Seminars in Speech and Language, 32*(1), 21–30.

Sapir, S., Spielman, J. L., Ramig, L. O., Story, B. H., & Fox, C. (2007). Effects of an extended version of the Lee Silverman Voice Treatment (LSVT) on voice and speech in Parkinson's disease. *American Journal of Speech Language Pathology, 16*(2), 95–107.

Schiratzki, H., & Fritzell, B. (1991). Treatment of spasmodic dysphonia by means of resection of the recurrent laryngeal nerve. *Acta Otolaryngolica. Supplementum, 449,* 115–117.

Schramm, V. L., May, M., & Lavorato, A. S. (1978). Gelfoam paste injection for vocal cord paralysis: Temporary rehabilitation of glottic incompetence. *Laryngoscope, 88*(8 Pt. 1), 1268–1273.

Sercarz, J. A., Berke, G. S., Ming, Y., Rothschiller, J., & Graves, M. C. (1992). Bilateral thyroarytenoid denervation: A new treatment for laryngeal hyperadduction disorders studied in the canine. *Otolaryngology-Head and Neck Surgery, 107*(5), 657–668.

Shindo, M. L., Herzon, G. D., Hanson, D. G., Cain, D. J., & Sahgal, V. (1992). Effects of denervation on laryngeal muscles: A canine model. *Laryngoscope, 102*(6), 663–669.

Smith, M. E., & Ford, C. N. (2000). Resistance to botulinum toxin injections for spasmodic dysphonia. *Archives of Otolaryngology-Head and Neck Surgery, 126*(4), 533–535.

Spielman, J., Ramig, L. O., Mahler, L., Halpern, A., & Gavin, W. J. (2007). Effects of an extended version of the Lee Silverman Voice Treatment (LSVT) on voice and speech in parkinson's disease. *American Journal of Speech Language Pathology*, *16*(2), 95–107.

Spielman, J. L., Borod, J. C., & Ramig, L. O. (2003). The effects of intensive voice treatment on facial expressiveness in parkinson disease: Preliminary data. *Cognitive Behavioral Neurology*, *16*(3), 177–188.

Stemple, J. C., Glaze, L. E., & Gerdeman-Klaben, B. (2000). *Clinical voice pathology: Theory and management* (3rd ed.). San Diego, CA: Singular.

Stemple, J. C., Lee, L., D'Amico, B., & Pickup, B. (1994). Efficacy of vocal function exercises as a method of improving voice production. *Journal of Voice*, *8*(3), 271–278.

Su, C. Y., Chuang, H. C., Tsai, S. S., & Chiu, J. F. (2007). Transoral approach to laser thyroarytenoid myoneurectomy for treatment of adductor spasmodic dysphonia: Short-term results. *Annals of Otology, Rhinology, and Laryngology*, *116*(1), 11–18.

The use of voice therapy in the treatment of dysphonia. Retrieved from http://www.asha.org/docs/html/TR2005-00158.html

Timmermans, B., De Bodt, M. S., Wuyts, F. L., & Van de Heyning, P. H. (2004). Training outcome in future professional voice users after 18 months of voice training. *Folia Phoniatrica et Logopaedica*, *56*(2), 120–129.

Titze, I. R. YouTube video, titze-straw.mp2 (http://www.youtube.com/watch?v=asDg7T-WT-0).

Tsunoda, K., Amagai, N., Kondou, K., Baer, T., Kaga, K., & Niimi, S. (2005). Autologous replacement of the vocal fold: A new surgical approach for adduction-type spasmodic dysphonia. *Journal of Laryngology and Otology*, *119*(3), 222–225.

Tucker, H. M. (1989). Long-term results of nerve-muscle pedicle reinnervation for laryngeal paralysis. *Annals of Otology, Rhinology, and Laryngology*, *98*(9), 674–676.

Van Riper, C. (1939). *Speech correction principles and methods*. Englewood Cliffs, NJ: Prentice-Hall.

Verdolini, K. (2000). Case study: Resonant voice therapy. In J. Stemple (Ed.), *Voice therapy: Clinical studies* (2nd ed., pp. 46–62). San Diego, CA: Singular.

Watts, C., Nye, C., & Whurr, R. (2006). Botulinum toxin for treating spasmodic dysphonia (laryngeal dystonia): A systematic cochrane review. *Clinical Rehabilitation*, *20*(2), 112–122.

Watts, C. C., Whurr, R., & Nye, C. (2004). Botulinum toxin injections for the treatment of spasmodic dysphonia. *Cochrane Database Systematic Review* (3), CD004327.

Welham, N. V., Lim, X., Tateya, I., & Bless, D. M. (2008). Inflammatory factor profiles one hour following vocal fold injury. *Annals of Otology, Rhinology, and Laryngology*, *117*(2), 145–152.

West, R., Kennedy, L., & Carr, A. (1937). *The rehabilitation of speech*. New York, NY: Harper and Brothers.

Whurr, R., Nye, C., & Lorch, M. (1998). Meta-analysis of botulinum toxin treatment of spasmodic dysphonia: A review of 22 studies. *International Journal of Language Communication Disorders*, *33*(Suppl.) 327–329.

Wilson, F. B., Oldring, D. J., & Mueller, K. (1980). Recurrent laryngeal nerve dissection: A case report involving return of spastic dysphonia after initial surgery. *Journal of Speech and Hearing Disorders*, *45*(1), 112–118.

Wingate, J. M., Ruddy, B. H., Lundy, D. S., Lehman, J., Casiano, R., Collins, S. P., . . . Sapienza, C. (2005). Voice Handicap Index results for older patients with adductor spasmodic dysphonia. *Journal of Voice*, *19*(1), 124–131.

Wolpes, J. (1987). *Essential principles and practices of behavior therapy*. Phoenix, AZ: Milton H. Erickson Foundation.

Wong, D. L., Adams, S. G., Irish, J. C., Durkin, L. C., Hunt, E. J., & Charlton, M. P. (1995). Effect of neuromuscular activity on the response to botulinum toxin injections in spasmodic dysphonia. *Journal of Otolaryngology*, *24*(4), 209–216.

Wood, K. W. (1991). Resolution of spasmodic dysphonia (focal laryngeal dystonia) via chiropractic manipulative management. *Manipulative Physiological Therapy*, *14*(6), 376–378.

World Health Organization. Retrieved from http://www.who.int/medicines/publications/essentialmedicines/en/

Zwirner, P., Murry, T., Swenson, M., & Woodson, G. E. (1992). Effects of botulinum toxin therapy in patients with adductor spasmodic dysphonia: Acoustic, aerodynamic, and videoendoscopic findings. *Laryngoscope, 102*(4), 400–406.

Zwirner, P., Murry, T., & Woodson, G. E. (1997). Effects of botulinum toxin on vocal tract steadiness in patients with spasmodic dysphonia. *European Archives of Otorhinolaryngology, 254*(8), 391–395.

Appendix 7–1
Voice Stimuli

The stimuli included in this Appendix are representative samples of clinical material to use with your patient in either your practice or for home-based therapy. There are a number of professional resources available that provide additional stimuli for use. See for example: Andrews, M. (1999). *Manual of Voice Treatment: Pediatrics to Geriatrics*, for a more comprehensive sample.

Phrases for Stimulating Frontal Focus/Resonance Training

- No no Nannette
- Many moons ago
- Nick never told me
- Mom made me noodles.
- Nate may move to Nevada.
- Never eat meat on Monday
- Mallory made me nut cookies
- Mike dislikes the noisy neighbors
- Last night the moon was magnificent
- Neil and Monica went to a movie at noon
- My mom saw a mouse in northern Maine
- Mom ate her meal with Nancy and Megan
- Mary took a 90-minute nap before making dinner
- Many members went up north to Missouri in November

Phrases for Stimulating Vocal Pitch Modulation

When making a statement, start the sentence at a slightly higher pitch so that the pitch can be brought down at the end. For example:

It's time to go home

I am happy to meet you

The dog had seven puppies

My son is a doctor

Let's try to meet at the store

My work day is busy today

I really like the way your car looks

Thank you for the time you spent with me today

When asking a question that could be answered "yes" or "no," do the opposite. Start lower and raise the pitch at the end. For example:

Are you ready to go?

Should we go to the movie today? Would you like more coffee?

Can you stay longer? What is your name? How are you today?

When asking a question that needs more than a "yes" or "no" answer, lower the pitch at the end of the question. For example:

Should we have soup or sandwich? What would you like for breakfast?

Do they live in Minneapolis or New York? How man eggs do you need for the recipe? What time did Matthew arrive home last night?

Strategies/Instructions to Use with Patients to Increase Vocal Loudness (A Clinical or Home Practice Routine)

1. Take a big breath before beginning to speak. This helps give enough air to speak on and will actually make the voice louder. Start by trying to hear the voice as soon as the breath is allowed to exhale. Begin by breathing in and then slowly exhaling. Try to control the air that is released when you exhale (slow and controlled). Next, say the vowels "ah" or "ee" with the lips slightly parted on a steady flow of exhaled air. Try to hold the sound for at least 15 to 20 seconds or make that an eventual goal as the practice continues. This can be done three times in a row with a 1 to 2-minute rest after each of the three sound productions. This should be done 3 to 4 times a day to help gain control of the breathing and develop an awareness of how speech is produced.

2. Make sure that the sentences/phrases that are spoken are not too long. The longer the phrase the more air that is used. If the amount of air runs out then it will require more physical effort to keep the voice loud. A phrase like: "The other day I went to the store," would be a phrase of adequate length. After finishing the phrase, another breath needs to be taken, if not it will be very difficult to make the voice stay loud.

3. Use the muscles in your abdomen to help force air out the lungs. This is especially true when the voice is used to yell or talk very loud over crowd noise. Try speaking aloud a short staccato counting phrase "hut, 2, 3, 4." Keep a hand on the abdomen and feel the in-and-out movement of the abdominal wall.

4. Maintain a good posture. It is most efficient if the body and head are facing straight. If the head is tilted to one side or the posture is slouched it does not allow the muscles that are working together to produce speech to be in an optimal position.

5. Open the mouth when speaking. If the mouth (jaw and lips) are not moving very much during speaking it actually makes the sound come out less loud. Try at first to overexaggerate lip and mouth movements when saying vowels such as "ah" or words. Hear and feel the difference when the mouth is open wide compared to trying to speak through nearly closed lips.

Voice Strategies: A Home Practice Routine for Your Patient (Useful for Patients with Hypofunctional Voice Disorders)

Integrating family members or friends is an important part of the therapy process. Having this type of support makes it easier to carry over the therapeutic strategies from a treatment session to daily activities. Also, family and friends can lend a hand by reminding you when the voice is not loud enough or clear enough. Sometimes a simple hand gesture can be a reminder to increase the loudness. These helpful reminders can help motivate a change in communication effectiveness. Below are some "homework routines" that can be completed. It's helpful to be consistent; therefore, try to choose a time of day to practice these exercises for 10 minutes without interruptions. You may wish to practice once in the morning and once in the afternoon. If you are unable to practice with a partner who can provide feedback then try to practice with a recording device so that you can play back and listen to the voice and speech production.

1. Take a big deep breath and say the vowel "ah" in a loud voice.
   Try to hold the vowel as long as possible;
2. Repeat step 1, except this time glide from the lowest possible tone (pitch) to the highest tone (pitch). Keep the voice loud and steady;
3. Practice reading short phrases, sentences, and reading paragraphs in a loud, high-energy voice;
4. Try talking in conversation in a high-energy voice;
5. Try making phone calls to friends or family members and be sure to use a high-energy voice; be aware of the number of times repetition is requested;
6. While driving or riding in a car, practice saying aloud the street signs or places passed,
7. Read short books or newspaper articles out loud. Read books to children or grandchildren in a loud voice.

Functional Sentences

1. Let's go out tonight.
2. How was your day?
3. Let's have chicken for dinner tonight.
4. It was nice to meet you.
5. Could you help me with this?
6. Did you get that?
7. I don't need any help.
8. Where are you going?
9. Who was that?
10. Have you met _____?
11. Have a good day!
12. What time is it?
13. Please pass the _____.
14. Would you do that for me?
15. Did _____ call today?
16. This is my friend, _____.
17. It's so good to see you!
18. Did you lock the door?
19. That was so nice of you!
20. Could you turn off the T.V.?
21. Are all of the windows closed?
22. Is the air conditioning on?
23. What do you have to drink?
24. I'd like to order a pizza.
25. What time will you be home?
26. What's the weather like outside?
27. I'm hungry. How about you?
28. Turn off the lights when you come up.
29. I can't find my glasses. Have you seen them?
30. I was wondering what time you would be home.
31. Could you direct me to the restrooms?
32. Would you like a cup of coffee? I could go for one.

Paragraphs for Reading (Adults)

These paragraphs can be used for oral reading exercises (with various treatment techniques)

Jane Austen, *Pride and Prejudice*

It is a truth universally acknowledged, that a single man in possession of a large fortune must be in want of a wife. However little known the feeling or views of such a man may be on his first entering a neighbourhood, this truth is so well fixed in the minds of the surrounding families, that he is considered the rightful property of some one or other of their daughters.

William Wordsworth, "Daffodils"

I WANDER'D lonely as a cloud

That floats on high o'er vales and hills,
When all at once I saw a crowd,

A host, of golden daffodils;

Beside the lake, beneath the trees,
Fluttering and dancing in the breeze.
Continuous as the stars that shine And
twinkle on the Milky Way,

They stretch'd in never-ending line

Along the margin of a bay:

Ten thousand saw I at a glance,

Tossing their heads in sprightly dance.
The waves beside them danced; but
they Outdid the sparkling waves in
glee:

A poet could not but be gay, In such a
jocund company:

I gazed — and gazed — but little
thought What wealth the show to me
had brought: For oft, when on my
couch I lie

In vacant or in pensive mood, They
flash upon that inward eye Which is
the bliss of solitude;

And then my heart with pleasure fills,
And dances with the daffodils.

Ralph Waldo Emerson, "The Amulet"

Your picture smiles as first it smiled,
The ring you gave is still the same,
Your letter tells, O changing child, No
tidings since it came.

Give me an amulet

That keeps intelligence with you, Red
when you love, and rosier red,

And when you love not, pale and blue.
Alas, that neither bonds nor vows

Can certify possession;

Torments me still the fear that love

Died in its last expression.

Ralph Waldo Emerson, "The Park"

The prosperous and beautiful

To me seem not to wear

The yoke of conscience masterful,
Which galls me everywhere.

I cannot shake off the god;

On my neck he makes his seat; I look
at my face in the glass, My eyes his eye-
balls meet. Enchanters! enchantresses!

Your gold makes you seem wise:

The morning mist within your grounds

More proudly rolls, more softly lies. Yet
spake yon purple mountain,

Yet said yon ancient wood,

That night or day, that love or crime

Lead all souls to the Good.

Thomas Jefferson, "On Slavery"

Deep rooted prejudices entertained by the
whites; ten thousand recollections, by the
blacks, of the injuries they have sustained;
new provocations; the real distinctions which
nature has made; and many other circumstances, will divide us into parties, and produce convulsions, which will probably never
end but in the extermination of the one or
the other race. — To these objections, which
are political, may be added others, which
are physical and moral. The first difference

which strikes us is that of colour.—Whether the black of the negro resides in the reticular membrane between the skin and scarf-skin, or in the scarf-skin itself; whether it proceeds from the colour of the blood, the colour of the bile, or from that of some other secretion, the difference is fixed in nature, and is as real as if its seat and cause were better known to us. And is this difference of no importance? Is it not the foundation of a greater or less share of beauty in the two races? Are not the fine mixtures of red and white, the expressions of every passion by greater or less suffusions of colour in the one, preferable to that eternal monotony, which reigns in the countenances, that immovable veil of black which covers all the emotions of the other race?

Susan B. Anthony, "Women's Suffrage"

Friends and fellow citizens: I stand before you tonight under indictment for the alleged crime of having voted at the last presidential election, without having a lawful right to vote. It shall be my work this evening to prove to you that in thus voting, I not only committed no crime, but, instead, simply exercised my citizen's rights, guaranteed to me and all United States citizens by the National Constitution, beyond the power of any state to deny.

The preamble of the Federal Constitution says:

> We, the people of the United States, in order to form a more perfect union, establish justice, insure domestic tranquillity, provide for the common defense, promote the general welfare, and secure the blessings of liberty to ourselves and our posterity, do ordain and establish this Constitution for the United States of America.

It was we, the people; not we, the white male citizens; nor yet we, the male citizens; but we, the whole people, who formed the Union. And we formed it, not to give the blessings of liberty, but to secure them; not to the half of ourselves and the half of our posterity, but to the whole people—women as well as men. And it is a downright mockery to talk to women of their enjoyment of the blessings of liberty while they are denied the use of the only means of securing them provided by this democratic-republican government—the ballot.

For any state to make sex a qualification that must ever result in the disfranchisement of one entire half of the people, is to pass a bill of attainder, or, an ex post facto law, and is therefore a violation of the supreme law of the land. By it the blessings of liberty are forever withheld from women and their female posterity.

To them this government has no just powers derived from the consent of the governed. To them this government is not a democracy. It is not a republic. It is an odious aristocracy; a hateful oligarchy of sex; the most hateful aristocracy ever established on the face of the globe; an oligarchy of wealth, where the rich govern the poor. An oligarchy of learning, where the educated govern the ignorant, or even an oligarchy of race, where the Saxon rules the African, might be endured; but this oligarchy of sex, which makes father, brothers, husband, sons, the oligarchs over the mother and sisters, the wife and daughters, of every household—which ordains all men sovereigns, all women subjects, carries dissension, discord, and rebellion into every home of the nation.

Webster, Worcester, and Bouvier all define a citizen to be a person in the United States, entitled to vote and hold office.

The only question left to be settled now is: Are women persons? And I hardly believe any of our opponents will have the hardihood to say they are not. Being persons, then, women are citizens; and no state has a right to make any law, or to enforce any old law, that shall abridge their privileges or immunities.

Hence, every discrimination against women in the constitutions and laws of the several states is today null and void, precisely as is every one against Negroes.

Patrick Henry, "Give Me Liberty, or Give Me Death"

Sir, we are not weak, if we make a proper use of the means which the God of nature hath placed in our power. Three millions of people, armed in the holy cause of liberty, and in such a country as that which we possess, are invincible by any force which our enemy can send against us. Besides, sir, we shall not fight our battles alone. There is a just God who presides over the destinies of nations, and who will raise up friends to fight our battles for us.

The battle, sir, is not to the strong alone; it is to the vigilant, the active, the brave. Besides, sir, we have no election. If we were base enough to desire it, it is now too late to retire from the contest. There is no retreat but in submission and slavery! Our chains are forged! Their clanking may be heard on the plains of Boston! The war is inevitable — and let it come! I repeat it, sir, let it come!

It is in vain, sir, to extenuate the matter. Gentlemen may cry, "Peace! Peace!" — but there is no peace. The war is actually begun! The next gale that sweeps from the north will bring to our ears the clash of resounding arms! Our brethren are already in the field! Why stand we here idle? What is it that gentlemen wish? What would they have? Is life so dear, or peace so sweet, as to be purchased at the price of chains and slavery? Forbid it, Almighty God! I know not what course others may take; but as for me, give me liberty, or give me death!

Open-Ended Questions (can be used with adult patients)

These questions can be used to stimulate spontaneous conversation with adult patients (to be used with various therapy techniques).

- Tell me about your job.
- Tell me about your family.
- Tell me about your hobbies.
- Tell me about your childhood.
- What did you do last weekend?
- What do you think you will be doing in 10 years?
- How did you decide what school/ college to attend?
- What do you think about the political climate in _____?
- What do you think about _____?
- Would you tell me more about _____?

Open-Ended Questions (can be used with pediatric patients)

These questions can be used to stimulate spontaneous conversation with children (to be used with various therapy techniques).

- What did you have for breakfast?
- Tell me about your favorite episode of _____?
- What did you do this morning?
- What did you do last weekend?
- Tell me how to play _____?
- Can you tell me how you brush your teeth?

Chapter 8

Management: Phonosurgery

On the DVD included with this text exist four video cases that are pertinent to this chapter: removal of a bilateral vocal fold nodules, removal of laryngeal papilloma with conventional and microdebrider techniques, CO_2 laser removal of a recurring squamous cell carcinoma postradiation, and management of Reinke's edema. Additionally, cases imaged via direct laryngoscopy pre- and postsurgery are included for a more complete library reference (see Cases 1–21).

After reading this chapter, you will:

■ Understand several phonosurgical procedures for removing vocal fold lesions/pathologies
■ Understand the difference between office-based procedures and those performed under anesthesia within the surgical suite
■ Understand the basic instrumental setups used in phonosurgical procedures of the larynx

by advancements in the diagnostic technology available in the voice lab, has driven much of this. Technologic advancements in the operating room have also played a role. Equally important, however, is the multidisciplinary and collaborative approach to voice disorders that pairs the otolaryngologist and voice pathologist in the diagnosis and management of these conditions.

The concept of phonosurgery was developed with the goal of preserving and enhancing the mucosal wave. Whereas older surgical approaches stressed removal of all apparently pathologic tissue, contemporary techniques treat many conditions based on the dictum that "less is more." This is particularly the case in those situations where mucosal or submucosal disease is reactive; abnormal looking tissue may be preserved to minimize scarring and preserve the layered ultrastructure of the vocal fold as much as possible. This chapter introduces the surgical options available to treat dysphonia, along with the postoperative considerations important to the voice pathologist.

Surgical Treatment of Dysphonia

The surgical management of dysphonia has undergone a significant transformation over the last few decades. An improved understanding of vocal physiology, made possible

Office-Based Procedures

Before those procedures performed in the operating room are addressed, the concept of office based laryngeal procedures is briefly discussed.

Indirect Laryngoscopy

Indirect laryngoscopy is the oldest technique for office examination of the vocal folds. In the hands of a skilled laryngologist, it can be used for procedural visualization. The mirror is placed near the soft palate to view the vocal folds, and topical anesthesia is produced by one of several techniques. Curved instruments are then introduced through the mouth to reach the vocal folds. This technique can be difficult to master and requires a very cooperative patient. Nonetheless, some laryngologists are quite successful in performing therapeutic injections, biopsies, and foreign body removals in the office by this approach.

Flexible laryngoscopes have been used more recently for visualization of the vocal folds in the office, and allow laryngeal inspection in patients whose anatomy or gag reflex precludes an adequate view with the indirect mirror. Newer versions of these scopes come equipped with operating channels that allow passage of small flexible instruments, laser fibers, or injection needles to the vocal folds under topical or local anesthesia. Placement of the video chip at the distal end of the scope can give image quality rivaling that of a rigid scope, and some of the newest scopes have combined this with an operating channel capability.

Alternatively, passing a needle transcutaneously through the cricothyroid membrane, while visualizing the injection progress with the flexible or rigid laryngoscope, can accomplish therapeutic injection of the larynx. The needle is usually introduced into the airway and then directed into the vocal fold at the desired point (Figure 8–1). The augmentation material or pharmacologic agent then can be securely placed. These procedures have been helpful in medializing a bowed or paralyzed vocal fold in order to immediately improve airway protection, or in treatment of laryngeal papillomatosis, when lesion recurrence is rapid and treatment is required between trips

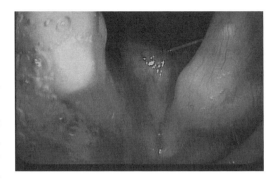

Figure 8–1. Image on injection needle introduced into the vocal fold. Courtesy of The Ear Nose Throat and Plastic Surgery Associates, Winter Park, Florida.

to the OR. In the case of Botox™ injection for spasmodic dysphonia, needle placement is often monitored by electromyography, rather than by visual inspection (see Chapter 6). This simplifies the procedure and allows the needle to be kept out of the airway, thereby reducing discomfort and the need for topical anesthesia.

All of these office-based procedures share the advantage of allowing approach to the larynx without general anesthesia, thereby reducing cost, anesthetic risk, and time required of the patient. The ability to assess glottic closure and phonation quality during the procedure is obviously beneficial. The degree to which tissue can be manipulated or resected is limited compared to those procedures performed in the operating room, but for many vocal conditions, office-based interventions are becoming a greater part of the laryngologists' armamentarium.

General Considerations in the Surgical Approach to the Larynx

In the majority of procedures, access to the vocal folds is accomplished by direct laryngoscopy (Figure 8–2). Basically, this involves the passage of a lighted, tubular scope that exposes

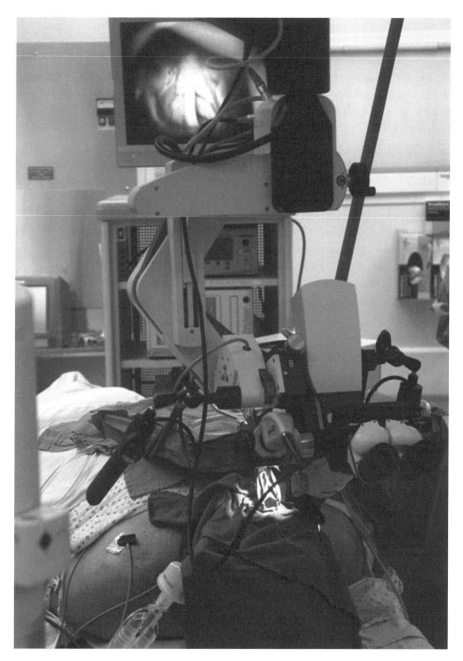

Figure 8–2. Surgical setup showing surgical microscope and suspension laryngoscopy. Vocal folds are projected above for surgeon viewing. Courtesy of The Ear Nose Throat and Plastic Surgery Associates, Winter Park, Florida.

the vocal folds by retracting the tongue base and supraglottic tissues out of the way. Several scope modifications are available, varying in their suitability for exposing different areas of the larynx and dealing with differing characteristics of patient airway anatomy. Other modifications facilitate suctioning of a laser plume (smoke), or allow distension of the scope lumen to allow for exposure of larger lesions.

Because of the significant stimulation of gag and autonomic reflexes associated with this exposure, general anesthesia is necessary. The airway is protected and secured by a small endotracheal tube that can usually be situated away from the area of dissection. The open lumen of the scope allows for visualization directly, by binocular microscopy, or by placement of a rigid-rod optic telescope (Figure 8–3). The laryngoscope is usually suspended in place mechanically, allowing a two-handed technique and stable exposure (Figure 8–4). Elongated instruments (Figure 8–5) can be easily introduced, allowing for direct manipulation of tissues, suctioning, and application of medications to the vocal tissues. Laser energy can be directed by micromanipulator along line of sight, or by optical fiber.

The glottis can also be approached externally through a midline vertical split of the thyroid cartilage, or through a lateral pharyngotomy. These approaches are used to deal with large tumors or difficult reconstructive challenges associated with injury or scarring. The specific considerations associated with these types of procedures go beyond the scope of this chapter, but they are generally associated with long hospital stays, need for a temporary tracheostomy, and a frequent need for stent placement during postoperative healing.

Laryngeal framework surgery to augment or reposition the vocal folds is important in the context of this chapter. Arytenoid and vocal fold edge position can be dramatically affected in order to address significant issues with glottic competence. This family of procedures involves an external approach to the thyroid cartilage, usually under local anesthesia with sedation, and the airway is not entered surgically.

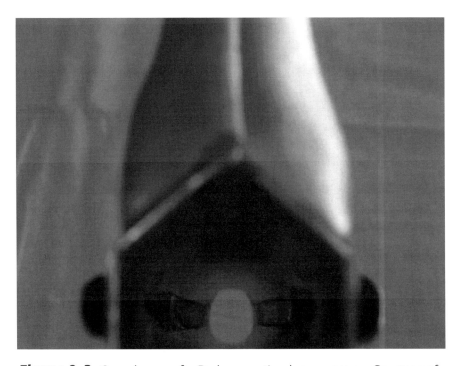

Figure 8–3. Open lumen of a Dedo operating laryngoscope. Courtesy of The Ear Nose Throat and Plastic Surgery Associates, Winter Park, Florida.

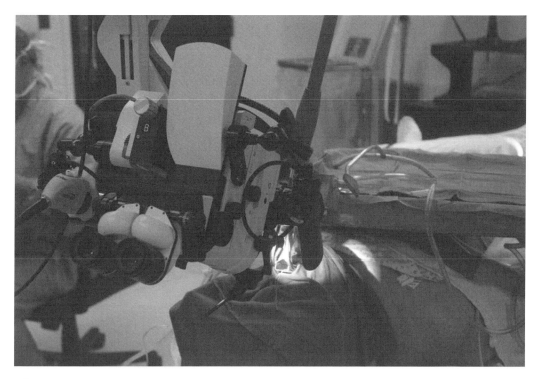

Figure 8–4. Suspended laryngoscope. Courtesy of The Ear Nose Throat and Plastic Surgery Associates, Winter Park, Florida.

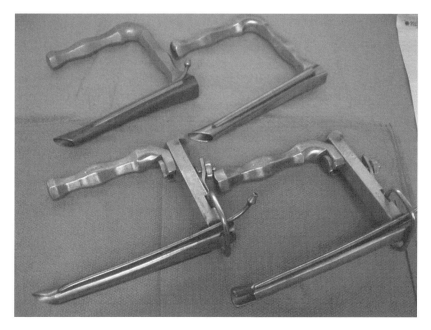

Figure 8–5. Laser laryngoscopes and instruments. Courtesy of The Ear Nose Throat and Plastic Surgery Associates, Winter Park, Florida.

Microlaryngoscopy with Nodule Removal

One of the most common procedures performed in the operating room is microlaryngoscopy with excision of nodular or small polypoid lesions causing dysphonia. This procedure involves suspension of the laryngoscope and use of the binocular microscope to enhance surgical precision. In most cases, microscissors and forceps are used in the dissection.

Laser application is usually limited to the cautery of any large feeding vessels, in the interest of limiting thermal injury to the adjacent tissues. The procedural time ranges between 10 and 20 minutes. The dissection is two-handed, using the forceps to mobilize and retract while the scissors are used to cut precisely and remove the desired tissue. The emphasis of the dissection in most of these cases is on removal of tissue that interferes with vocal edge contact and propagation of mucosal wave, while minimizing the surface area of the uncovered vocal fold that must heal by secondary means.

When dealing with small vocal nodules, surgical intervention usually is not needed, as most cases will respond to voice therapy. In refractory cases, the decision to proceed is made after much deliberation regarding compliance with vocal rest, control of aggravating factors, and the degree of dysphonia present. The persistence of visible nodular change will often be tolerated by the physician and patient, as long as voice is acceptable and remains so within the patient's daily vocal activity. If a surgical option is chosen, it is kept as pinpoint in scope as possible.

Recovery after this type of procedure is usually rapid, with improved vocal quality often noted immediately. Voice rest is ordered to minimize mechanical trauma to tissues during early healing. However, the length and degree of restriction prescribed will vary from surgeon to surgeon (Appendix 8–1). Three days of complete vocal rest is typically prescribed in my practice, followed by another 10 days of modified vocal rest. Singing or other more strenuous vocal activity is usually reintroduced gradually at 3 weeks postoperatively, with close monitoring by the voice pathologist during the process. Instruction in proper vocal hygiene is a very important part of postoperative counseling, to prevent against recurrence of nodules. Ideally, this instruction has been ongoing throughout the treatment process, making its incorporation into the patient's lifestyle more seamless.

Microflap Dissection

For larger polyps or more diffuse polypopid degeneration, the microflap dissection technique is best employed. In this application the approach is based on the creation of an initial incision on the upper vocal fold surface, usually just lateral to the edge of the lesion, followed by dissection in Reinke's space to mobilize areas of firm pathology and evacuate Reinke's edema that affect the vocal fold contour. The mucosa is then redraped over the vocal fold body, and excess portions are excised, along with areas of hyperkeratosis or other mucosal pathology unlikely to resolve without removal. The goal is to leave as little of the vocal fold body uncovered as possible, and achieve a more normal vocal fold contour. Complete operating room time ranges from 20 to 30 minutes. Microsurgical scissors, spatula-shaped flap dissectors, and microforceps are usually used in the dissection. Pre-injection of Reinke's space with vasoconstrictive local anesthetic solution is often performed. Laser use is usually limited to control of larger blood vessels, as previously noted.

Vocal fold cysts are ideally treated by a microflap approach. The incision is usually placed over the top of the cyst, which is then mobilized with careful submucosal dissection.

With the cyst wall entirely removed, normal vocal contour is restored leaving the mucosal covering intact (Figure 8–6 and Color Plate 19). Voice improvement is usually dramatic and immediate.

Postoperative recovery can range from a week or two, in cases of smaller polyps, to six weeks or more in the more extensive polypoid degeneration cases. The amount of time and degree of dysphonia experienced by the patient depends largely on the breadth of the submucosal dissection ultimately necessary. In other words, a large polyp arising from a relatively slender base on the vocal fold is associated with a much quicker and easier postoperative recovery than a smaller lesion of polypoid degeneration that has a wider base.

In addition to providing instruction in vocal hygiene and short-term vocal rest, the voice pathologist plays a very important role in those cases where vocal recovery is slow. Positive attitude is quite important in achieving patient compliance with treatment plans, and a patient's perception of how well recovery is proceeding can be influenced by the feedback of serial laryngostroboscopic exams. Careful counseling in vocal use and technique is very important in ensuring that an optimal result occurs. In cases of more extensive pathologic change, where it may not be possible to

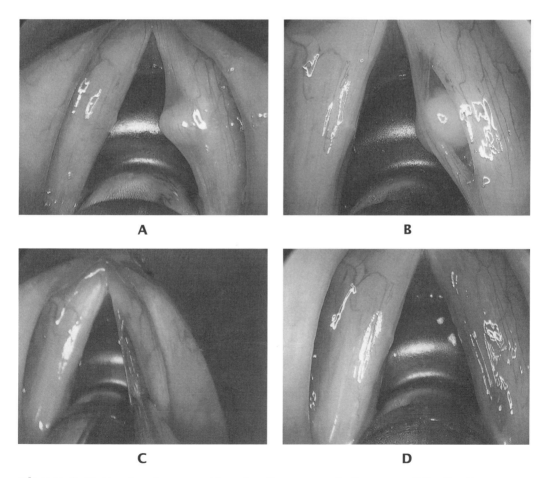

A

B

C

D

Figure 8–6. Vocal cyst removed by microflap approach. Courtesy of The Ear Nose Throat and Plastic Surgery Associates, Winter Park, Florida. See Color Plate 19 for a color version of this figure.

achieve "normal" tissue characteristics, the voice pathologist's efforts can make all the difference in the patient's perception of how successful surgery was.

Laser Laryngoscopy

Mention the word "laser" to a patient, and you usually get a satisfied and knowing nod, coming from the patient's thought that they are being treated with the most advanced and cutting-edge technology available. There is a common misperception that lasers can achieve magical results, without the need to cut or traumatize tissues in the process. When dealing with smaller vocal fold lesions, the laser often is not the ideal tool from the standpoint of limiting collateral tissue trauma.

The frequency of the laser light, the absorption characteristics of the target, the size and focus of the spot, and the time course of energy delivery determine the effect of laser energy on tissues. Of the lasers available for clinical use, the one that is by far the most widely used in laryngeal surgery is the CO_2 laser (Case 4 on DVD). This distinction owes to its small thermal spread at the target site, resulting from the high absorption of the energy by water. Translated, this means a more precise cut or ablation of tissue, while limiting burn injury to the adjacent tissue. Careful application of surgical steel, however, results in less collateral tissue damage. In view of the phonosurgical objective of preserving or enhancing the voice giving characteristics of the tissues, this makes the laser less desirable in dealing with most small vocal fold lesions.

That being said, the CO_2 laser is very useful when dealing with larger and more vascular lesions, precisely because it produces a zone of thermal energy spread. Vessels can be sealed and blood coagulated by this energy, improving visualization during dissection and limiting the need for electrocautery, which

can be difficult to apply and less precise in its effect. The range of pathologies that can be resected laryngoscopically has certainly been expanded by the CO_2 laser. The recent introduction of a small fiber delivery system enhances the application CO_2 laser energy in difficult cases.

Because of its short wavelength, CO_2 laser light does not travel well through a conventional optical fiber. This has limited its delivery to line of sight, as directed by a mirror micromanipulator at the objective end of the operating microscope. Though precise, this has the disadvantage of a tangential approach to the subglottic surfaces. The new fiber system allows for direction of the laser energy at an angle from the line of vision by inserting the fiber through a curved guide to the area of dissection (see Case 4, DVD).

Operating room setup is more complex in laser cases, due to the need to observe safety protocols. There is a very real risk of airway fire when using laser energy in proximity of an oxygen-rich environment. Special endotracheal tubes (Figure 8–7) must be utilized

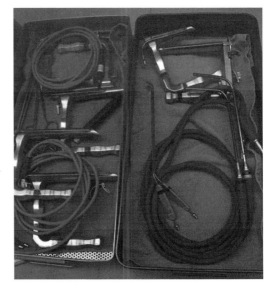

Figure 8–7. Types of laryngoscopes. Courtesy of The Ear Nose Throat and Plastic Surgery Associates, Winter Park, Florida.

and additional precautions taken to avoid any chance of ignition. As a result, laser cases take 30 to 40 minutes and are more costly than conventional cases.

Postoperative recovery varies greatly depending on the type of lesion treated, but may be prolonged in those cases where large areas of vocal fold surface are affected, or when deeper dissection becomes necessary. The role of the voice pathologist is similar to that associated with the more extensive microflap cases.

Before moving on, the pulsed dye laser should be briefly discussed. The wavelength of this laser makes it absorbed preferentially by vascular tissue. It can be delivered through a thin conventional fiber, making it usable in the office through the channel of a flexible fiberoptic scope. Some laryngologists successfully treat papillomatosis and other vascular lesions in this way.

Laryngeal Microdebrider Dissection

Adapted from use in orthopedics and endoscopic sinus surgery, the microdebrider has made a recent impact in the laryngoscopic resection of papillomata and bulky laryngeal tumors (Figures 8–8, 8–9, and Color Plate 20; see also Phonosurgical Case 3 on DVD). Basically, the microdebrider blade consists of an external sheath enclosing another, hollow tube. Both have openings at the side of the tip, and the movement of one relative to another creates a scissors action. Suction is applied to the inner tube, drawing tissue to be cut into the openings. The aggressiveness of the dissection is controlled by size, shape, and sharpness of the openings.

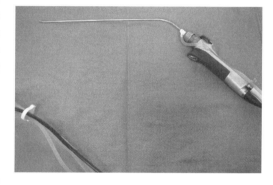

Figure 8–8. Microdebrider. Courtesy of The Ear Nose Throat and Plastic Surgery Associates, Winter Park, Florida.

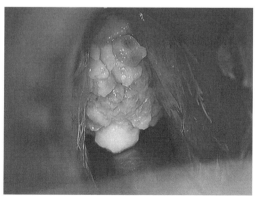

Pre

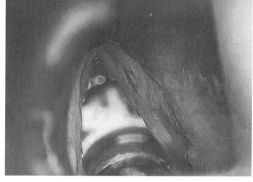

Post

Figure 8–9. Surgical removal of laryngeal papilloma by microdebrider approaches. Courtesy of The Ear Nose Throat and Plastic Surgery Associates, Winter Park, Florida. See Color Plate 20 for a color version of this figure.

In its laryngeal form, the microdebrider blade is very long and angled to allow insertion through the laryngoscope. The openings in the tip are small and round, producing a less aggressive, skimming action over the vocal folds. Advantages of this form of dissection include continuous suctioning of blood for improved visualization, precise resection of tissue by gradual "nibbling away" of pathology, and less potential for collateral tissue injury over laser techniques when the microdebrider is used with care.

Injection Augmentation

Weak, breathy phonation due to vocal fold atrophy or neurolaryngeal dysfunction can be treated by augmenting one or both vocal folds to achieve better glottic closure. Teflon paste has been used in the past, but has several drawbacks, including potential development of a granulomatous foreign body reaction; with associated vocal fold stiffness and distortion.

Fat, obtained from a small incision or a microliposuction technique, can be injected into the vocal fold as an autologous graft. Placed within the thyroarytenoid muscle, it provides good augmentation, without risk of rejection reaction, and with very good vibratory mass characteristics relative to the vocal fold body. On the down side, intentional overcorrection of at least 50% is necessary to account for the breakdown and mobilization of a portion of the injected fat cells. Delayed atrophy of the injected fat is also possible. The technique requires operating room resources and general anesthesia, but has been useful in treating presbylaryngis, small glottic gaps due to paralysis, and for "touching up" laryngeal framework surgical results. Operating room time is about 30 minutes. After shrinkage of the fat graft in the first four to six weeks, long-term stability of the augmentation results is good.

Injection substrates used for cosmetic tissue augmentation are being used in the vocal folds as well. Cymetra™ and Radiesse™ can both be injected by direct laryngoscopic approach, or in an office-based transcutanous technique. Radiesse™ has better long-term stability than Cymetra™, making it better suited for long term correction of glottic closure deficits. Cymetra™ has been used for short-term augmentation in my practice. One such application is in the correction of symptomatic glottis gaps during the initial waiting period after new onset paralysis. Because eventual nerve function recovery is anticipated in many of these cases, a less permanent form of augmentation is usually desired.

Laryngeal Framework Surgery

For long-term correction of more severe glottic closure issues, medialization thyroplasty is, generally, the procedure of choice. There are commercially available implant kits (Figure 8–10). The operating surgeon can, alternatively, hand carve an implant out of block silicone. Regardless, the surgical goal is to achieve midline correction of the paralyzed

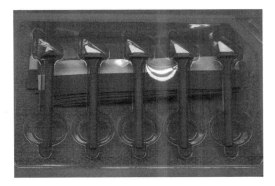

Figure 8–10. Montgomery implant sizers. Courtesy of The Ear Nose Throat and Plastic Surgery Associates, Winter Park, Florida.

vocal fold by placing the implant through a rectangular window created in the thyroid cartilage. In the interest of precise correction, the procedure is usually performed under local anesthesia with sedation so that the patient can phonate at the time of implant sizing (Figures 8–11 and 8–12). Glottic closure is usually observed by flexible fiberoptic laryngoscopy in the operating room, and voice quality as well as maximum phonation time can be assessed (see DVD for pre- and postlaryngostroboscopic exam following thyroplasty surgery).

Surgical time is usually one hour, but can be longer if the implant is handmade/fashioned. The patient is usually observed overnight, and discharged after wound drain removal. Vocal recovery is immediate in terms of the ease of phonation, although the voice usually has a pressed, harsh quality initially that resolves over 4 weeks or so as postoperative vocal fold stiffness and swelling resolve. The voice pathologist is often called on to help the patient "unlearn" compensatory vocal behaviors developed during the course of the course of the paralysis, that become detrimental once the augmentation has been accomplished.

Other framework modifications are possible, the most common being medialization of the arytenoid cartilage. This can be performed in conjunction with medialization thyroplasty, and is used in the most severe cases of glottic incompetence, such as that seen with high lesions of the vagus nerve.

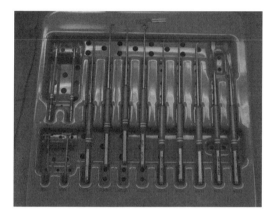

Figure 8–11. Thyroplasty surgical tools. Courtesy of The Ear Nose Throat and Plastic Surgery Associates, Winter Park, Florida.

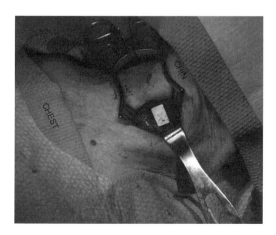

Figure 8–12. Placement of the implant through the rectangular window of the thyroid cartilage. Courtesy of The Ear Nose Throat and Plastic Surgery Associates, Winter Park, Florida.

Selected Clinical Cases

Patient A presented to the office with a long history of considerable hoarseness, associated with phonotraumatic vocal behaviors as well as smoking. During the initial assessment, the voice pathologist described the patient's vocal quality as rough. The patient's laryngostroboscopic exam yielded a large, pedunculated polyp arising from the right vocal fold, which alternately moved from the subglottic to the supraglottic space during inspiratory and phonatory efforts. Opposite this lesion, on the left vocal fold, was a smaller hemorrhagic lesion that appeared to be a hematoma (Figures 8–13 through 8–16 and Color Plates 21 through 24).

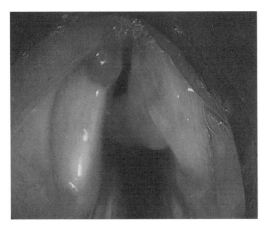

Figure 8-13

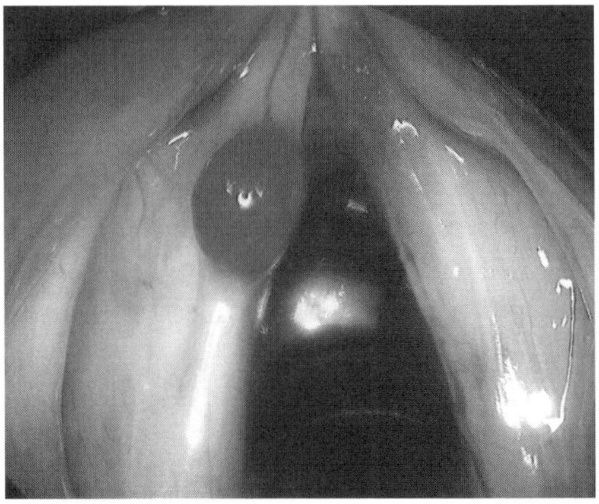

Figure 8-14

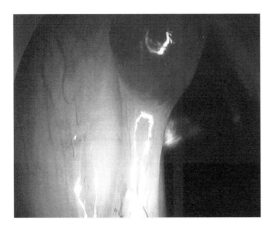

Figure 8-15

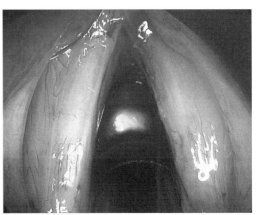

Figure 8-16

Figures 8-13 through 8-16 show surgical removal of left hemorrhagic polyp based within a mucosal band isolated by an underlying sulcus vocalis. Courtesy of The Ear Nose Throat and Plastic Surgery Associates, Winter Park, Florida. See Color Plates 21 through 24 for color versions of these figures.

In this case the decision to proceed to surgery was made quickly, as there was no reasonable expectation of recovery with conservative treatment. Instruction in vocal rest and vocal hygiene was initiated at the diagnostic visit, however, only in the interest of improving postoperative recovery.

At surgery, the findings on the right vocal fold were as expected from the laryngostro-boscopic examination, but those on the left were somewhat surprising. Instead of a simple hematoma, the lesion on the left proved to be a hemorrhagic polyp, based within a mucosal band isolated by an underlying sulcus vocalis. This area was difficult to assess on the pre operative study due to the larger right-sided polyp's tendency to obscure the view of this area, and to interfere with generation of a mucosal wave that would have allowed assessment of tissue motion (see Phonosurgical images on DVD, Cases 1A and 1B).

Operative management consisted of microflap excision of the right-sided polyp, followed by simple excision of the mucosal band on which the left-sided polyp was based. This patient's recovery was rapid and her change in vocal quality was dramatic. She came back for only one postoperative laryngostroboscopic study, and did that only with insistence. In addition to documenting surgical results, it provided the voice pathologist an opportunity to perform postoperative counseling, in the interest of preventing recurrent pathology. This illustrates the concept that size of pathology and degree of preoperative dysphonia matter less in vocal prognosis than the extent of dissection at or beneath the vocal fold surface.

Patient B presented to the office with dysphonia, characterized by a low pitch, and concern regarding the possibility of cancer. She did have a history of smoking, which had raised the latter concern in the mind of her primary physician. Her laryngostroboscopic assessment showed a picture of moderate polypoid degeneration of the right vocal fold, with minimal polypoid change noted on the left (Figure 8–17 and Color Plate 25; see also Phonosurgical images on DVD, Cases 13A and 13B, and DVD video, Microflap Resection, Reinke's Edema). Mucosal appearance was unremarkable, with the exception of some hypervascularity. This patient was given the option of surgical intervention after a brief trial of conservative management.

Even though the vocal quality was more normal in this case compared to that of patient A, and the pathology was less dramatic, the surgical dissection required was actually more extensive. Micro-flap dissection involved the entire, right, vocal fold length. The decision to leave the left vocal fold alone was based on the minimal Reinke's edema present on that side, along with the normal appearance of the mucosal surface.

The recovery for this patient was somewhat slower than in the case of patient A, and the vocal result, although very satisfying, was somewhat less dramatic. Her pathology was negative for cancer or premalignant change, consistent with the smooth and translucent appearance of the mucosa in the laryngostroboscopic study. In terms of her postoperative

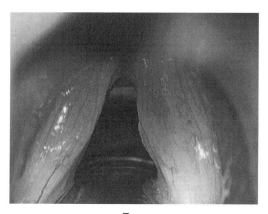
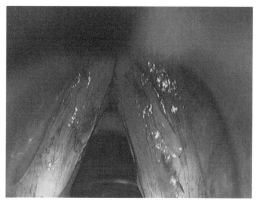

Pre   **Post**

Figure 8–17. Microflap dissection of moderate polypoid degeneration. Courtesy of The Ear Nose Throat and Plastic Surgery Associates, Winter Park, Florida. See Color Plate 25 for a color version of this figure.

care, more input from the voice pathologist was needed to assure the patient that her recovery was proceeding optimally. The postoperative laryngostroboscopic studies helped significantly, to show the patient the objective improvement in tissue appearance and the characteristics that were occurring throughout the period of relative vocal restriction. These visits also provided more opportunity to emphasize the importance of smoking cessation, key to the prevention of recurrent pathology in this case.

Patient C presented with milder dysphonia affecting his singing voice more so than the speaking voice. This had been a gradually developing condition, and was treated with conservative measures for months before the patient was prepared to go ahead with sur-

gical intervention (Figure 8–18 and Color Plate 26; see also Phonosurgical images Cases 8A and 8B and DVD video, Nodules). The laryngostroboscopic assessment showed bilateral nodular change, with a broader base and stiffer characteristic to the nodule on the right side. Extensive preoperative preparation was given, in terms of vocal rest and hygiene as well as a realistic expectation of the operative result.

The findings at surgery were those of a firm nodule, although small on each vocal fold. Precise excision was performed with gentle retraction and a microscissor was used to cut and minimize dissection and mucosal gap. Healing was rapid and uneventful, with involvement of the voice pathologist directed at long-term prevention of recurrence.

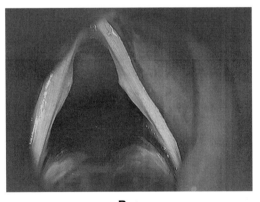
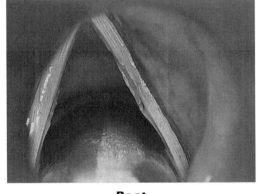

Pre   **Post**

Figure 8–18. Pre- and postsurgical removal of bilateral vocal fold nodules. Courtesy of The Ear Nose Throat and Plastic Surgery Associates, Winter Park, Florida. See Color Plate 26 for a color version of this figure.

Suggested Readings

Altman, K. W. (2007). Vocal fold masses. *Otolaryngology Clinics of North America*, *40*, 1091–1108.

Bastian, R. W., & Delsupehe K. G. (1996). Indirect larynx and pharynx surgery: A replacement for direct laryngoscopy. *Laryngoscope*, *106*, 1280–1286.

Bouchayer M., & Cornut G. (1991). Instrumental microscopy of benign lesions of the vocal folds. In C. Ford & D. Bless (Eds.), *Phonosurgery* (pp. 25–41) New York, NY: Raven.

Hirano, M. (1975). Phonosurgery: Basic and clinical investigations. *Otologia (Fukuoka)*, *21*, 239–442.

Hirano, M. (1981). Structure of the vocal fold in normal and diseased states: Anatomic and physical studies. Proceedings of the Conference on the Assessment of Vocal Pathology. *ASHA*, *11*, 11–27.

Hochman, I. I., & Zeitels, S. M. (2000). Phonomicrosurgical management of vocal fold polyps: The subepithelial microflap resection technique. *Journal of Voice*, *14*, 112–118.

Jako, G. J. (1972). Laser surgery of the vocal cords. *Laryngoscope*, *82*(12), 2204–2216.

Mortenson, M., & Woo, P. (2006). Office steroid injections of the larynx. *Laryngoscope*, *116*, 1735–1739.

Scalco A. N., Shipman, W. F, & Tabb, H. G. (1960). Microscopic suspension laryngoscopy. *Annals of Otology, Rhinology and Laryngology*, *69*, 1134–1138.

Strong, M. S., & Vanghan, C. W. (1971). Vocal cord nodules and polyps—the role of surgical management. *Laryngoscope*, *81*, 911–922.

Zeitels, S. M. (1996). Laser versus cold instruments for microlaryngoscopic surgery. *Laryngoscope*, *106*, 545–552.

Appendix 8–1

Postoperative Vocal Fold Microlaryngoscopy Surgery Instruction

This patient handout is a compilation of recommendations common to many clinical practices. These recommendations were not written specifically by the authors or by the affiliated clinical settings they practice with.

This guide is intended for patients who have had vocal fold surgery (phonosurgery). How you use your voice directly after surgery (and several weeks thereafter) may significantly affect the "final result" of your voice. As an analogy, an injured athlete who undergoes knee or shoulder surgery and then does not rest properly or enroll in physical therapy, but instead tries to ski two days after surgery, will not have a very good result regardless of the "success" of the surgery.

The amount of voice rest recommended may vary depending on the type of surgery you had. Voice rest is not a penalty. Also, we do not want you to change your personality, just the manner in which you use your voice socially and/or occupationally. Our voice pathologist will assist you in this therapeutic process.

For all postoperative vocal fold microsurgery patients: Drink plenty of noncaffeinated fluids daily; ideally, 8 to 10 8-oz glasses of water daily.

Swelling, Nodules, or Polyp Surgery

Week 1: For the first 72 hours (unless specified differently by your physician) following surgery, we advocate complete voice rest. Beginning on days 4 to 7, you are asked to use a softly engaged–low impact voice (quiet, relaxed, and breathy) for no more then 1 hour per day. If you choose not to engage in conversation, a vocalized sigh (i.e., yawn-sigh) may be helpful. This keeps the vocal folds flexible without taxing them. Your voice will sound hoarse (like laryngitis). Do not worry, this is normal. During this time your voice may be inconsistent and variable in quality. Do not be concerned; just allow the voice to do what it wants. For singers, you may add humming: mmm-ah, mmm-oh, mmm-ee (using a forward, more resonant focus). All vocalizations should be made using a quiet, relaxed, and breathy voice (i.e., your low-impact voice). Remember, you should never whisper— this is not a therapeutic option.

Weeks 2 to 3: This is still considered the early healing phase; try to be patient. By the end of week 3 you may be seen by the voice pathologist to visualize your vocal folds, interpret the healing process with the physician, and begin lifting some of your voice restrictions. During this time you may begin humming: mmmm . . . ; mm-ah, mm-oh, mm-ee; uhm-hmm (singers: scales up and down—stay in a 1-octave comfortable range on a lip trill, sigh, or hum using a low-impact voice). These vocalizations should be done no more than 3 times daily for 3 to 5 minutes. Your speech pathologist and physician will help devise an appropriate vocal rehabilitation program for you. Voice therapy may be completed both office and home based.

Note: Between weeks 3 and 5, your voice usage may be gradually increasing so developing an awareness of the phonotraumatic behaviors that may have been responsible for the initial injury is important.

Surgery for Reinke's Edema (Smoker's Polyps)

The immediate outcome of your postoperative voice will be dependent on how large your polyps were prior to the surgery. In some cases you will have almost no voice for the first 5 days or up to 4 to 5 weeks. This is not uncommon. Your vocal folds were damaged by years of cigarette smoke and will take some time to recover. Your initial voice rest time will be for
_____.

There should be **no smoking** following surgery. During weeks 2 to 3 you may be able to vocalize in a low-impact voice (quiet, relaxed, and breathy; yawn-sigh) only for 3 to 5 minutes of every hour. Remember, do not whisper. By the end of week 3 you should be seen by the voice pathologist to visualize your vocal folds, interpret the healing process with the physician, and begin lifting some of your voice restrictions. Your voice pathologist and physician will help devise an appropriate vocal rehabilitation program for you. Voice therapy may be recommended both office and home based.

Cyst or Sulcus Surgery

As mentioned during your office visits, surgery for cysts and sulci may require a small incision into the vocal folds. The healing time is most likely going to take longer and the final out-come is determined in large part by whether your vocal folds scar or not. The final voice may not be evident for 3 to 9 months. Follow the guidelines listed for Swelling, Nodules, or Polyp Surgery listed above.

Additional Instructions:

Chapter 9

Management of
Head and Neck Cancer

Head and Neck Cancer Statistics

The American Cancer Society estimated that in 2011, nearly 12,740 (10,160 men and 2,580 women) new cases of laryngeal cancer and 39,400 (27,710 men and 11,690 women) cases of oral and pharyngeal cancer would be diagnosed in the United States with an estimated 11,460 deaths from disease occurring at these sites. Overall, head and neck cancer accounts for approximately 3% of new cases of cancer in the United States. The male to female ratio for head and neck cancer is estimated as 4 to 1 (Jemal, Siegel, Xu, & Ward, 2010).

A wealth of peer-reviewed information and updated quarterly reports can be found under the head and neck section on the National Cancer Institute Web site at http://www.cancer.gov. Specific information is provided on the site for the clinician working with patients with cancer as well as a separate section for patients.

The Surveillance Epidemiology and End Results section of the National Cancer Institute website provides the SEER Cancer Statistics Review which reports incidence, mortality, survival, prevalence and lifetime risk statistics (http://seer.cancer.gov/csr/1975_2008/index.html).

Five-year survival rates from 2001 to 2007 indicated a 60.8 % survival rate for laryngeal cancer and a 60.8% survival rate for cancer of the oral cavity and pharynx (http://seer.cancer.gov/csr/1975_2008/results_merged/topic_survival.pdf).

After reading this chapter, you will:

- Understand the primary causes of head and neck cancer
- Understand the make-up of the multidisciplinary clinical and research team involved in the assessment and treatment of patients with head and neck cancer
- Understand the variety of head and neck cancer types and the disease staging process
- Understand the variety of surgical options for treating head and neck cancer
- Understand the primary modes of alaryngeal communication following a total laryngectomy

Causes of Head and Neck Cancer

Cancer is a class of diseases characterized as the uncontrolled growth of malignant cells. Cancer cells can grow and divide beyond normal limits; cells may accumulate and form tumors, invade adjacent tissue or structures, and/or spread to other locations in the body via blood or the lymphatic system (metastasis). The primary risk factors linked to the development of head and neck cancer are inhaled cigarette or marijuana smoke, pipe and cigar smoke, as well as chewing tobacco. The greatest risk occurs when anatomical areas and their susceptible epithelium are directly exposed to these toxins. The risk level is dependent on daily consumption, type, toxicity, and manner of tobacco use (Casper & Colton, 1998). A synergistic effect exists when tobacco use is combined with consumption of alcohol, creating a higher risk of cancer development compared to if each was consumed independently. Although tobacco use and alcohol have consistently been implicated as a causative factor for head and neck cancer, head and neck cancer can develop in their absence, although it is significantly less common (Spitz, 1994). Additionally, although laryngopharyngeal reflux (LPR) has been largely implicated in esophageal disease, a recently identified relationship between severe LPR and head and neck disease exists (Lipan, Reidenberg, & Laitman, 2006). Recent research shows that a portion of head and neck squamous cell cancers test positive for the Human Papilloma Virus (HPV). There are numerous types of HPV; the type most frequently associated with oropharyngeal cancer is HPV-16. HPV-18 has also been associated with this cancer. (Kreimer, Clifford, Boyle & Franceschi, 2005). Studies have also found that oral HPV infections can be acquired through sexual contact (D'Souza et al., 2007). The incidence of these HPV-positive squamous cell carcinomas has increased in recent decades, especially in younger individuals. HPV-positive tumors have been associated with better survival rates than non-HPV-positive tumors. (Ang et al., 2010)

Mechanisms and Sites of Laryngeal Cancer

Chapter 2 described the different anatomic parts of the supraglottis (the epiglottis, false vocal folds, ventricles, aryepiglottic folds, and arytenoids), the glottis (the true vocal folds and the anterior and posterior commissures) and the subglottic region which begins about 1 cm below the true vocal folds and extends to the lower border of the cricoid cartilage or the first tracheal ring. Cancer can develop and spread to any of these anatomic regions. Cancer can spread readily through the lymphatic system from the supraglottic area due to the density in lymphatic tissue and richness in lymphatic drainage (Spaulding, Hahn, & Constable, 1987).

> The lymphatic system is closely related to the circulatory system and functions to deliver nutrients, oxygen, and hormones to cells as well as carry away waste.

Conversely, the true vocal folds are devoid of lymphatics. As a result, early stage laryngeal cancer confined to the vocal folds rarely presents with involved lymph nodes. Cancer extended above or below the vocal folds may, however, lead to lymph node involvement (Spaulding, Hahn, & Constable, 1987).

Primary subglottic cancers (which are rare) drain through the cricothyroid and cricotracheal membranes to the pretracheal, paratracheal, and inferior jugular nodes, and occasionally to the mediastinal nodes (Spaulding, Hahn, & Constable, 1987).

Multidisciplinary Team

A team of professionals is critical for the successful and coordinated rehabilitation plan for the patient diagnosed with head and neck cancer.

Team Members

Head and Neck Surgeon

The surgeon acts as the case manager. Responsibilities include diagnosis of the disease and organization of the treatment plan including the medical management of the condition. The surgeon is also responsible for making referrals to other physicians as well as members of the rehabilitation team so the patient can acquire all of the information needed to sort through the treatment options.

Radiation Oncologist

The radiation oncologist is responsible for studying the stages of the tumor development and the potential involvement of the surrounding tissues or structures. The radiation oncologist decides if radiation therapy is a viable treatment option for the patient. If treatment is recommended, the radiation oncologist decides the optimal treatment, dosage levels, and type.

Medical Oncologist

As a nonsurgical cancer specialist, the medical oncologist is responsible for the administration of chemotherapeutic agents, often used in conjunction with radiation therapy in more advanced tumors. He is also involved in general aspects of patient care when disease is advanced, including staging of the cancer,

supportive care, psychological aspects, and palliative or pain care.

Radiologist/Nuclear Medicine Specialist

The radiologist performs and determines the results of imaging including magnetic resonance imaging (MRI), computer tomography (CT), and positive emission tomography (PET) scans, or ultrasound for the diagnosis or post-treatment assessments. Radiologists work with the surgeon to plan appropriate treatment approaches based on imaging findings.

Pathologist

The pathologist examines any tissue that has been removed during the patient's course of management to evaluate it for anatomical abnormalities. A report is sent to the treating physician as to the type of tissue (i.e., squamous cell carcinoma) and the completeness of surgical excision, which then guides the treating physician to the next step in management.

Internal Medicine

The internal medicine physician(s) may be part of the health care team for pre and postoperative management of medical comorbidities, such as heart disease, diabetes, and high blood pressure. They work with patients preoperatively to identify those who are at risk for postsurgical complication(s) and also help with treatment complications following radiation or surgery including hypothyroidism, metabolic imbalance due to nutritional inadequacy, and cardiovascular events such as myocardial infarction or stroke. Internal medicine subspecialists are involved as needed to contribute to specific issues. For example, an infectious disease specialist is often consulted to help in treatment of postoperative infections, especially those due to difficult to treat bacteria such as MRSA.

> MRSA stands for *Methicillin-Resistant Staphylococcus aureus* and is also referred to as "staph" infection. It can result in serious skin and soft tissue infections and/or serious pneumonia.

> The stoma is a surgically created opening in the neck in order to allow for breathing.

Plastic Surgeon

The plastic surgeon performs any reconstructive surgery that may be necessary after the cancer treatment to lessen the appearance of scarring or removal of structures. Some extensive surgical resections are performed with a two team approach, utilizing a reconstructive specialist to perform microvascular free-flap transfer after the tumor is resected by the head and neck surgical team.

Dental/Maxillofacial Prosthodontist

The dentist who is specialized in making replacements for removed teeth or other oral cavity structures helps in restoring the patient's comfort, health, and appearance. In some cases, prosthesis placement can provide functional and cosmetic restoration superior to results obtainable by surgical reconstruction.

Nurse

Nursing personnel care for the patient in all phases of inpatient diagnosis and treatment, and are often involved in case coordination in the outpatient setting. Nurses collaborate with other team members to implement an individualized care plan. They assist and support the patients during any procedure, administration of therapies, surgery, hospital stays, and so forth. The nurse is also responsible for patient education prior to release from the hospital, particularly for stoma care for those patients experiencing a total laryngectomy, including how to suction and clean the stomal area.

Speech/Voice Pathologist

The voice pathologist's role is to evaluate and provide treatment for head and neck cancer patients with short-term and long-term communication needs. The voice pathologist is also responsible for evaluating the dysphagia that may occur as a result of surgical intervention and/or radiation treatments. For the patient who has had a total laryngectomy, the voice pathologist will show the patient how to use devices to substitute for the loss of the vocal folds and restore vocal communication.

Registered Dietitian

A registered dietician is responsible for evaluating the patient's nutritional health prior to and following surgery, radiation, or other intensive treatments. Dietitians make recommendations regarding caloric intake to gain or maintain a patient's weight, and counsel the patient and caregivers regarding nutritional health and well-being.

Mental Health Counselor/Social Worker/Case Manager

These rehabilitation team members are responsible for providing counseling to the patient or family to help them cope with issues surrounding: potential death, serious illness, end of life care, postoperative depression, role of family or caregivers, self-image, anger, anxiety, and so forth.

Physical/Occupational Therapist

Both the physical and occupational therapists work to restore movement or skills that have been impaired due to surgery. Patients who have undergone extensive surgery to the head or neck can develop limited mobility of the shoulder, neck, arm, or hand on the same side as the surgical site. Physical therapists work with the patients to rehabilitate gross motor movement, and occupational therapists concentrate on fine motor movements of the hand.

Lymphedema Therapist

Lymphedema therapists come from varied backgrounds including physical therapy, occupational therapy, massage therapy and nursing. Specialty training is required for certification in this specialty. Patients who have undergone removal of lymphatic structures, such as dissection of lymph nodes in the neck, or who have sustained damage to these areas from a tumor or radiation therapy can experience reduced drainage of lymphatic fluid which can result in swelling and discomfort of the head and neck area. Lymphedema therapy promotes drainage of lymphatic fluid into the bloodstream and results in decreased swelling in the head and neck region.

Respiratory Therapist

The respiratory therapist evaluates, treats, and cares for breathing or respiratory disorders. These disorders can include ventilator management, tracheostomy care, and delivery of nebulized medications to treat asthma or other pulmonary diseases.

The Laryngectomized Visitor

Finally, an important nonprofessional team member is the person who has experienced the patient's situation (or similar). This is referred to as a laryngectomized or laryngectomee visitor. The laryngectomized/laryngectomee visitor serves to help boost the patient's morale by showing ease of communication through mastered alaryngeal speech. In many cases, the visit

provides motivation to become engaged in the rehabilitation process. Often, the visitor's spouse or caregiver will visit with the patient's spouse/ caregiver providing support. These interactions are valuable as patient-to-patient support (Stemple, Glaze, & Klaben, 2000).

Primary Symptoms Associated with Head and Neck Cancer

Patients with supraglottic cancers typically present with symptoms of sore throat, painful and effortful swallowing, referred ear pain, change in voice quality, and so forth. Early vocal fold cancers are associated with chronic and progressive hoarseness. Cancers arising in the subglottic area commonly involve the vocal fold(s) once they become symptomatic and thus, symptoms usually relate to a contiguous spread (Castellanos, Spector, & Kaiser, 1996).

Head and Neck Cancer Sites

- Oral cavity: lips, floor of mouth, oral tongue, buccal mucosa, gingival, retromolar trigone, hard palate
- Oropharynx: tonsil, soft palate, base of tongue, lateral/posterior pharyngeal wall
- Nasopharynx
- Hypopharynx: pyriform sinus
- Larynx: glottic, subglottic
- Nasal and paranasal sinuses
- Salivary glands: parotid, submandibular, sublingual, minor salivary glands
- Ear
- Neck
- Regional soft tissues and supporting bones

> The retromolar trigone is a small mucosal area behind the last molar of the lower jaw. Cancer identified in this location often rapidly spreads to adjacent oral structures.

Head and Neck Cancer Types

Ninety percent of head and neck cancers are of squamous cell histology (Hsu et al., 2008; Spitz, 1994). A portion of squamous cell cancers test positive for the Human Papilloma Virus (HPV-16). Squamous cell subtypes include keratinizing and nonkeratinizing and well-differentiated to poorly differentiated grade, a system used by pathology. Variants of squamous cell types can include undifferentiated carcinoma, lymphoepithelioma, spindle cell carcinoma, and vererrucous carcinoma. Other less common head and neck cancer types include (Mendenhall, Riggs, & Cassisi, 2005):

- Sarcoma—arises from connective tissue
- Adenocarcinoma—develops in the glandular lining of an organ
- Mucoepidermoid carcinoma—develops in the salivary glands, minor or major aggressiveness; major aggressiveness is associated with higher grade tumors. Lower grade, as determined by the pathologist, is often associated with a more benign natural history
- Adenoid cystic carcinoma—occurs in major or minor salivary glands. It may recur many years after treatment, and has a tendency to follow nerves
- Acinic cell carcinoma—found in the glands of head and neck
- Lymphoma—begins in cells of the immune system: There are many subtypes, and the tumor behavior varies significantly depending on the precise classification. Broadly, lymphomas are divided into Hodgkins and non-Hodgkins categories
- Melanoma—arises from the melanocytic system of the skin or other organs

Staging of Head and Neck Cancers

Cancer staging is described using a numbered system from I to IV that denotes how the cancer spreads. The stage takes into account the size of a tumor, how deep it has penetrated, whether it has invaded adjacent organs, if it has metastasized to lymph nodes, and whether it has spread to distant organs. Management is typically prescribed and/or changed based on the stage of diagnosis and remains a powerful predictor of survival. The staging system is clinical, based on the best possible estimate of disease extent recorded before treatment. The assessment of the primary tumor is based on inspection and palpation, when possible, and by visual endoscopic/stroboscopic examination. In order to accurately stage the cancer, the tumor must be confirmed histologically by biopsy. Radiographic studies such as CT, MRI, or PET scans help delineate the degree of local extent, as well as potential regional lymphatic and distant metastatic spread (Mendenhall, Riggs, & Cassisi, 2005).

Defining the TNM System

The staging system, developed by the American Joint Committee on Cancer (AJCC) Staging (http://www.nci.gov), is as follows:

T: Tumor (extent of primary tumor)

N: Nodal disease (lymphatic spread; regional metastasis)

M: Metastasis (distant; spread outside head and neck region)

TNM Definitions

Primary tumor (T)

- TX: Primary tumor cannot be assessed
- T0: No evidence of primary tumor
- Tis: Carcinoma in situ

Staging Supraglottic Cancer

- T1: Tumor limited to one subsite of supraglottis with normal vocal fold mobility
- T2: Tumor invades mucosa of more than one adjacent subsite[1] of supraglottis or glottis or region outside the supraglottis (e.g., mucosa of base of tongue, vallecula, or medial wall of piriform sinus) without fixation of the larynx
- T3: Tumor limited to larynx with vocal fold fixation and/or invades any of the following: postcricoid area, pre-epiglottic tissues, para-glottic space, and/or minor thyroid cartilage erosion (e.g., inner cortex)
- T4a: Tumor invades through the thyroid cartilage, and/or invades tissues beyond the larynx (e.g., trachea, soft tissues of the neck including deep extrinsic muscle of the tongue, strap muscles, thyroid, or esophagus)
- T4b: Tumor invades prevertebral space, encases carotid artery, or invades mediastinal structures

Subsites include the following:

- False vocal folds
- Arytenoids
- Suprahyoid epiglottis
- Infrahyoid epiglottis
- Aryepiglottic folds (laryngeal aspect)

Note: Supraglottis involves many individual subsites.

Staging Glottic Cancer

- T0: No evidence of primary tumor
- Tis: Carcinoma in situ: confined to tissues lining the larynx
- T1: Tumor limited to the vocal fold(s), which may involve anterior or posterior commissure, with normal mobility
  - T1a: Tumor limited to one vocal fold
  - T1b: Tumor involves both vocal folds
- T2: Tumor extends to supraglottis and/or subglottis and/or with impaired vocal fold mobility
- T3: Tumor limited to the larynx with vocal fold fixation and/or invades paraglottic space, and/or minor thyroid cartilage erosion (e.g., inner cortex)
- T4a: Tumor invades through the thyroid cartilage and/or invades tissues beyond the larynx (e.g., trachea, soft tissues of neck, including deep extrinsic muscle of the tongue, strap muscles, thyroid, or esophagus)
- T4b: Tumor invades prevertebral space, encases carotid artery, or invades mediastinal structures

---

[1]Determination varies for different parts of the head and neck.

Note: Glottic presentation may vary by volume of tumor, anatomic region involved, and the presence or absence of normal vocal fold mobility.

Staging of Subglottic Cancer

- T1: Tumor limited to the subglottis
- T2: Tumor extends to vocal fold(s) with normal or impaired mobility
- T3: Tumor limited to larynx with vocal fold fixation
- T4a: Tumor invades cricoid or thyroid cartilage and/or invades tissues beyond the larynx (e.g., trachea, soft tissues of neck, including deep extrinsic muscles of the tongue, strap muscles, thyroid, or esophagus)
- T4b: Tumor invades prevertebral space, encases carotid artery, or invades mediastinal structures

Definition of Regional Lymph Nodes (N)

- NX: Regional lymph nodes cannot be assessed
- N0: No regional lymph node metastasis
- N1: Metastasis in a single ipsilateral lymph node 3 cm or smaller in greatest dimension
- N2: Metastasis in a single ipsilateral lymph node, larger than 3 cm but 6 cm or smaller in greatest dimension, or in multiple ipsilateral lymph nodes 6 cm or smaller in greatest dimension, or in bilateral or contralateral lymph nodes 6 cm or smaller in greatest dimension:
  - N2a: Metastasis in a single ipsilateral lymph node larger than 3 cm but 6 cm or smaller in greatest dimension

- N2b: Metastasis in multiple ipsilateral lymph nodes 6 cm or smaller in greatest dimension
- N2c: Metastasis in bilateral or contralateral lymph nodes 6 cm or smaller in greatest dimension
- N3: Metastasis in a lymph node larger than 6 cm in greatest dimension

In the clinical evaluation, the actual size of the nodal mass is measured to complete staging, and allowance should be made for intervening soft tissues.

Defining Distant Metastasis (M)

- MX: Distant metastasis cannot be assessed
- M0: No distant metastasis
- M1: Distant metastasis

American Joint Committee on Cancer Staging (AJCC)

Stage 0

- Tis, N0, M0

Stage I

- T1, N0, M0

Stage II

- T2, N0, M0

Stage III

- T3, N0, M0
- T1, N1, M0
- T2, N1, M0
- T3, N1, M0

Stage IVA

- T4a, N0, M0

- T4a, N1, M0
- T1, N2, M0
- T2, N2, M0
- T3, N2, M0
- T4a, N2, M0

Stage IVB

- T4b, any N, M0
- Any T, N3, M0

Stage IVC

- Any T, any N, M1

Treatment Options for Head and Neck Cancers

Small superficial cancers without laryngeal fixation or lymph node involvement are successfully treated by radiation therapy or surgery alone, including laser excision surgery (see Chapter 8). Radiation therapy may be selected, instead of surgery, with the goal being to preserve the larynx and vocal function (also referred to as organ preservation). The radiation oncologist determines the radiation field and dose based on the location and size of the primary tumor.

Radiation is energy in the form of waves or moving subatomic particles emitted by an atom or other body as it changes from a higher energy state to a lower energy state.

Chemotherapy refers to treatment of a disease by chemicals that kill cells, specifically those of microorganisms or cancer.

A variety of curative surgical procedures are also recommended for laryngeal cancers, some of which preserve vocal function (Carew & Shah, 1998; Maddox & Davies, 2012).

If surgery is required, an appropriate surgical procedure must be considered for each patient, given the anatomic problem, stage of cancer, voice and swallowing status, cognitive status, motor function and coordination, quality of life factors, and clinical expertise of the treatment team. Advanced laryngeal cancers are often treated by combining radiation, chemotherapy, and/or surgery (Fowler, 1992; Mendenhall et al., 2005; Silver & Ferlito, 1996; Thawley, Panje, Batsakis, et al., 1999; Wang, 1997).

There are at least three types of combined management approaches for treating head and neck cancer.

Definitive: an approach where radiation is administered alone as a curative method. Chemotherapy is not considered a definitive treatment for the management of head and neck cancer.

Concomitant: an approach that is administered in conjunction with another treatment such as chemotherapy and radiation.

Sample of Types of Combined Management

The selection of treatment modality is usually dependent on the site and extent of tumor:

- Surgery followed by radiation or chemoradiation
- Chemotherapy followed by surgery, radiation, or chemoradiation
- Chemoradiation followed by surgery

In making these choices the rehabilitation team considers the potential functional outcomes of each treatment choice and the patient's preference.

Adjuvant: an approach which typically follows surgery and enhances the outcome response. Although radiation therapy and chemotherapy may be considered organ preservation approaches, preservation of the anatomic structure does not equal improved function, and in most cases organ preservation frequently results in significant sequelae and a decrease in quality of life (Logemann et al., 2008).

> Sequelae are morbid conditions following the consequences of disease and could include pain, bleeding, ulcerations to mucosa, bone damage, permanent damage to salivary glands, chewing difficulty, and/or dysphagia.

Organ Preservation Options

Radiation and combined chemoradiation protocols are used to successfully treat selected patients with head and neck tumors who wish to attempt to retain organ function (Figures 9–1 and 9–2); however, the adverse impact of radiation may equal or exceed that associated with surgery because of the long-term sequelae including fibrosis, tissue changes, and altered sensory awareness (Forastiere et al., 2003; Stupp, Weichselbaum, & Vokes, 1994; Taylor, 1987). For example, radiation-induced fibrosis restricts laryngeal movements, can reduce tongue and jaw movements, and diminish pharyngeal wall motion when the larynx is in the radiation field (Fung et al., 2005). Although uncommon, in some instances, a patient may undergo a salvage total laryngectomy when the larynx is rendered nonfunctional as a result of radiation treatment if dysphagia is severe and vocal quality is poor. In this case, the cancer has not recurred, but

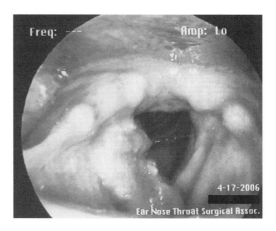

Figure 9–1. Depiction of T-3 carcinoma pre-chemoradiation. Courtesy of The Ear Nose Throat and Plastic Surgery Associates, Winter Park, Florida.

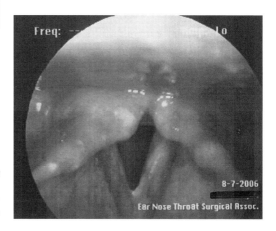

Figure 9–2. Depiction of 3-month post-chemoradiation. Courtesy of The Ear Nose Throat and Plastic Surgery Associates, Winter Park, Florida.

a total laryngectomy following an organ preservation approach that results in failure to maintain function could result in improved swallowing function and an alaryngeal form of communication might be more effective than the voice that the patient can produce with altered structure/function post treatment. New methods of intensity-modulated radiation therapy (IMRT) have been developed to reduce the postradiation morbidity by targeting the tumor with set radiation doses while limiting the dose to other structures.

The voice pathologist plays a significant role in helping patients through the radiation treatment while targeting minimization of long-term effects on speech and swallowing. The goals of therapy should be to prevent or reduce the formation of fibrosis and maintain the range of motion of the oropharynx and larynx through maneuvers such as sliding glissandos, falsetto phonation, and the Mendelsohn manuever (Kielbassa, Hinkelbein, Hellwig, & Meyer-Luckel, 2006; Logemann et al., 2008).

Typical Schedules of Radiation Therapy

Radiation dosage is measured in gray (Gy). One gray is equal to 100 rads. A rad defines the rate of absorption of radiation energy. One rad results in the absorption of 100 ergs of energy per gram of target tissue. Fractionation refers to dosing radiation in small increments over a specific time period with intervals between the small dose fractions (Bastholt & Berthelsen, 1997; Clifford Chao, Ozyigit, Low, Wippold, & Thorstad, 2002). Figures 9–1 and 9–2 depict an example of pre- and postradiation treatment for a case of laryngeal cancer.

- Conventional dosages
  - Dose per fraction (treatment) 1.8 to 2 Gy
  - Doses to gross disease 66 to 70 Gy
  - Subclinical doses 50 to 54 Gy
  - Postoperative doses 56 to 63 Gy

Methods of Delivering Radiation

- Hypofractionation: fewer fractions, higher doses, shorter treatment duration

- This approach divides the daily dose into less than one per day, resulting in a less overall daily dose. The smaller fractions allow greater doses without increased morbidity
- Accelerated fractionation: "concomitant boost," conventional progressing to hyperfractionation
- Hyperfractionation: more than one dose of radiation within the same day but in smaller dosage amounts

---

Postradiation Symptoms:

- Dental loss and tooth decay (caries)
- Dysgeusia: Bad taste in the mouth
- Dysphagia: Difficulty swallowing
- Dysphonia: Difficulty producing voice, including hoarseness and change in pitch, loudness, or quality
- Edema: Swelling caused by excess fluid in body tissues
- Erythema: Redness of the tissue
- Fatigue: Condition marked by extreme tiredness and inability to function due lack of energy. Fatigue may be acute or chronic
- Fibrosis: The growth of fibrous tissue
- Fistulas: An abnormal passage, opening, or connection between two internal organs or from an internal organ to the surface of the body
- Hypersensitive gag/oral aversion: increased/exaggerated response to oral stimuli due to increased sensitivity
- Inflammatory reactions: Local response to cellular injury that is marked by capillary dilatation, redness, heat, pain, swelling, and often loss of function

- Loss of appetite
- Mucositis: Complication of some cancer therapies in which the lining of the digestive system becomes inflamed, resulting in sores in the mouth
- Nausea: Feeling of sickness or discomfort in the stomach that may come with an urge to vomit
- Necrosis: Death of living tissues
- Odynophagia: Pain produced by swallowing
- Stricture/stenosis: Narrowing (stricture) of a duct or canal
- Thick secretions: Heavy substance of mucus
- Thrush: Type of yeast (*Candida*), grows out of control in moist skin areas of the body including the oral and laryngeal cavities.
- Trismus: Spasm of the muscles of mastication resulting from any of various abnormal conditions or diseases. Postradiation fibrosis can also cause trismus which results in decreased jaw opening.
- Xerostomia: Dry mouth

Role of the Voice Pathologist In Organ Preservation Protocols

The voice pathologist is involved, on an as-needed basis, in the care of head and neck cancer patients prior to treatment, during treatment and post-treatment. Prior to chemoradiation, the voice pathologist performs a clinical evaluation of speech, voice and swallowing, including an instrumental assessment with endoscopy, laryngostroboscopy, fiberoptic endoscopic evaluation of swallowing (FEES), and/or modified barium swallow (MBS), as indicated.

Patient counseling includes explaining the normal anatomy and physiology of the head and neck to the patient while providing information about the potential changes that may occur from chemoradiation as well as possible changes that may be evident upon examination due to the presence of the tumor itself. The voice pathologist provides realistic expectations for recovery and return to work, reducing fears or misconceptions about the process and outcomes associated with radiation. Prior to chemoradiation the patient should be provided with a swallow rehabilitation plan and vocal hygiene protocol to minimize side effects. It is critical that the patient understands their responsibility in complying with the rehabilitation program. During treatment, and in the post-treatment phase of chemoradiation, the voice pathologist may recommend saliva substitutes as needed, or provide suggestions to alleviate symptoms of xerostomia, introduce swallow strategies or diet modification as needed, and establish a swallowing schedule, reinforce swallow exercises, vocal hygiene, and oral care.

Surgical Options for Laryngeal Cancer

There are a number of surgical procedures used in the management of head and neck cancers including various processes involving laser technology (Zeitels & Burns, 2005), and microflap reconstruction (Anthony, Singer, & Mathes, 1994; Aryan, 1979). A new surgical technique, transoral robotic surgery (TORS), was approved by the FDA for use in the head and neck cancer population in 2009. With the use of this system, a specially trained surgeon sits at a robotic console and controls robotic arms that hold miniaturized surgical tools. This allows for effective resection of tumors via the mouth and thus, surgery can be completed without large incisions in the head and or neck regions. This less invasive surgical technique can be utilized to remove lesions of the mouth or throat. Studies have shown that effective resection of head and neck lesions can be completed with TORS while preserving function. Additionally, the en bloc surgical resection completed by this system may eliminate the need for radiation therapy following surgery or if radiation therapy is required, the dosage that needs to be administered can be reduced. By eliminating radiation therapy or decreasing the dosage necessary following surgery, organ function following surgical resection can be maximized, (Leonhardt, Quon, et al., 2012). Currently, TORS can be utilized for resection of lesions in the oral and supraglottic regions; resection of lesions in the glottic or subglottic regions cannot currently be completed with TORS. The increased accessibility to anatomic locations that were previously only managed by open surgical techniques holds great promise (Van Abel & Moore, 2012).

Although voice pathologists do not make surgical decisions, their involvement in the surgical process is critical to patients overall rehabilitation. The voice pathologist must have an understanding of the exact nature and extent of the resection and reconstruction that will occur during surgery so that accurate and informative counseling is administered and effective communication for the patient occurs prior to and following surgery.

Laryngectomy Types

Total Laryngectomy

A total laryngectomy is when the entire larynx is removed. The hyoid bone is cut from the suprahyoid musculature and the thyroid and cricoid cartilages are removed from the pha-ryngeal muscles and trachea. With a total laryngectomy, communication is dependent on alaryngeal speech modes. Figure 9–3 depicts the normal anatomic orientations prior to a total laryngectomy. Figure 9–4 depicts a total laryngectomy. As a result of this procedure, the trachea is redirected to form a stoma; an opening in the front of the neck. A total laryngectomy is performed when the extent of the laryngeal carcinoma is not amenable to conservation surgical or nonsurgical procedures.

Prior to laryngectomy, normal anatomy allows air to be filtered via the nose hairs and warmed and humidified by the mucous membrane of the nose and pharynx. Postlaryngectomy, there is an alteration to the normal head and neck anatomy resulting in air flowing directly into the trachea via the stoma without being filtered or warmed by the nose. This change in the filtration system of the respiratory tract results in irritation, inflammation, and possibly bacteria formation in the airway passages. In addition, the loss of heat and humidity results in more viscous mucus. The decreased resistance to airflow results in a reduction in tissue oxygenation and lung function, decreased olfaction (loss of smell), and increased mucus production and decreased mobilization of secretions.

Postlaryngectomy, the patient adjusts to breathing through the stoma. As the laryngectomized patient breathes in and out of the stoma, not the nose, the natural filtration system is no longer in place. Instruction regarding this important change following surgery is provided by the voice pathologist and ways to filter the air being breathed into the lungs should be discussed. Stoma covers, worn over the stoma, can provide some filtration of air. Cloth stoma covers can be homemade or purchased by the patient; disposable foam stoma covers are also available (Figures 9–5 and 9–6).

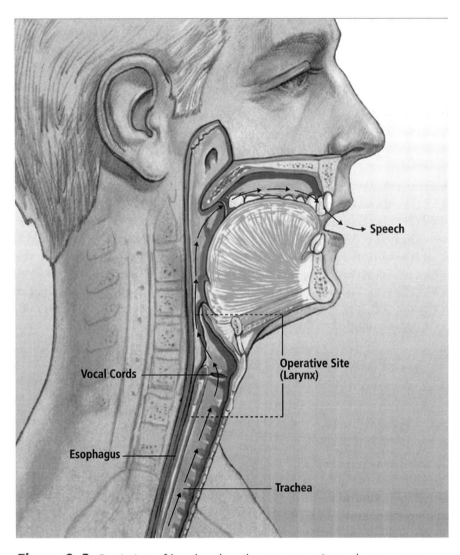

Figure 9–3. Depiction of head and neck anatomy prior to laryngectomy. Courtesy of InHealth Technologies (www.inhealth.com).

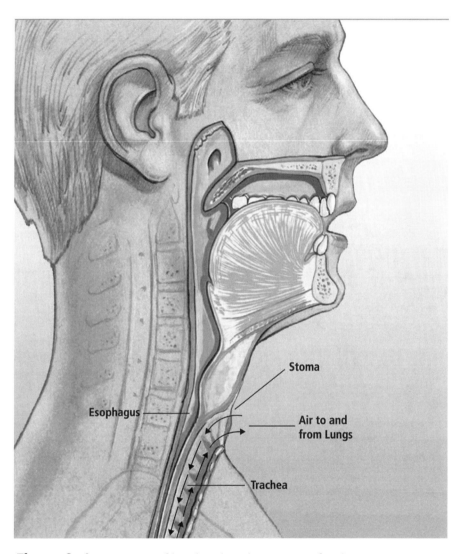

Labels in figure:
- Stoma
- Esophagus
- Air to and from Lungs
- Trachea

Figure 9–4. Depiction of head and neck anatomy after laryngectomy. Courtesy of InHealth Technologies (www.inhealth.com).

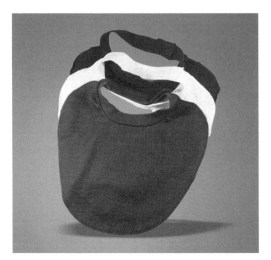

Figure 9–5. Cloth stoma covers.

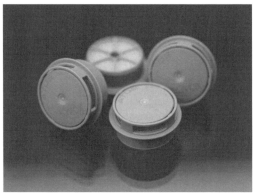

Figure 9–7. HME cassette. Courtesy of Atos Medical.

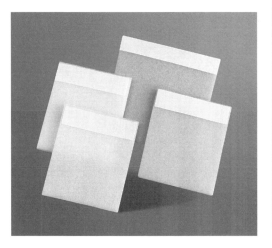

Figure 9–6. Disposable foam stoma covers.

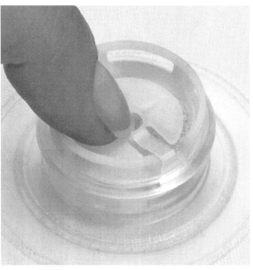

Figure 9–8. HME Easy Touch Speech Button. Courtesy of InHealth Technologies (www.inhealth.com).

Another method to warm and filter the air entering via the stoma is through us of a heat and moisture exchange (HME) system. There are several products commercially available. They involve use of a disposable filter cassette that attaches to the stoma with an adhesive base plate, laryngectomy button, or laryngectomy tube (Figures 9–7 through 9–11).

The HME device works on the principle that during exhalation, heat and moisture will be absorbed by the filtering mechanism and transferred back to the incoming air on inhalation (Hilgers et al., 1991). Although these products vary in design, airflow resistance, and in their efficiency of use, HME use increases the air temperature and the humidity of air entering the body thereby promoting function

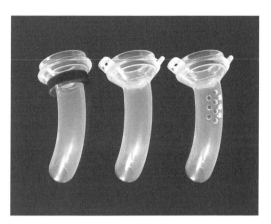

Figure 9–9. Provox larytubes, which can be used to hold an HME device within the stoma. Courtesy of Atos Medical.

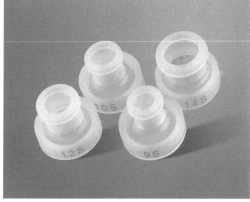

Figure 9–10. Barton-Mayo buttons, which can be used to hold an HME device within the stoma. These buttons are custom sized for individual patients by the voice pathologist. Image courtesy of InHealth Technologies (www.inhealth.com).

of cilia in the lungs. This process decreases significantly following total laryngectomy as a result in the physiologic changes in breathing. Return of cilia function allows for improved pulmonary hygiene resulting in the ability to expectorate secretions decreasing the amount of mucus, coughing, and the likelihood of mucus becoming encrusted in the bronchial pathways.

> Pulmonary hygiene, also called pulmonary toilet, refers to the ability of an individual to clear secretions from the airway.

In addition to the changes in filtration and humidification of air being breathed as described above, the presence of a stoma also has an impact on safety. As the stoma leads directly into the trachea, a barrier from water is necessary. Special care is necessary for bathing/showering to keep water from entering into the stoma. A shower shield or collar that is made of a substance that will not allow water to penetrate can be utilized to provide a barrier while permitting the patient to breathe (Figure 9–12). Other safety recommenda-

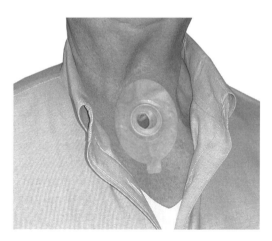

Figure 9–11. View of a stoma with a disposable adhesive base plate holding an HME device in place. Image courtesy of InHealth Technologies (www.inhealth.com).

tions include refraining from swimming and becoming aware of the changes in the instructions for giving and receiving cardiopulmonary resuscitation (CPR) which include specific details on how to administer mouth to stoma resuscitation.

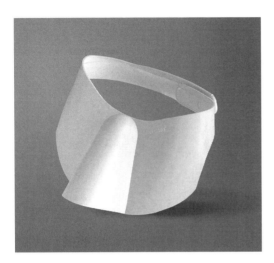

Figure 9–12. Rubber shower collar. Image courtesy of InHealth Technologies (www.inhealth.com).

Types of Partial Laryngectomy Procedures

Smaller laryngeal cancers can be removed without complete removal of the larynx. There are several different types of partial laryngectomy procedures. For supraglottic cancers, only the portion of the larynx above the vocal folds may be removed. This procedure, called supraglottic laryngectomy, allows the patient to retain normal speech. With small cancers of the vocal folds the surgeon may be able to remove the cancer by taking out only a portion of the vocal folds, with efforts in preserving voice production. This procedure is referred to as a partial cordectomy.

Hemilaryngectomy: Vertical. This procedure involves removal of one vertical half of the larynx including one false vocal fold, ventricle, true vocal fold, and portion of the thyroid cartilage on the involved side. Typically, this procedure excludes the removal of the hyoid and epiglottis. In some cases it can be extended to include a portion of the anterior commissure and vocal fold anteriorly (this puts the patients at a greater risk for airway stenosis).

In this procedure, reconstruction with tissue bulk on the operated side provides a means in which the nonoperated side can achieve closure for airway protection and sound production (Mohr, Quenelle, & Shumrick, 1983). There are several variations of this procedure depending upon the extent of cancer invasion.

Supraglottic Laryngectomy. In this procedure, usually part or all of the hyoid and epiglottis, aryepiglottic folds, and false vocal folds are removed. The goal is maintenance of airway protection, respiration, and phonation. Reconstruction usually elevates the thyroid cartilage by attaching the thyroid perichondrium to the tongue base. This is referred to as a laryngeal suspension procedure. The larynx is released by dividing the infrahyoid strap muscles. An extended supraglottic laryngectomy that includes resection of one arytenoid with re-approximation of the true vocal fold edge to the cricoid cartilage. The vallecula and base of tongue may be resected superiorly including the superior and anterior wall of the pyriform sinus. Following surgery, the patient must be taught how to protect their airway during swallowing. Therapeutic compensations can include supraglottic and super-supraglottic swallow, and tongue base retraction exercises.

Supracricoid Laryngectomy. A supracricoid laryngectomy, also known as a horizontal partial laryngectomy, is a type of laryngectomy designed with speech reconstruction in mind. This surgery typically includes removal of the supraglottic structures including the true and false vocal folds, and the thyroid cartilage including the paraglottic and preepiglottic spaces. The hyoid bone, cricoid cartilage, and at least one arytenoid are salvaged. Phonation and swallowing is aided by the arytenoid left in place (see video on DVD corresponding to this chapter).

Subtotal Laryngectomy. A subtotal laryngectomy is a modified technique with removal of half of the larynx vertically and the upper half of the contralateral larynx, including the ventricle and upper margin of the vocal fold. The most important structure needed to prevent postoperative dysphagia is the posterior laryngeal wall, which is reconstructed with the use of the infractured superior thyroid horn (Iwai, Tamura, Yoshioka, Okuizara, & Yanagihara, 1970). A permanent tracheostomy is necessary. The residual laryngeal tissue serves as tracheoesophageal speech shunt.

Cordectomy. A cordectomy involves removing part or all of a vocal fold. It can be used to treat very limited or superficial glottic cancers.

Postoperative Strategies

A variety of therapeutic compensations to aid voice, speech or swallowing posthemilaryngectomy may be used. Some of these can include:

- Chin-down technique: this helps by pushing the epiglottis posteriorly, narrowing the airway entrance (Shanahan, Logeman, Rademaker, Pauloski, & Kahrilas, 1993)
- Head-rotation technique: rotation to the operated side is used to achieve airway closure; this may be combined with a chin-down technique (Ertekin et al., 2001)
- Supraglottic or super-supraglottic swallowing therapy procedure or other swallowing procedure (Lazarus, Logemann, & Gibbons, 1993)
- Vocal fold adduction exercises: effortful focus on closing the vocal folds during nonphonatory or phonatory tasks

> Due to the extent of resection during a cordectomy for carcinoma, this type of surgery is usually completed for a unilateral vocal fold carcinoma. A bilateral cordectomy for cancer resection could result in impaired voice and swallowing function.

Role of the Voice Pathologist

Presurgical Counseling

Similar to the counseling techniques used with the patient undergoing organ preservation, the voice pathologist plays a key role with the patient in counseling prior to surgery. Patient counseling is completed by the voice pathologist. The timing of when the counseling is completed is typically determined by the surgeon and or the circumstances of the surgery (routine versus urgent). During the counseling session, psychosocial issues are addressed which include identifying the patient's unique learning needs, discussing their cultural preferences, teaching coping skills, developing and investigating their support systems, and discussing their financial situation. Also, an explanation of anticipated swallowing deficits, an explanation about the alterations in anatomy that will occur with the surgery and their impact on voice, speech, and swallow function are provided as well as discussion and practice with alternative modes of communication. Baseline measures such as quality of life scales, scales related to voice and swallowing function, and instrumental assessment including videoflouroscopy or endoscopic methods for imaging laryngeal and pharyngeal function are collected during the presurgical counseling session in order to assess patient's functional outcomes pre- and post-treatment.

Postsurgical Counseling and Management

Postsurgical counseling and management focuses on readdressing psychosocial issues, talking about patient and family support systems, available community resources, lifestyle changes, and nutritional changes that will need to occur as a result of the surgery. Patients are encouraged to participate in support groups to aid in coping with the postsurgical outcomes, facilitate socialization, and assist in the emotional recovery. Management should focus on practicing with voice, speech, and swallowing strategies (if necessary). During the preoperative consultation for the patient undergoing a total laryngectomy, use of an electrolarynx may be introduced and the patient can initiate use of the device (without use of their vocal folds) to begin to learn techniques to communicate effectively with the device including: overarticulation, proper phrasing, and proper placement of the device on the neck. The voice pathologist maintains close collaboration with the physician, nurse, dietitian, social worker, physical therapist, psychiatric professional, and other team members to ensure comprehensive care of the patient (Stemple, Glaze, & Klaben, 2000).

The rehabilitation goal for a laryngectomized individual is to learn to communicate with whatever multiple options of communication he or she may want to use as well as know how to use a backup method. The next section provides an overview of the modes of communication for those post total laryngectomy.

Offering Modes of Communication Following Total Laryngectomy

There are several rehabilitation options available following a total laryngectomy, including artificial/electromechanical, esophageal, or prosthetic. The "best" technique for the patient to use as an alternative mode of communication depends on a number of factors including: the person's age, cognitive status, motor coordination, cultural and personal preferences. The goal of rehabilitation for a laryngectomized individual is to learn to communicate with whatever option is best to improve functional communication and quality of life (Table 9–1).

Electromechanical Speech

An electromechanical device (also referred to as an artificial larynx or electrolarynx) is a useful treatment option in the early postoperative phase when the patient cannot use other voice rehabilitation techniques, thereby limiting the frustration as they adjust to experiencing voicelessness. The voice pathologist (along with the patient), selects the most appropriate device, teaches basic use/care of device in acute care (including the use of an intraoral adaptor which must be used in the immediate postoperative phase since on the neck placement of the device is not possible while the patient is healing from the surgery in the neck region), assesses for on the neck placement of the electrolarynx (when appropriate to do so in the healing process), and trains the patient how to use the device in all communicative settings (including in one to one communication, communication in a noisy environment and over the telephone).

Types of electrolarynges include transcervical and intraoral devices. Most of the artificial larynges available today are able to be used for both intraoral and on the neck placement. They have a vibrating head that can be used for on the neck placement, and a cap with attached oral tube that can be placed on the vibrating head of the device for intraoral use. All of these devices rely on the principle of introducing an electromechanical vibration that can be heard as a tone or buzz.

Table 9–1. Description of Primary Alaryngeal Modes of Communication

Type	Production	Disadvantages	Advantages	Troubleshooting for SLPs	Outcome Studies
Artificial Larynx	An electrical powered vibration that functions as a sound source Types: *Transcervical:* vibratory device is placed against the neck *Transoral:* vibration/sound is delivered directly to the mouth via tube *Intraoral:* remote controlled operated device that is custom built into the upper denture or orthodontic retainer	▪ A monopitch sound with metallic quality that may sound unusual and distracting ▪ Requires clear articulation skills ▪ Hand-held device ▪ Difficult to use with the telephone	▪ Fast and easy way to communicate after surgery (portable) ▪ Can be used as a backup to another means of communicating ▪ Battery operated ▪ Volume and pitch control features	▪ Find the right placement ▪ Work on eliminating distracters such as: on/off timing, body movement, and stance ▪ Increase intelligibility by teaching appropriate articulation, rate, phrasing, pitch, loudness, and stress	▪ Adaptive filtering and subtractive-type algorithms will reduce the noise level associated with electrolarynx and improve the speech quality and intelligibility (Liu & Ng, 2007) ▪ Breathiness during speech had a higher acceptability rating than during quick breathing and exhalation. The results showed that newer electrolarynxes can control pitch by expiration pressure (Liu, Wan, Wang, & Niu, 2004)

continues

Table 9–1. *continued*

Type	Production	Disadvantages	Advantages	Troubleshooting for SLPs	Outcome Studies
Esophageal Speech	Air is trapped into the mouth and then forced back up, causing the walls of the esophagus and pharynx to vibrate. The sound is then shaped into speech using the remaining articulators.	• Low pitch sound, derived from a controlled belch or burp. • Difficult to learn how to do. • Articulation must be clear • Reduced length of utterance	• No devices are needed to produce speech. • It is possible to produce a "normal" sounding voice (may improve quality of life)	Build skill level of patient: • Voice: increase length of utterance and develop appropriate stress patterns • Develop consistency and duration of speech • Eliminate distracters: stoma noise, lip smacking, intruding consonants	• Most preferred by laryngectomee patients, however, least intelligible during 5 dB and 10dB message-to-competition ratios (Clark & Stemple, 1982)
Tracheo-Esophageal Speech (TEP)	A small surgical passage is created inside the stoma, from the back wall of the trachea into the esophageal wall. A small valved tube (voice prosthesis) is placed into this passage to enable tracheoesophageal speech. Voice is produced by blocking the stoma	• Requires a good seal around the perimeter of the stoma • Requires ability to maintain prosthesis • Costly: some equipment needs to be replaced daily	• More natural speech • Improved intelligibility • Greater sound duration	Monitor for: • Leakage of liquids through or around the TEP • Candida • Poor cleaning: brushing and flushing device • Wrong size prosthesis • Muscle tension of overall body	• Research shows that there is a normal air-stream source in speech production using a TEP device, which contributes to speech timing and intelligibility of alaryngeal speakers

The transcervical device is placed against the neck (in an area of soft tissue, not in contact with bone) and a vibration is transmitted as a tone/buzz to the oral cavity (Figures 9–13, 9–14, and 9–15). The remaining intact structures of the vocal tract (tongue, lips, and teeth) modulate the tone. This articulation produces speech. Most devices available are rechargeable and have loudness and pitch control.

The intraoral device, which is used in the immediate postoperative period for most patients and can be a continued method of usage for some patients, introduces the sound source by placing a tube directly into the oral cavity. Voice/sound generation occurs in the same way as the transcervical device. The major advantage of both devices is that the production of basic speech is learned quickly by the majority of laryngectomy patients and will not interfere or delay progress mastering other forms of alaryngeal speech. The devices can also help facilitate other forms of alaryngeal speech and serves as an immediate form of communication. There can be certain patient conditions that prevent the use of these devices. Some examples include patients who underwent extensive surgery and radiation therapy, which may result in fibrosis of the neck, or may hamper the transmission of the tone/buzz toward the oral cavity. Limited dexterity and limited cognitive function may also inhibit the successful use of these devices.

The major disadvantage associated with electromechanical devices is the sound quality that results from its use. The sound produced is mechanical, even when a pitch variation mechanism is built into the device. The sound output is robotic, which can be distracting to some listeners' attention. Yet, Hillman and colleagues (1998) reported that artificial larynx use was the predominant mode of alaryngeal communication at follow-up. Eighty-five percent of patients in their study used an artificial larynx at 1-month postoperative treatment and 55% still used it as their primary means of communication 24 months

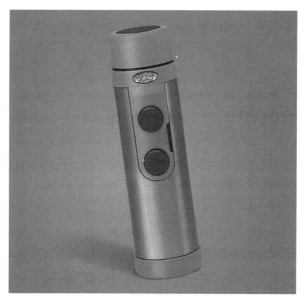

Figure 9–13. Depiction of Servox electrolarynx. Courtesy of InHealth Technologies (www.inhealth.com).

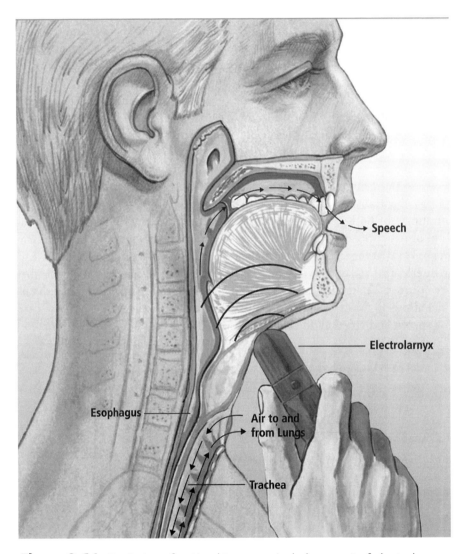

Figure 9-14. Depiction of optimal transcervical placement of electrolarynx. Courtesy of InHealth Technologies (www.inhealth.com).

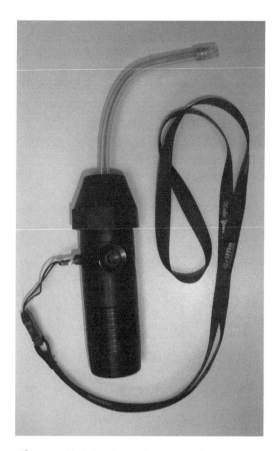

Figure 9–15. Electrolarynx with intraoral adapter in place.

post-treatment. Other surveys (Carr, Schmid-bauer, Majaess, & Smith, 2000) found similar results that report more than half of the individuals undergoing total laryngectomy continue to use electromechanical means of communication.

Esophageal Speech

Esophageal speech (Figure 9–16) is another option of alaryngeal communication for an individual post total laryngectomy. When the larynx is removed the upper portion of the trachea is pulled forward and attached superiorly to the sternum. The reconstructed pharynx is joined directly to the esophageal opening. The junction at which the hypopharynx joins the esophagus is called the pharyngoesophageal (PE) segment. The PE segment is composed of striated muscle: the cricopharyngeeus muscle, the lower strands of the inferior pharyngeal constrictor, and the superior esophageal sphincter (Zemlin, 1998). During esophogeal speech, sound is produced by the vibration of the pharyngoesophageal (PE) segment (Zemlin, 1998).

Esophageal speech can be produced when the individual transports a small amount (75 ml) of air from the oral and pharyngeal cavity into the esophagus. The air is redirected back past the PE segment to force vibration of the tissue. Rapid repetition of the air transport can ultimately produce intelligible esophageal speech. This process is similar to a controlled belch or burp (Salmon, 1986).

The patient then forms this sound into words with the tongue, lips, teeth, and palate. There are two primary techniques that can be used to transport air from the oral cavity to the esophagus to produce esophageal speech: injection (a positive pressure approach) and inhalation (a negative pressure approach). These techniques of esophageal speech are based on how the PE segment opens to allow air intake (Salmon, 2005).

Injection Method

The injection method requires the use of the tongue to force air back into the pharynx and esophagus. During this technique the lip and tongue movements increase the already positive air pressure in the oral cavity, forcing air through the closed PE segment and into the upper portion of the esophagus (Duguay, 1999; Graham, 2005). The tightening of the thoracic and abdominal muscles prevents the air from moving farther down the esophagus. The trapped air moves upward through the PE segment, setting the surrounding musculature (pharyngeal-esophageal) into vibration, thereby producing sound (Graham, 2005). As

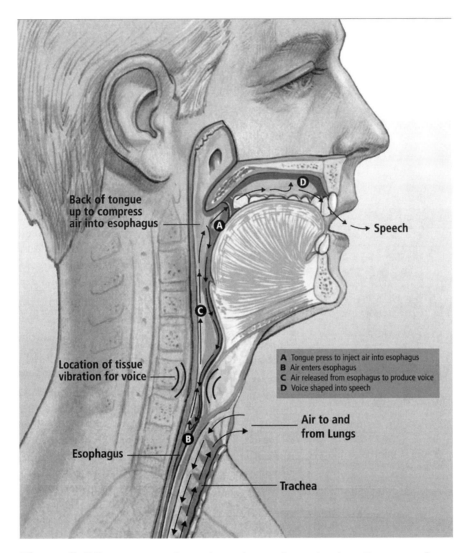

Back of tongue
up to compress
air into esophagus

Speech

Location of tissue
vibration for voice

A Tongue press to inject air into esophagus
B Air enters esophagus
C Air released from esophagus to produce voice
D Voice shaped into speech

Air to and
from Lungs

Esophagus

Trachea

Figure 9–16. Depiction of esophageal speech production. Courtesy of InHealth Technologies (www.inhealth.com).

the laryngectomee articulates, the vibrations are then further shaped with resonance in the nasal and oropharyngeal cavities (Edels, 1983).

This method is further described by two techniques used to inject air into the esophagus: the consonant press injection method and the glossopharyngeal press (Graham, 2005). The consonant press injection method (also referred to as injection method for obstruents or consonant injection) uses the natural intraoral air pressures created by plosive and fricative sounds to inject air into the esophagus. When a patient produces sounds such as /t/, /p/, /k/ or words such as "poach," "toad," or "kick" the strength of contact in the lips and tongue musculature builds and compresses intraoral air pressure sufficient enough to overcome the resistance of the closed PE segment (Edels, 1983; Graham, 2005). Sound is produced as the air is redirected to vibrate the PE segment. As not all syllables begin with a plosive, fricative, or affricate a proficient esophageal speaker learns the injection method. This method is also known as the tongue pump or glossopharyngeal press (Graham, 2005; Salmon 1994). For this method, lips and tongue seal are used to increase intraoral air pressure to move the air toward the PE segment. The tongue creates a pumping action that reduces the size of the oral cavity, compressing the air, which, in turn, increases intraoral air pressure causing the PE segment to open and vibrate.

Inhalation Method

The inhalation method uses a rapid expansion of the thoracic cavity during inspiration to draw air into the esophagus. To accomplish this task, the laryngectomized patient is instructed to take a quick, short breath through the stoma. As the diaphragm moves downward, there is an increase in the negative pressure within the thoracic cavity (where the esophagus is located). A vacuum effect is created in the esophagus as the negative air pressure begins to increase. This allows air from the oral and pharyngeal cavities to be drawn passively into the esophagus. Once the air has entered the upper esophagus, the PE sphincter closes, thereby trapping the air in the esophagus. The procedure for returning the air to the oropharynx parallels that of the consonant press injection method (Graham, 2005).

Advantages for esophageal speech are that it does not require expensive electromechanical devices and prostheses and is a hands-free speech technique. The main disadvantage is its limited success rate for acquiring useful voice production, which is reported to be only as high as 20 to 25% (Gates, Ryan, Cooper, et al., 1982) and in recent studies as low as 7 to 10%

(Hillman, Walsh, & Heaton, 2005). Furthermore, esophageal speech results in low-pitched (50–80 Hz) and low-intensity speech that can result in poor speech intelligibility.

The factors that have been associated with successful acquisition of esophageal speech include: type and extent of surgery, positive attitude, psychosocial adjustment, frequency of therapy, and positive family support. Failures in developing esophageal speech have been associated with poor attitude, lack of patient motivation, limited physical strength, postoperative radiation effects, dysphagia, and limited therapy (Gates, Ryan, Cantu, & Hearne, 1982; Graham, 2005).

Patients who master esophageal speech should also be provided with training on a backup method of communication that is typically the use of an electrolarynx. If a patient becomes ill or is feeling fatigued, ability to produce esophageal speech may deteriorate and having a backup method of communication can become necessary.

Tracheoesophageal Puncture (TEP)

Another option for speech rehabilitation following a total laryngectomy is tracheoesophageal voice production. This method was first introduced by Singer and Blom (1980) and since that time has gained popularity as a major rehabilitation option for voice and speech production in patients following a total laryngectomy (Webster & Duguay, 1990). Similar to esophageal speech, patients who utilize a TEP should also be provided with training on a back-up method of communication. If the prosthesis malfunctions, an alternate means of communication can become necessary. Typically, patients will utilize an electrolarynx, and thus training with this method of communication is an important part of the rehabilitation process even if the patient plans to use their TEP as a primary means of voice production.

The tracheoesophageal puncture (TEP) is performed either at the time of the laryngectomy surgery (referred to as a primary TEP), in an uncomplicated laryngectomy case, or at a later time when sufficient healing has occurred (referred to as a secondary TEP). The secondary TEP can occur approximately 6 weeks postlaryngectomy or post radiation therapy, or anytime thereafter. After the puncture is produced, a balloon catheter is directed downward through the fistula from the trachea and into the esophagus (Gress & Singer, 2005) or an indwelling prosthesis can be placed at the time of surgery. When a primary TEP is performed and a balloon catheter is placed in the TE tract, the catheter serves as a feeding tube which is ultimately replaced by the voice prosthesis after sufficient healing has occurred. In cases where a surgeon places an indwelling prosthesis during a primary TEP, another means of nonoral nutrition such as a nasogastric tube or percutaneous gastrostomy tube will be necessary until the patient has healed sufficiently to initiate oral intake.

> The tracheoesophageal puncture creates a surgical opening (fistula) between the posterior wall of the trachea and the anterior wall of the esophagus for insertion of a voice prosthesis.

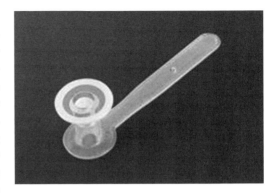

Figure 9–17. Depiction of InHealth voice prosthesis. Courtesy of InHealth Technologies (www.inhealth.com).

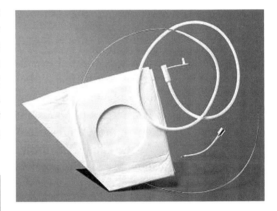

Figure 9–18. Depiction of tracheoesophageal puncture set. Courtesy of InHealth Technologies (www.inhealth.com).

The TEP procedure, involves surgically creating a small puncture through the posterior tracheal wall into the esophagus. A small one-way valve (prosthesis) is inserted into the puncture in order to prevent its spontaneous closure and prevent the aspiration of pharyngoesophageal contents into the trachea (Figures 9–17 and 9–18). Once in place, the voice prosthesis allows for a one-way flow of air from the trachea into the region below the PE segment. The puncture permits diversion of pulmonary air to drive pharyngoesophageal vibration for the production of tracheoesoph-ageal speech (also referred to as TE voice and speech) (Gress & Singer, 2005).

Tracheoesophageal (TE) Sound Generation

To produce the TE sound, the laryngectomized individual will be able to inhale then exhale as the tracheostoma is occluded. The occlusion can be made by a finger placed over the tracheostoma. In this case, the TE speaker needs to be able to coordinate finger occlusion of the tracheostoma and the associated release to meet the alternation of inhalation and exhalation. Stoma occlusion can also be achieved through the use of a tracheostoma valve to allow for hands-free speech production. The valve opens under positive pressure as the air enters the esophagus and closes by elastic recoil. Therefore, when pulmonary air enters the prosthesis, it opens the one way valve and releases air into the pharyngoesophagus, setting these tissues into vibration for sound generation. As the sound enters the oral and nasopharyngeal cavities, articulation and resonance shape the sounds for speech (Gress & Singer, 2005). Figure 9–18 depicts TE speech production.

Types of Prostheses for TEP Voice

The voice prosthesis is a cylindrical shaped tube, usually made from medical grade silicone. Two categories of devices are available; the indwelling prosthesis (placed by the clinician) and the non-indwelling prosthesis (placed by the patient). The neck strap on the indwelling prosthesis is usually cut following insertion and thus, taping to the neck is not necessary. For both types of prostheses, at the distal end, a slit, hinged, or ball valve is placed through front wall of the esophagus. The tracheal flange of the prosthesis is flush with the back wall of the stoma/trachea. During voice production, pulmonary air flows through the opening at the tracheal flange of the prosthesis, when the stoma is occluded. Air enters into the esophagus through the prosthesis and then flows through the PE segment producing audible vibration (voice). Cleaning of the prosthesis can be completed via the opening of the device at the back wall of the stoma; tools for cleaning the prosthesis are provided by the prosthesis manufacturer. Keeping the prosthesis free of debris is very important as food debris that collects at the level of the esophageal flange of the prosthesis can lead to yeast (*Candida*) growth. When this occurs, the *Candida* will invade the surface of the pros-

thesis valve and will result in malfunction of the valve. This causes leakage, initially of fluids, through the prosthesis when the patient drinks. Once this occurs, the prosthesis must be replaced due to aspiration risk.

Types of commercially available prostheses include:

Non-Indwelling Devices:

Duckbill Style: Original prosthesis designed by Singer and Blom (1980) with use of a slit-type valve (Figure 9–19)

Low Pressure/Low Resistance: Hinged valve with a lower opening pressure. This design requires less respiratory effort for sound generation to occur as compared with the duckbill devices (Gress & Singer, 2005; Pauloski, 1998) (Figure 9–20)

Indwelling Prosthesis: Refers to an extended wear clinician inserted prosthesis thereby minimizing prosthesis maintenance (Gress & Singer, 2005) (Figures 9–21, 9–22, and 9–23)

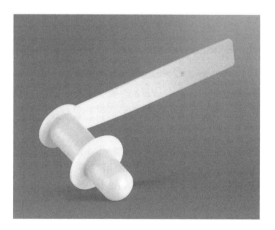

Figure 9–19. The duckbill style of non-indwelling devices, with use of a slit-type valve. Image courtesy of InHealth Technologies (www.inhealth.com).

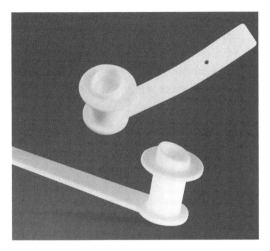

Figure 9–20. The low pressure/low resistance style of non-indwelling devices, with a hinged valve with a lower opening pressure. Image courtesy of InHealth Technologies (www.inhealth.com).

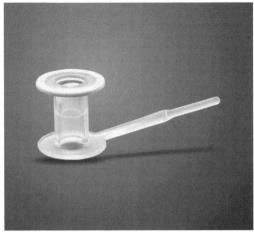

Figure 9–21. Classic indwelling device. Courtesy of InHealth Technologies (www.inhealth.com).

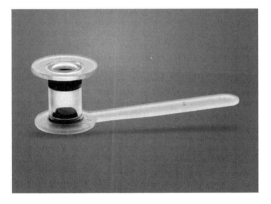

Figure 9–22. Blom Singer dual valve prosthesis. Courtesy of InHealth Technologies (www.inhealth.com).

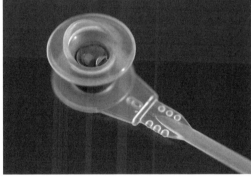

Figure 9–23. Provox 2 voice prosthesis. Courtesy of Atos Medical (www.atos medical.com).

Prosthesis length and methods for sizing vary by each manufacturer. Prosthesis product literature should be consulted to determine proper sizing tools, protocol, and other specifications of the selected prosthesis. Voice prostheses length ranges in size from 4.5 mm to 28 mm; prosthesis diameters range from 16 French to 22.5 French. There are several manufacturers of voice prostheses.

French is a unit of measure in medicine for the outer diameter of a tube. 1 Fr = 0.33 mm.

The main advantages of the TEP method of voice production include a relatively good voice quality when compared to the other alaryngeal methods. Although similar in quality to voice produced with esophageal speech, the duration of TEP voice production on one breath is often greater than with production of esophageal speech. Disadvantages of TEP can include postoperative complications, the daily maintenance of the prosthesis by the patient, recurrent leakage of the prosthesis after a period of time requiring replacement by the clinician, the cost, and, as mentioned, for some patients the need to use a finger to occlude the tracheostoma.

Some of the more current voice prostheses tend to be more reliable and safe to use, have a frontloading insertion technique, indwelling fixation and low resistance to airflow. Overall, satisfaction with speech quality, fluency of speech, overall intelligibility, ease of phone use, satisfaction with social interactions, and quality of life tends to be high with the TEP method in comparison to artificial and esophageal methods (Clements et al., 1997; Hillman, Walsh, & Heaton, 2005).

Prosthesis Placement

Various prosthetic products are available and selection of a prosthesis type and style are not uniform, rather they are patient specific. If the surgeon does not place a prosthesis during the TEP surgical procedure, prosthesis placement can occur as soon as the tissue in the TEP site has healed. This can be completed by the surgeon or the voice pathologist. The catheter is removed and the TEP tract diameter can be dilated as necessary. Dilation occurs by insertion of catheters of increasing diameter until the puncture is approximately a size 2 French greater in diameter than that of the selected TEP prosthesis. This gradual process helps to decrease tissue trauma when the prosthesis is inserted. Using a measuring device provided by the prosthesis manufacturer, the depth of the TE party wall (this is the union of the posterior tracheal wall and the anterior esophageal wall) is assessed. There are conditions when

the TE party wall separates which can result in impaired voice production and/or further medical complications.

An accurate measurement is critical for determining the proper length for the prosthesis. If a prosthesis that is placed is too short in length, it may not be fully in place in the esophageal wall. If this occurs, the back wall of the tract will close and the TEP tract will be lost. If a prosthesis that is placed is too long, a pistoning (back and forth) movement of the prosthesis can occur with use and this can result in inadvertent dilation of the tract diameter and tissue irritation. As a result, the patient may begin to experience leakage of fluids when drinking around the outer diameter of the prosthesis. The prosthesis is typically inserted from the tracheal side using a standard insertion tool supplied by the manufacturer (Gress & Singer, 2005). The clinician needs to orient themselves to the position of TE tract, "line it up," and firmly insert the prosthesis until it is positioned flush with the back wall of the trachea. The methods for insertion will vary based on the type and manufacturer of the prosthesis (Gress & Singer, 2005).

Evaluation of and treatment for patients utilizing the TEP method of alaryngeal speech requires training and clinical practice beyond what is traditionally offered in graduate level programs in speech pathology. There are a number of voice institutes throughout the country offering courses in laryngectomy rehabilitation; for example, the International Association of Laryngectomees Voice Rehabilitation Institute offers a yearly training conference; another option would be to apprentice at a facility offering laryngectomy rehabilitation. Furthermore, the American Speech-Language-Hearing Association has published a position statement of practice policy entitled *Roles and Responsibilities of Speech-Language Pathologists With Respect to Evaluation and Treatment for Tracheoesophageal Puncture and Prosthesis* (ASHA, 2004).

The role of the voice pathologist in the multidisciplinary care of laryngectomized individuals is dependent on facility guidelines and/or surgical team preference. In some facilities the voice pathologist aids the surgeon in evaluation of a patient's suitability to use a voice prosthesis, sizing and fitting; prosthesis placement, trains the patient how to fit and care for their prosthesis, and implements therapy to maximize the patient's ability to communicate while using the voice prosthesis (Stemple, Glaze, & Klaben, 2000).

Safety

After laryngectomy the patient is classified as a neck breather. Special considerations and safeguards are necessary particularly in an emergency situation. Typically, when someone stops breathing, a rescuer may blow air into the individual's mouth. Mouth-to-mouth rescue breathing is a quick and effective way to provide oxygen to an individual. This technique will no longer work if the person is a neck breather since the individual now breathes through an opening in their neck (stoma), and no longer through their mouth or nose. The only way the individual will get oxygen is if it is provided through the neck opening and not through the mouth or nose. It is critical that the rescuer is knowledgeable about the difference in breathing mechanisms as this can present a life-threatening situation. The voice clinician should plan to share this information in the pre- and postoperative counseling sessions. Laryngectomees may decide to obtain a brightly colored emergency card with them on their person or to keep in their vehicle or on their vehicle window. Some individuals may choose to wear a special "medic alert" bracelet or necklace. These items identify the person as a total neck breather and provide vital medical

information in an emergency situation. Clinicians should also advocate that their patients contact their local EMS following surgery to alert the local responders of their address and register that they are a neck breather. Lastly, patients and their families should be educated about purchasing an Ambu bag at a local medical supply store. Should the laryngectomee require CPR by a family member the Ambu bag can be utilized with a pediatric mask that can be placed on the stoma for CPR administration. The ambu bag can be utilized with a regular sized CPR mask for the laryngectomee to use on others as the laryngectomee cannot administer mouth-to-mouth breathing.

Web Sites Helpful for Head and Neck Cancer Information and Support

Support for People With Head and Neck Cancer
http://www.spohnc.org/
http://www.oralcancersupport.org

Scott Hamilton CARES initiative
http://www.chemocare.com

The Head and Neck Cancer Alliance
http://www.headandneck.org

Oral Cancer Foundation
http://www.oralcancerfoundation.org

National Cancer Institute
http://www.cancer.gov

American Cancer Society
http://www.cancer.org

The International Association of Laryngectomees
http://www.theial.com

CancerCare
http://www.cancercare.org

Webwhispers
http://www.webwhispers.org

Developing a System to Track Outcomes with the Head and Neck Cancer Population

Evaluation of treatment outcome in the head and neck cancer population can be reported in a variety of ways: locoregional control, disease-free survival, overall survival at 2 to 5 years, functional outcomes related to activities of daily living, and quality of life. Outcomes should be reported after initial surgery, initial radiation or planned combined treatment, and at specified landmarks in the post-treatment time period. Databases used to track outcomes with this population typically include data on survival rates for all patients with information on cancer grade and stage, age, and other noteworthy features of the case or primary treatments. From the perspective of the voice pathologist, a database can be developed to include the following information:

- ■ Functional outcomes following surgery
  - ▪ Differentiate type of surgery
  - ▪ Medical management
- ■ Functional outcomes following radiotherapy
  - ▪ Audit of complications of radiation therapy via clinical and instrumental exam
- ■ Proportion of patients undergoing laryngectomy who receive surgical voice restoration or use other methods of alaryngeal speech

- ■ Patient satisfaction with medical and behavioral support services during therapy period
- ■ Audit of patient performance status (based on specified time intervals)
- ■ Audit of therapy protocol/ therapy compliance
- ■ Quality of Life (QOL) outcomes
  - ▪ QOL related to swallowing function
  - ▪ QOL related to vocal function

Summary

The successful restoration of function in those with head and neck cancer requires a team effort including a knowledgeable and skilled voice pathologist. The voice pathologist is involved in the rehabilitation of speech and swallowing, which are critical life-sustaining behaviors that must be maintained. Therefore, clinicians must continue to objectively evaluate management results to improve functional outcomes and allow evidence-based comparisons of different forms or combinations of cancer management.

References

American Cancer Society. (2008). *Cancer Facts and Figures 2008*. Atlanta, GA: Author.

American Speech-Language-Hearing Association. (1992, March). Position statement and guidelines for evaluation and treatment for tracheoesophageal fistulization/puncture. *American Speech and Hearing Association*, *34*(Suppl. 7), 17–21.

Ang, K. K., Harris, J., Wheeler, R., Weber, R., Rosenthal, D. I., Nguyen-Tân, P. F., . . . Gillison, M. L. (2010). Human papillomavirus and survival of patients with oropharyngeal cancer. *New England Journal of Medicine*, *363*(1), 24–35.

Anthony, J. P., Singer, M. I., & Mathes, S. J. (1994). Pharyngoesophageal reconstruction using the tubed free radial forearm flap. *Clinics in Plastic Surgery*, *21*(1), 137–147.

Aryan, S. (1979). The pectoralis major myocutaneous flap. A versatile flap for reconstruction of cervical esophagus by revascularized isolated jejunal segment. *Annals of Surgery*, *149*, 162.

Bastholt, L., & Berthelsen, A. (1997). Importance of overall treatment time for the outcome of radiotherapy of advanced head and neck carcinoma: Dependency on tumor differentiation. *Radiotherapy and Oncology: Journal of the European Society for Therapeutic Radiology and Oncology*, *43*(1), 47–51.

Carew, J. F., & Shah, J. P. (1998). Advances in multimodality therapy for laryngeal cancer. *Cancer Journal for Clinicians*, *48*(4), 211–228.

Carr, M. M., Schmidbauer, J. A., Majaess, L., & Smith, R. L. (2000). Communication after laryngectomy: An assessment of quality of life. *Otolaryngology-Head and Neck Surgery*, *122*(1), 39–43.

Casper, J., & Colton, R. (1998). *Clinical manual for laryngectomy and head/neck cancer rehabilitation* (2nd ed.). San Diego, CA: Singular.

Castellanos, P., Spector, G., & Kaiser, T. (1996). *Tumors of the larynx and laryngopharynx: Otorhinolaryngology-head and neck surgery* (15th ed., pp. 585–652). Baltimore, MD: Williams & Wilkins.

Clements, K. S., Rassekh, C. H., Seikaly, H., Hokanson, J. A., & Calhoun, K. H. (1997). Communication after laryngectomy. An assessment of patient satisfaction. *Archives of Otolaryngology-Head and Neck Surgery*, *123*(5), 493–496.

Clifford Chao, K. S., Ozyigit, G., Low, D. A., Wippold, F. J., & Thorstad, W. L. (2002). *Intensity modulated radiation therapy for head and neck cancers*. St. Louis, MO: Lippincott Williams & Wilkins.

D'Souza, G., Kreimer, A. R., Viscidi, R., Pawlita, M., Fakhry, C., Koch, W. M., . . . Gillison, M. L. (2007). Case-control study of human papillomavirus and oropharyngeal cancer. *New England Journal of Medicine*, *356*(19), 1944–1956.

Duguay, M. J. (1999). Esophageal speech training: The initial phase. In S. J. Salmon (Ed.), *Alaryngeal speech rehabilitation: For clinicians by clinicians* (2nd ed., pp. 155–201). Austin, TX: Pro-Ed.

Edels, Y. (1983). Pseudo voice theory and practice. In Y. Edels (Ed.), *Laryngectomy: Diagnosis rehabilitation* (pp. 107–141). London, UK: Croom Helm.

Ertekin, C., Keskin, A., Kiylioglu, N., Kirazli, Y., On, A. Y., Tarlaci, S., & Ayodogu, I. (2001). The effect of head and neck positions on oropharyngeal swallowing: A clinical and electrophysiologic study. *Archives of Physical Medicine and Rehabilitation*, *82*(9), 1255–1260.

Forastiere, A. A., Goepfert, H., Maor, M., Pajak, T. F., Weber, R., Morrison, W., . . . Cooper, J. (2003). Concurrent chemotherapy and radiotherapy for organ preservation in advanced laryngeal cancer. *New England Journal of Medicine*, *349*(22), 2091–2098.

Fowler, J. F., & Lindstrom, M. J. (1992). Loss of local control with prolongation in radiotherapy. *International Journal of Radiation Oncology, Biology, and Physics*, *23*(2), 457–467.

Fung, K., Lyden, T., Lee, J., Urba, S., Worden, F., Eisbruch, A., . . . Wolf, G. T. (2005). Voice and swallowing outcomes of an organ preservation trial for advanced laryngeal cancer. *International Journal of Radiation Oncology Biology and Physiology 63*(5), 1395–1399.

Gates, G., Ryan, W., Cantu, E., & Hearne, E. (1982). Current status of laryngectomee rehabilitation: II. Causes of failure. *American Journal of Otolaryngology*, *3*(1), 8–14.

Gates, G., Ryan, W., Cooper, J., Lawliss, G., Cantu, E., Hayashi, T., Luder, E., Welch, R., & Hearne, E. (1982). Current status of laryngectomee rehabilitation: I. Results of therapy. *American Journal of Otolaryngology*, *3*, 1–7.

Graham, M. (2005). Esophageal speech: Taking it to the limits. In P. Doyle & R. Keith (Eds.), *Contemporary considerations in the treatment and rehabilitation of head and neck cancer voice speech and swallowing* (pp. 379–430). Austin, TX: Pro-Ed.

Gress, C., & Singer, M. (2005). Tracheoesophageal voice restoration. In P. Doyle & R. Keith (Eds.), *Contemporary considerations in the treatment and rehabilitation of head and neck cancer voice speech and swallowing* (pp. 431–452). Austin, TX: Pro-Ed.

Hilgers, F., Aaronson, N., Ackerstaff, A., Schouwenburg, P., & VanZanwijk, N. (1991). The influence of a heat and moisture exchanger (HME) on the respiratory symptoms after total laryngectomy. *Clinical Otolaryngology*, *16*, 152–156.

Hillman, R., Walsh, M., & Heaton, J. (2005). Laryngectomy speech rehabilitation. In P. Doyle & R. Keith (Eds.), *Contemporary considerations in the treatment and rehabilitation of head and neck cancer voice speech and swallowing* (pp. 75–90). Austin, TX: Pro-Ed.

Hsu, Y. B., Chang, S.Y., Lan, M. C., Huang, J. L., Tai, S. K., & Chu, P.Y. (2008). Second primary malignancies in squamous cell carcinomas of the tongue and larynx: An analysis of incidence, pattern, and outcome. *Journal of the Chinese Medical Association*, *71*(2), 86–91.

Iwai, H., Tamura, M., Yoshioka, A., Okuizara, H., & Yanagihara, N. (1970). Subtotal laryngectomy. *European Archives of Oto-Rhino-Laryngology*, *197*(2), 85–96.

Jemal, A., Siegel, R., Xu, J., & Ward, E. Cancer statistics, 2010. *CA: A Cancer Journal for Clinicians 2010*, *60*(5), 277–300

Kielbassa, A., Hinkelbein, W., Hellwig, E., & Meyer-Lückel, H. (2006). Radiation- related damage to dentition. *Lancet Oncology*, *7*(4), 326–335.

Kreimer, A. R., Clifford, G. M., Boyle, P., & Franceschi, S. (2005). Human papillomavirus types in head and neck squamous cell carcinomas worldwide: A systematic review. *Cancer Epidemiology, Biomarkers, and Prevention*, *14*(2), 467–475.

Larynx. (2002). *American Joint Committee on Cancer: AJCC cancer staging manual* (6th ed., pp. 47–57). New York, NY: Springer.

Lazarus, C., Logemann, J. A., & Gibbons, P. (1993). Effects of maneuvers on swallowing function in a dysphagic oral cancer patient. *Head and Neck*, *15*(5), 419–424.

Leonhardt, F. D., Quon, H., Abrahão, M., O'Malley, B. W. Jr., & Weinstein, G. S. (2010). Transoral robotic surgery for oropharyngeal carcinoma and its impact on patient-reported quality of life and function. *Head and Neck*, *34*(2), 146–154.

Lipan, M. J., Reidenberg, J. S., & Laitman, J. T. (2006). Anatomy of reflux: A growing health problem affecting structures of the head and neck. *Anatomical Record Part B: The New Anatomist*, *289*(6), 261–270.

Logemann, J. A., Pauloski, B. R., Rademaker, A.W., Lazarus, C. L., Gaziano, J., Stachowiak, L., . . . Mittal, B. (2008). Swallowing disorders in the first year after radiation and chemoradiation. *Head and Neck*, *30*(2), 148–158.

Maddox, P. T., & Davies, L. (2012). Trends in total laryngectmy in the era of organ preservation: A population based study. *Otolaryngology-Head and Neck Surgery*, *27* [Epub ahead of print].

Mendenhall, W. M., Riggs, C. E., Jr., & Cassisi, N. J. (2005). Treatment of head and neck cancers. In V. T. DeVita Jr., S. Hellman, & S. A. Rosenberg (Eds.), *Cancer: Principles and practice of oncology* (7th ed., pp. 662–732). Philadelphia, PA: Lippincott Williams & Wilkins.

Mohr, R. M., Quenelle, D. J., & Shumrick, D. A. (1983). Vertico-frontolateral laryngectomy (hemilaryngectomy). Indications, technique, and results. *Archives of Otolaryngology: Head and Neck Surgery*, *109*(6), 384–395.

Pauloski, B. (1998). Acoustic and aerodynamic characteristics of tracheosophageal voice. In E. D. Blom, M. I. Singer, & R. C. Hamaker (Eds.), *Tracheoesophageal voice restoration following total laryngectomy* (pp. 123–141). San Diego, CA: Singular.

Salmon, S. J. (1986). Adjusting to laryngectomy. *Seminars in Speech and Language*, *7*, 67–94.

Salmon, S. J. (1994). Methods of error intake and associated problems. In R. L. Keith & S. L. Darley (Eds.), *Laryngectomee rehabilitation* (3rd ed., pp. 219–234). Austin, TX: Pro-Ed.

Salmon, S. J. (2005). Commonalities among alaryngeal speech methods. In P. Doyle & R. Keith (Eds.), *Contemporary considerations in the treatment and rehabilitation of head and neck cancer voice speech and swallowing* (pp. 59–74). Austin, TX: Pro-Ed.

Shanahan, T. K., Logeman, J. A., Rademaker, A.W., Pauloski, B. R., & Kahrilas, P. J. (1992). Chin-down posture effect on aspiration in dysphagia patients. *Archives of Physical Medicine and Rehabilitation*, *74*(7), 736–749.

Silver, C. E., & Ferlito, A. (1996). *Surgery for cancer of the larynx and related structures* (2nd ed.). Philadelphia, PA: Saunders.

Singer, M., & Blom, E. (1980). An endoscopic technique for restoration of voice after laryngectomy. *Annals of Otology, Rhinology and Laryngology, 89,* 529–533.

Spaulding, C. A., Hahn, S. S., & Constable, W. C. (1987). The effectiveness of treatment of lymph nodes in cancers of the pyriform sinus and supraglottis. *International Journal of Radiation Oncology, Biology, and Physics, 13*(7), 963–968.

Spitz, M. R. (1994). Epidemiology and risk factors for head and neck cancer. *Seminars in Oncology, 21*(3), 281–288.

Stajner-Katusic, S., Horga, D., Musura, M., & Globlek, D. (2006). Voice and speech after laryngecotomy. *Clinical Linguistics and Phonology, 20*(2–3), 195–203.

Stemple, J. C., Glaze, L. E., & Klaben, B. G. (2000). *Clinical voice pathology: Theory and management* (3rd ed.). San Diego, CA: Singular.

Stupp, R., Weichselbaum, R. R., & Vokes, E. E. (1994). Combined modality therapy of head and neck cancer. *Seminars in Oncology, 21*(3), 349–358.

Taylor, S. G., IV. (1987). Integration of chemotherapy into the combined modality therapy of head and neck squamous cancer. *International Journal of Radiation Oncology, Biology, and Physics, 13*(5), 779–783.

Thawley, S. E., Panje, W. R., Batsakis, J. G., & Lindberg, R. D. (Eds.). (1999). *Comprehensive management of head and neck tumors* (2nd ed.). Philadelphia, PA: W. B. Saunders.

Van Abel, & Moore, E. J. (2012). The rise of transoral robotic surgery in the head and neck: Emerging applications. *Expert Review of Anticancer Therapy, 12*(3) 373–380.

Wang, C. C. (Ed.). (1997). *Radiation therapy for head and neck neoplasms* (3rd ed.). New York, NY: Wiley-Liss.

Webster, P., & Duguay, M. (1990). Surgeons reported attitudes and practices regarding alaryngeal speech. *Annals of Otology, Rhinology, and Laryngology, 99*(3, Pt. 1), 1727–1736.

Zeitels, S., & Burns, J. A. (2006). Laser applications in laryngology: Past, present, and future. *Otolaryngologic Clinics of North America, 39*(1), 159–172.

Zemlin, W. R. (1998). *Speech and hearing science* (4th ed.). Boston, MA: Allyn & Bacon.

Appendix 9–1

Voicing Practice Exercises:
Handout for the Laryngectomized Patient

Regardless of which method of voice restoration is chosen by the patient and voice pathologist, there are a few basic exercises that can be performed immediately after the surgery.

The following sounds are unvoiced consonants: /p, t, k, ch, f, sh, th, and s/. These are sounds that people make without using their voice. The louder and clearer you can produce these sounds the better others will be able to understand what is being said by you. The following exercises are designed to get your lips, teeth, tongue, and jaw moving. All of these structures should be able to move as well as they did before your surgery. The next few steps will help prepare your articulators for whichever of the new voice methods work best you.

Single Sound Drills

Say the following sounds slowly and carefully, as though they were being overemphasized. It is important to hear each sound. Rate of production can be increased only when the sounds are produced accurately. It may be a good idea to practice the sounds in front of a mirror. This will help you to monitor the production of each sound and understand the importance of overemphasizing each sound. Say each of the following sounds from the beginning to the end of the line.

1. /p p p/ /p p p/ /p p p/ /p p p/
2. /t t t/ /t t t/ /t t t/ /t t t/
3. /k k k/ /k k k/ /k k k/ /k k k/
4. /ch ch ch/ /ch ch ch/ /ch ch ch/ /ch ch ch/
5. /f f f/ /f f f/ /f f f/ /f f f/ /f f f/
6. /sh sh sh/ /sh sh sh/ /sh sh sh/ /sh sh sh/
7. /th th th/ /th th th/ /th th th/ /th th th/
8. /s s s/ /s s s/ /s s s/ /s s s/

Mixed Sound Drills

Practice each group of sounds. Be sure to overemphasize each sound so that each sound can be distinctly heard. Increase the rate as production of each sound becomes easier.

/p, t, k/	/p, t, k/	/p, t, k/	/p, t, k/
/t, ch, f/	/t, ch, f/	/t, ch, f/	/t, ch, f/
/sh, p, f/	/sh, p, f/	/sh, p, f/	/sh, p, f/
/t, s, ch/	/t, s, ch/	/t, s, ch/	/t, s, ch/
/k, th, p/	/k, th, p/	/k, th, p/	/k, th, p/
/th, s, p/	/th, s, p/	/th, s, p/	/th, s, p/

Word Drills

Just like the single sound drill, practice these words slowly and carefully, and overemphasize them. Be sure that others can clearly hear the beginning and ending of each word.

P		
PAT	POT	PAP
PICK	PITCH	PUP
PART	PUSH	PEP
PIT	POP	PUFF

K		
CUP	CASH	KEEP
CAP	CORK	CAT
CAB	CAKE	CUT
COKE	COOP	KIT

F		
FEET	FAT	FUDGE
FUSS	FAD	FAKE
FIT	FAST	FISH
FORK	FORT	FIFTH

T		
TOP	TOCK	TOUCH
TIP	TOT	TAP
TAKE	TROT	TAPE
TICK	TOOT	TEACH

S		
SOAP	SICK	SOUP
SIT	SAP	SIP
SOCK	SAUCE	STOP
START	STOCK	STAFF

TH		
THICK	FOURTH	THOUGHT
THINK	THANK	THROUGHOUT
PATH	THROAT	THREW

SH		
SHIP	SHAPE	SHOT
SHOOT	SHEIK	SHOCK
SHOWS	SHREK	SHAKE

CH		
CHAT	CHALK	CHEAT
CHIP	CHAMP	CHECK
CHOP	CHEW	CHURCH

Chapter 10

Vocal Performance

The extreme anatomic, physiologic, and vocal demands of professional voice users challenges our research and clinical skills, leading to new questions about assessment and the development of unique techniques to aid their rehabilitation.

Professional voice users span a broad range of vocal sophistication and their livelihood relies heavily on producing exceptional vocal quality and sustaining vocal endurance. The vocal needs of all types of performing artists are frequently comparable to Olympic athletes (Sataloff, 1998).

After reading this chapter, you will:

- Understand the uniqueness of professional voice; its assessment and care

The Singing Voice

Categories/Levels of Vocal Performance

Amateur singers. Amateur singers typically have no formal training and sing primarily for enjoyment.

Community choral singer and theater performer. Community choral singers are found in church or community-based choral ensembles. These singers are typically untrained or have a limited amount of vocal training and enjoy singing for community/social interaction. Community theater performers are community-based programs that organize and perform musical theater and traditional theater. Some performers have formal training yet most have little to none.

Semiprofessionals. Semiprofessional singers are typically trained vocalists, and perform occasionally for monetary compensation.

Music educators. Music educators are a professional group of singers by occupation. Their job encompasses both the singing and the speaking voice.

Professional singers. Professional singers perform vocally for their primary occupation (Bunch & Chapman, 2000).

From an artistic standpoint, singing is the act of using the human voice as a musical instrument, creating melodies combined with artistry and emotion. In singing, the instrument, in this case, is the whole person. That is why singing is such a human and moving activity, both for those who perform the music and for those who listen to it. From a physiologic standpoint the production of song requires physical work. Laryngeal configuration must be manipulated to meet the demands of the singing task. These demands include producing rapid changes in frequency, intensity, and sound duration, which are ultimately controlled through an interaction of respiratory volumetric and pressure adjustments (Watson, & Hixon, 1985, 1991).

The Voice Care Team

Professional voice care necessitates a clinical skill set that combines artistic abilities and scientific inquiry. Therefore, a team approach to the care of the voice is highly recommended. Otolaryngologists, voice pathologists, music educators, vocal coaches, and voice scientists represent the type of professionals interested in assessing, caring and treating the professional voice. Ancillary clinical team members can also include directors, stage managers, producers, agents/managers, and so forth. Although the latter individuals may not take part in the direct clinical management of the professional voice user, their cooperation is critical for the successful rehabilitation process. In some cases the voice care team may prescribe a modified performance schedule, change in tour schedule, change in amplification, change in costume (due to physical constraints), and so forth. With the cooperation of these ancillary team members, therapeutic regimens can be met with less resistance, and in most cases a faster recovery time will result for the vocal performer.

Performer Classifications

Vocal Performer

"Vocal performer" is a label used to classify a large number of individuals who earn a living using their voices. However, each type of performer uses their voice in a different manner. The country/pop singer may use a breathy or "rough" type of voice quality, whereas an opera or classically trained singer strives for a very specific balance of clarity and tone. Musical theater performers typically sing during a highly exhausting choreographed production with a "chest" or belting style and actors may strictly use their voices for projected dialogue. Many performers have attributes that make them exciting and electric on stage (high levels of habitual energy, ability to communicate a large range of strong emotions, high degree of sensitivity, awareness, and concentration). These attributes also make them susceptible to voice difficulties (Raphael, 1998).

The relationship between type and style of vocal use or vocal performance (choral, opera, country, rock, theater), on laryngeal function and degree of vocal effort has been examined in the literature. These studies have documented the relationship between degree of vocal use and the severity of the resulting pathology (Kitch & Oats, 1994; Sataloff, 1987). It appears that the degree of "incapacity" experienced by each performer varies with the vocal occupational demands and severity of the voice disorder. This "incapacity" can affect the performer's ability to efficiently function in daily activities. As indicated previously, dysphonia is a disruption in vocal fold vibration that results in a voice quality that is perceived as abnormal (see Chapter 5). Dysphonia, then, can interfere with and detract from the performance.

It is widely agreed that dysphonia in professional voice users can have a devastating effect on vocal performance (Sataloff, 1998).

It may also create occupational, emotional, and morale problems. Poor vocal performance, caused by dysphonia, has the potential to hinder an entire show because the performer's vocal stamina may be limited or inefficient. As a result it becomes necessary for other members of the performance group to work more hours, cover for the "weak" cast member, or in the worst case scenario, cancel scheduled performances (Sataloff, 1985, 1998) (Figure 10–1).

High-Risk Performers

"High-risk" performer is a term we use to describe performers who work in major theme parks or similar venues (Hoffman-Ruddy, Lehman, Crandell, Ingram, & Sapienza, 2001). The style of performance is typically musical theater. It is not uncommon for these individuals to complete five to seven shows per day in a five-day work week; in a working environment not optimum for producing healthy voice. In addition to their vocal performance demand, other contributing environmental variables they encounter include physical interference with costumes, poor stage acoustics, and improper amplification, ranging from inferior microphone placement to no amplification at all (Hoffman-Ruddy et al., 2001) (Figures 10–2 and 10–3). These constraints can also be a challenge for performers in touring companies and bands placing them "at risk" for vocal injury. Common complaints from high-risk performers are breathlessness, decreased vocal output, and a change in voice quality characterized primarily by loss of vocal range and difficulty sustaining song duration.

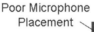

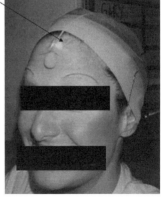

Figure 10–2. Depiction of poor microphone placement due to costume constraints.

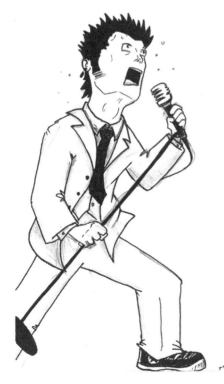

Figure 10–1. Weekend warrior seeking the American Idol dream.

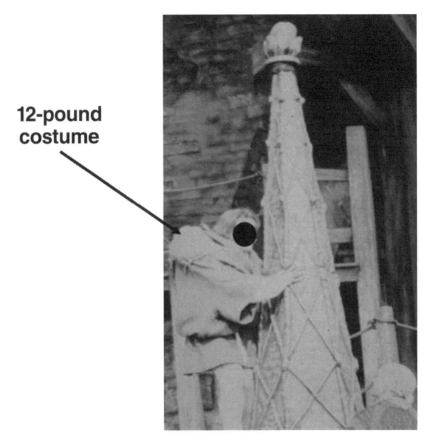

12-pound costume

Figure 10–3. Depiction of a costume constraint characterized by a heavy physical load on the back.

The types of voice disorders that "high-risk"/"at-risk" performers present with typically include vocal fold nodules, vocal fold polyps, edema, and hemorrhagic conditions. These Performers are typically unprepared for the type of vocal and environmental demands placed on them, regardless of the type of training they have participated in.

Vocal Percussionists

Vocal percussionists are another unique "high-risk" group of performers. Their performance requires sound to be produced from both the larynx and/or the supraglottic articulators.

A substantial amount of subglottal or intraoral air pressure is required to produce the glottal stops, oral fricatives or laryngeal fricatives that create the percussion-like sounds and other instrumental effects. The problems that vocal percussionist have, as a result of the performance type, include dysphonia, vocal fatigue, globus sensation, dyspnea, difficulty maintaining a work schedule, and lack of endurance. The voice pathologist must present treatment options and strategies that can be used to prevent vocal fold injury while maintaining or enhancing their performances. These options may have to go beyond traditional vocal hygiene counseling and behavioral therapies.

Etiology of Dysphonia in Vocal Performers

Causes of dysphonia in vocal performers can include physical overcompensation of the voice/speech production mechanism as a result of infection and irritation to the larynx, excessive muscle tension typically localized to the larynx, engaging in phonotraumatic behaviors such as yelling, screaming, or talking too loud, inadequate vocal training, singing in an unnatural pitch or tense, poor amplification, poor environmental conditions, and emotional reaction stemming from the stresses of one's daily lifestyle (Sataloff, 1985, 1998). All of these causes can create an "imbalance" of the respiratory, laryngeal, and supralaryngeal systems (power supply, voice source, and filter) and create an unnatural voice quality (Stemple, 1984).

Compensatory/Cover Techniques Used by Vocal Performers

Compensatory behavior during song production can manifest in several ways. For example, a common laryngeal response when singing forcefully is activation of the extrinsic laryngeal muscles (see Chapter 2). This extrinsic compensatory strategy results in an intrinsic overpressure of the ventricular folds impeding vocal fold movement (Sataloff, 1988). As a result, vocal fold vibration is limited, and the perception of "work" involved in producing sound is far greater. This can even be visualized as tension and constriction in neck, face, shoulders, and other areas of the body. This form of habitual behavior may result in vocal fatigue and often diminishes vocal quality. Singing or speaking in an inappropriate range is another compensatory behavior.

Researchers such as Hollien (1974), Moore (1975), Miller (1986), Sundberg (1987), Hixon (1987), Aronson (1990), Titze (1994), Hirano and Bless (1993), and many others have spent the past 3 to 4 decades using objective measures to define the distinctions between the speaking and singing voice, the registers of the singing voice, the effects of vocal intensity changes on the singing voice, and the effect of age-related anatomic changes on the singing voice. One distinguishing finding from the above-mentioned studies is how a change in one's respiratory cycle can affect acoustic features of voice and can change the configuration of the laryngeal structure.

Singers and "Support"

"Support" is a respiratory term that is commonly used by many disciplines that work with singers (see Chapter 1). Although each discipline has slightly different definitions for the word, all recognize that the respiratory system is integral in the production of a healthy and efficient voice production (Sataloff, 1988). The combination of thoracic, rib cage, and abdominal muscle function provide the physiologic support for any activity that requires high vocal demand (i.e., singing, acting, public speaking) (Sataloff, 1987). Although the exact modes and methods of training programs are not typically explained in much detail, particularly in the vocal coaching/vocal pedagogy literature, it is accepted that proper training of the thoracic and abdominal mechanism is essential for adequate vocal quality and maintenance of the singing voice. A keen understanding of respiratory system anatomy is fundamental for understanding respiratory physiology associated with speech and song (Hixon, 1987). Deficiencies in vocal technique or anatomy (due to diseases undermining the effectiveness of the respiratory system) often result not only in unacceptable vocal quality and projection, but also in phonotraumatic compensatory behavior and possible laryngeal injury (Carroll, Sataloff, Heuer, Spiegel, Randionoff, & Cohn, 1996).

Empirical evidence of inadequate laryngeal function in singers relates to anteroposterior laryngeal press (Shipp & Izdebski, 1975; Sundberg & Askenfelt, 1981). A high laryngeal position during singing may be related to excessive tension in both extrinsic and intrinsic laryngeal muscle groups and it may be related to a disturbance in intrinsic laryngeal muscle function. Sundberg and Askenfelt (1981) suggest "the muscles used for raising the larynx also may affect the way in which the vocal folds vibrate" (p. 24). Shipp (1977) addressed this same relationship and reported that an increase in vocal fold stiffening results from the upward stretch of vocal fold tissues created by laryngeal height elevation. It is not unusual for singers with this particular pattern of compensation to report sensations of pain and soreness in the neck just lateral to the larynx (Colton & Casper, 1996). These singers typically report that their voice quality deteriorates throughout the day, characterized by breathy and hoarse phonation with a significant loss of vocal range and vocal intensity.

Clinical Assessment of Vocal Performers

A comprehensive voice assessment generally includes most, if not all, of the following components: a thorough medical history, behavioral/social history, laryngostroboscopic assessment of the larynx using both the rigid and flexible scope with sustained vowel, speaking and singing tasks, objective voice measures, and auditory/visual perceptual assessment of the speaking and singing voice. There are several ways to enhance each of these components to effectively evaluate singers and other types of performers (Sandage & Emerich, 2002).

The Medical, Social, and Singing History

Compared to the nonsinger who experiences dysphonia, the singer often requires additional detail to be gathered during the interview process (Sataloff, 2006). The Singer's Voice Handicap Index (SVHI) is a recommended tool to help the clinician understand the performer's perception of their singing difficulties (Cohen et al., 2007). Additionally, detailed information about the singer's performance or rehearsal environment should be gathered. Also, information should be gathered about use of amplification (i.e., whether or not it exists or is used), the sound levels required of the song production, presence and type of sound monitors, types of costumes worn, and stage and back stage/green room setting, which may be full of dust and/or mold. Additional history of any singing training, singing style(s), performance schedule, and warm-up/cool-down practice should be discussed with the performer.

> Dust and molds can cause allergic reactions affecting vocal fold health.

Speaking Voice Assessment

The speaking voice assessment is a critical element of the complete evaluation process. And, while many singers are very careful about their technique, the placement of their tone, and breath management this is not always the case with the production of their speaking voice. It should not be assumed that the causative factors leading to voice difficulty in singers is due only to the singing voice production. That is why during the speaking voice assessment, the voice pathologist should evaluate the appropriate speaking pitch(es), pitch used at the end of a phrase, phrase duration, rate of speech, breath management, breath-holding maneuvers/posturing, anatomic posture, muscle tension, resonance/resonant focus, persistence of glottal fry, and features of vocal loudness (Sandage & Emerich, 2002; Sataloff, 2006).

Singing Voice Assessment

Interestingly, many singing voice disorders can be a challenge for the voice pathologist to "hear" and/or detect. However, patients may describe perceived "air" in the tone or a "sticky" feeling, particularly in the upper register or only on the highest 2 to 3 notes (Sandage & Emerich, 2002). Singers may also report fatigue and/or increased effort without associated hoarseness. They may express concerns about an unstable midrange, difficulty singing softly, loudly, loss of vocal flexibility, shortness of breath, decreased phrase duration, physical discomfort, and increased physical effort and strain. All of these symptoms should be addressed in the singing voice assessment. The voice pathologist should closely observe the extent of vocal range that can be produced with ease versus those notes that are produced with increased effort. The voice pathologist should try to document the effort that is produced during the song production, evaluating perceived strain, anatomic posture, maladaptive postures of the neck, jaw, or spine, poor phrasing, lengthy phrase duration, changes in breath management, and so forth. Conclusion of the assessment should involve the patient singing selected music that is both easy and challenging and/or part of their current performance repertoire in order to fully assess the various features of the singing voice.

See the Glossary of common singing terms at the end of this chapter.

Training and Techniques Specific to Performance Voice

The Alexander Technique

The Alexander technique is based on the discoveries of F. Matthias Alexander (1869–1955), an Australian actor and teacher. The Alexander Technique was originally developed as a method of vocal training for singers and actors in the 1890s. While Alexander was developing his method of voice training, he realized that the basis for all successful vocal education was an efficient and naturally functioning respiratory mechanism. So, in teaching voice, Alexander focused primarily on helping the breathing mechanism to function more effectively. Alexander evolved a method for learning how to consciously change maladaptive habits of coordination (i.e., posture, breathing, and tension patterns). He believed that the mind and body functioned as an integrated entity, a rather unusual realization for that time. Alexander found that habits, whether "physical" habits or "mental" habits, were all psychophysical in nature. His observations suggested that how people thought about activities determined how they coordinated themselves to do those activities, and, equally, how long-held habits of excessive tension and inefficient coordination affected how they felt and thought. In a relatively short period of time, Alexander evolved his technique from a method of vocal training into a method of breathing re-education and then into a comprehensive technique of psychophysical re-education. His technique deals with the psychophysical coordination of the whole person. See http://www.alexandertech nique.com/at.htm for complete details and history of the technique.

Feldenkrais Method

The Feldenkrais Method was developed by Moshé Feldenkrais, D.Sc. (1904–1984), who synthesized information from physics, motor development, biomechanics, psychology, and martial arts to develop an application demonstrating the lack of separation between thought, feeling, perception and action. The Feldenkrais method teaches singers to ameliorate (or improve) problems of tension, muscle strain, and illness in order to obtain optimal vocal performance. See http://www.feldenkrais.com/ for more detail on the method.

Estill Voice Training

Estill Voice Training™ and Figures for Voice™ were founded by Jo Estill in 1988. Estill was a classically trained singer who was well known for her work with a form of musical theater style singing called "belting." The Estill method is taught through a series of workshops led by certified instructors. In Estill Voice Training there are 13 vocal exercises or "Figures for Voice." Each exercise or "figure" establishes control over a specific structure of the vocal mechanism, in isolation, by moving the structure through a number of positions. For example, the figure for velum (soft palate) control involves moving the velum through raised, partially lowered and lowered positions. The 13 Figures for Voice include: True Vocal Folds: Onset/Offset Control, False Vocal Folds Control, True Vocal Folds: Body-Cover Control, Thyroid Cartilage Control, Cricoid Cartilage Control, Larynx Control, Velum Control, Tongue Control, Aryepiglottic Spincter Control, Jaw Control, Lips Control, Head and Neck Control, and Torso Control (http://www.estillvoice.com/).

Singing Health

Warm-Ups

Warm ups are hypothesized to improve vocal performance and help prevent vocal injury. Scientific data associated with the benefits of vocal warm-ups is lacking therefore, much of what we know about vocal warm-ups are primarily beliefs or accepted "truths" that have been shared among singers, singing voice specialists, voice scientists, and others. In general, it is believed that warming up the voice improves the performance of the individual muscles of the lung/thorax unit, larynx, and vocal tract as well as help coordination between the subsystems of voice production (respiration, phonation and resonance). Most vocal warm-up routines are approximately 20 minutes or less in duration, contain a variety of different exercises (some voiced, some unvoiced) to focus upon respiratory and laryngeal muscles activation and coordination. Regular use of vocal warm-ups even on days when a person is not rehearsing or performing is considered good "singing health." Samples of vocal warm-ups are provided in Figure 10–4; however, there are many different types of exercises that singers can use to build a healthy singing technique.

Cool-Downs

After rigorous singing activity "cooling down" the voice may be helpful. Similar to athletes who cool down with gentle stretches after an athletic event, singers may elect to vocalize on a gentle and softly engaged hum gliding down in a relaxed manner, much like a slow stretch of a leg muscle Use of sounds such as /la/ /na/ or /blah/ may help reduce tension in the base of tongue and other articulators. The purpose of any type of relaxation or "cool-down" exercise is to make coordination easier and in particular for the performer, to reduce the sound of strain and harshness in the voice as well as help prevent vocal injury. Another goal during the "cool down" is to allow the jaw to remain relaxed, loose, and open. Singers should begin by allowing the jaw to release in a comfortably open position, allow the tongue to remain loose and able to move freely, and keep the face relaxed by releasing their facial expression. Clinicians can instruct the singer to breathe in and allow the sound to feel like the beginning of a yawn. Allow the onset of the sound to be instantaneous and effortless. For the first exercise in Figure 10–5, after the /b/ and /l/ are articulated, the singer should allow the tongue to gently hang out over the bottom lip. Like all

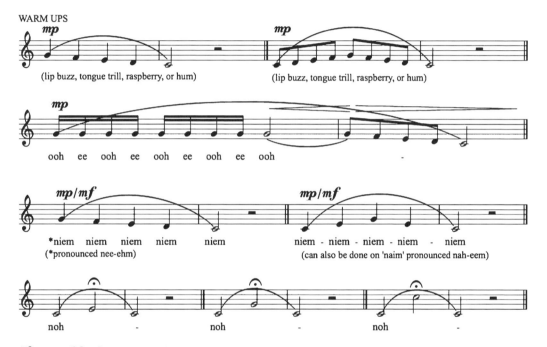

Figure 10–4. Sample of vocal warm-up exercises.

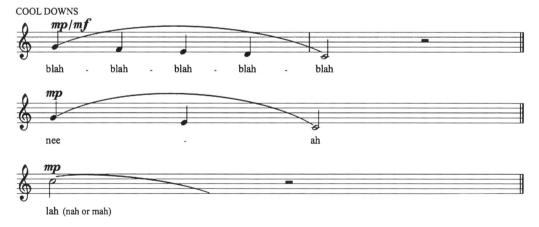

Figure 10–5. Sample of vocal cool-down exercises.

other exercises, this exercise should be done in a comfortable range with a soft voice focusing on ease of production.

Breath Coordination

Breathing exercises are used to help coordinate respiratory effort and laryngeal configuration for singing and speaking tasks. In some cases, these exercises are used to eliminate hyperfunctional or hypofunctional behaviors (i.e. a strained voice versus a breathy voice). Other strategies are implemented to improve sound duration, singing dynamics (soft voice versus loud voice) or stylistic enhancements. Singers have to extend the length of sound production more than typical voice users. Singers will typically use more variations in frequency and intensity when singing pitches that are high and low, soft and loud, and with varying emotions. Therefore, it is necessary to be able to develop and control various levels of sub glottal pressure. An example, is the singer who is performing the phrase *for the land of the free* in the "Star Spangled Banner"; most singers will attempt to perform this phrase loudly, hold the phrase longer on one breath, and sing the word *free* with a higher pitch. Coordinating subglottic air pressure is essential in order to accomplish this task. An example of breath coordination exercises are found in Figure 10–6.

Professional Associations

NATS

National Association of Teachers for Singers (NATS) is the largest professional association of teachers of singing in the world with more than 7,000 members. NATS is dedicated to encouraging the highest standards of singing through excellence in teaching and the promotion of vocal education and research. NATS provides a variety of learning experiences to its members, with workshops, intern programs, master classes, and conferences, all beginning at the chapter level and progressing to national events. NATS supports the publication of *Journal of Singing*, a scholarly journal comprised of articles, written by distinguished experts, on all aspects of singing and the teaching of singing. (http://www.nats.org/).

VASTA

The mission of the Voice and Speech Trainers Association, Inc (VASTA) "is to practice and encourage the highest standards of voice and speech use and artistry in all professional arenas; serve the needs of voice and speech teachers and students in training and practice; promote the concept that the art of the voice

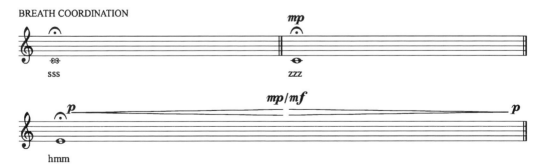

Figure 10–6. Sample of exercises to improve breath coordination during singing.

and speech specialist is integral to the successful teaching of acting and to the development of all professional voice users; and encourage and facilitate opportunities for ongoing education and the exchanging of knowledge and information among professionals in the field" (http://www.vasta.org/Organization/mission.html).

The Voice Foundation

The Voice Foundation is the world's oldest and leading organization dedicated to voice medicine, science, and education. The Voice Foundation brings together physicians, scientists, speech-language pathologists, performers, and teachers to share their knowledge and expertise in the care of the professional voice user. The Mission of The Voice Foundation is to enhance knowledge, care and training of the voice through educational programs and publications for voice care professionals, the public and professional voice users, and through supporting and funding research. The Voice Foundations supports the *Journal of Voice* which is a peer-reviewed journal for voice medicine and research. (http://www.voicefoundation.org/).

The evaluation and management of singers and various types of vocal performers is complex, requiring knowledge beyond the typical graduate level training. For voice pathologists who want to improve knowledge or specialize in this area of the field, a few suggestions for continued study include:

- Taking singing/acting voice lessons
- Exploring techniques used by singing and acting teachers, such as the Alexander technique, Feldenkrais method, Lessac method, McClosky Method, Speech Level Singing, and Estill Voice Training
- Apprenticing with a mentor Participate in the National Center

for Voice and Speech Vocology Institute
- Becoming involved with professional associations (i.e., NATS, VASTA, Voice Foundation, etc.)

As the management of the vocal performer is dynamic and includes multiple management approaches, this next section discusses medical, surgical, and behavioral management of this population through case examples of various vocal performers.

Case Studies

When reviewing the cases try to identify the causative factors, determine the intrinsic and extrinsic variables that may be related to the maintenance of the condition and determine if the therapeutic strategies employed were positive in remediating the condition. Would you change any of the procedures? Why or why not?

Case 1: Touring Performer

This case focuses on an opera singer, mezzo-soprano who is recognized worldwide. Her performance career took her to some of the world's greatest opera houses and concert halls, some of which included: the Metropolitan Opera, Vienna Staatsoper, Royal Opera—Covent Garden, San Francisco Opera, Opera Nationale de Paris, The Washington Opera, Bayerische Staatsoper, Arena di Verona, Deutsche Oper Berlin, Opernhaus Zurich, Houston Grand Opera, Dallas Opera, Teatro Coln in Buenos Aires, Los Angeles Music Center Opera, and the Festival Maggio Musicale in Florence. Her repertoire includes, at the very minimum, 20 operatic roles as well as regular performances in concert and recitals.

Course of Referral

She was referred to our clinic for a voice evaluation for symptoms of dysphonia, which occurred upon arrival to our local area. She was referred by the management/administration of the opera company.

She had been touring extensively and performing an average of three performances a week. She developed symptoms of dysphonia, especially in the upper notes of her range, following an upper respiratory infection she had a week prior to visiting our clinic. She maintained her performance schedule during this time period and was treated for upper respiratory infection symptoms with over-the-counter medication including Advil, aspirin, and decongestants on a daily basis. She experienced vigorous sneezing with this illness and some coughing. Most of these symptoms resolved just prior to her visit to our clinic.

Her past medical history was remarkable for a right vocal fold hematoma (see Chapter 5), which developed 4 months prior to presenting to our clinic. She was seen in New York, prior to the onset of her tour, by an otolaryngologist and treated with one month of voice rest and a course of prednisone for approximately six days. She was treated again with the prednisone one and a half months later to help ensure an optimal performance for an important singing engagement. The physician in New York followed her progress with a series of laryngeal examinations and the hematoma improved but did not fully resolve.

In addition to the laryngeal symptoms she claimed a history of cluster headaches, which were causing some current discomfort. These headaches had been occurring for the past two to three weeks. She also complained of symptoms associated with gastro-esophageal reflux, pain during chewing, located near the temporomandibular joint, and jaw clenching during sleep. She also related feeling general body swelling during a recent airplane flight with the swelling more notable on long international travel. She stated that 2 weeks ago she had returned to the United States from performing in London and recalled that these symptoms were even more exaggerated.

Time Line

She came to our clinic regarding symptoms of dysphonia just after completing a series of performances in neighboring cities. She was scheduled to perform opening night, the leading role in an opera, three days later. The opera was due to run one week and she was scheduled to perform every other day. In the mean time, she was scheduled for various interviews and press parties as well as daily dress rehearsals with the entire cast.

Evaluation

Perceptual Impressions. Conversational voicing during the initial interview was perceived as slightly breathy with a few observable strained/pressed voicing segments. She demonstrated a minimal amount of difficulty with loudness and pitch in the speaking voice. The singing evaluation revealed a reduction in vocal range with a loss of the top four to five notes in the upper range. She stated that her current role was a classic mezzo soprano and that she was comfortable with the range of the score to be performed.

Results of Laryngostroboscopy

- Vocal fold edge: Very slight swelling in the area of the anterior one-third and posterior two-thirds on the left true vocal fold, and a hemorrhagic polyp in the general area of the anterior one-third and the posterior two-thirds of the right vocal fold. This polypoid change was fairly wide based and appeared to be somewhat red and soft

- Glottic closure: Complete only during lower pitches. As pitch range increased, there was hourglass closure
- Phase closure: Generally, the open phase predominated
- Vertical level: Equal
- Amplitude: Slightly decreased in the left true vocal fold; slightly to moderately decreased in the right true vocal fold
- Mucosal wave: Slightly decreased in the left true vocal fold; slightly to moderately decreased in the right
- Vibratory behavior: Vibratory characteristics were observed to be slightly limited
- Phase symmetry: Mostly irregular
- Hyperfunction: Not present

Intervention

The treatment was a combination of medical/pharmacologic and behavioral management. She was immediately prescribed another trial of an anti-inflammatory for a 12-day dosage. She was also prescribed a mucosal thinner, Mucinex, because of her complaints of "thick" drainage. It was strongly suggested by the voice care team that she discontinue aspirin to avoid further development of vocal hemorrhage (see Chapter 11). Our physician reviewed her current medications including her prescriptions and over the counter drug use to ensure there were no adverse interactions. She was told to begin modified voice rest. She was concerned that she would not be able to warm up her voice and prepare for the performance. A very light vocal warm-up was advocated. She was supervised in our clinic and engaged in therapeutic vocal exercises that promoted respiratory strategies and a forward tone focus in order to decrease overcompensation in the larynx as a result of the laryngeal condition. All vocalizations were maintained at a low impact/soft engaged voice in order to decrease the collision force of the vocal folds to maximize vocal recovery. Laryngeal relaxation strategies such as lowering jaw position and tongue release strategies were covered. She was encouraged to use these strategies as part of her daily routine even when she was not experiencing vocal difficulty in order to prevent any musculoskeletal tension. In addition to the light vocal warm-up session, she was counseled on vocal health and hygiene. Emphasis was placed heavily on proactive vocal health during travel and maintaining her busy schedule. Inadequate hydration was readdressed as she was already experiencing symptoms of swelling and dehydration during airline travel. Additionally, it was recommended that during long and frequent airline flights that she wear a portable humidifier around her neck. Use of a humidifier in the hotel room was also recommended. She understood the importance of diet especially just prior to performance and during airline travel. The use of a portable amplification system when touring and speaking with large groups was highly advocated. Typically, she maintained modified vocal rest just prior to performance however, when traveling to a new city she became bombarded with interviews and reporters. These conversational interactions were quite demanding on her voice and most of the time they occurred in settings with loud background noise such as back stage parties or speaking to larger group of 15 to 20 press people. Because of the current limitations of her voice at this point, she obtained a personal amplification device immediately and wore this during the current dress rehearsals (just in case she did need to speak, even though the director and manager of the opera company agreed to let her walk through the rehearsal silently), back stage, and during press parties for the remainder of her time in our local area.

We referred her for an evaluation with a prosthodontist for the temporomandibular joint and headache symptoms. She indicated that she was instructed to wear a mouth guard when she slept. She did not currently have this mouth guard with her. General body relaxation was reviewed to help with the general body tension, headache, and fatigue symptoms.

For the next 2 days, just prior to opening night, she maintained modified voice rest and was seen in our clinic for a half-hour session of light vocal warm-ups with continuation of vocal health counseling. During our sessions she analyzed her upcoming performance for areas where she was straining or using compensatory techniques in order to reduce the laryngeal tension.

On the evening of her opening night, a representative from our clinic accompanied her back stage during warm-ups and through the duration of the performances. After the performance she wore the amplification device because there was a mandatory backstage party, which included interviews from the local press. The very next morning she was seen in the clinic again and another laryngeal examination was performed to check laryngeal status post performance. Our physician viewed her laryngeal examination. The hemorrhagic (redness) portion in the right true vocal fold was observed to have dissipated somewhat and the remainder of the vocal folds and vocal fold function showed little to no change from her previous examination. Modified voice rest was maintained. The schedule remained the same for the duration of her stay in town. Laryngeal examination followed each evening performance.

She was seen again by our clinic for another examination on the day she was scheduled to return to her hometown. The results continued to show slight improvement of the hemorrhagic polyp. It was highly recommended that she take the next two months to follow through with vocal rest and rehabilitation without any interruptions. She was scheduled to leave for a month-long international tour; however, she understood the importance and the impact of this condition to her career so she canceled the tour and returned home. The physician and voice care professionals saw her immediately in her local area. Our clinic followed up with her local voice care team on our clinical findings, medical management, and plan of care that was incorporated in this part of her tour.

Case 2: Theme Park Performer—Street Theater

This case study is a 26-year-old singer/actor street theater performer in a major theme park. Street theater is a unique setting where the performance site is outside with no covering or barrier walls. The performers sing and project dialogue with no amplification and typically perform 5 to 9 (30-minute) shows daily.

Course of Referral

The referral came from the stage manager to the theme park's first aid station, an association that was formed by the theme park to protect the performer from injuring themselves and/or refer the performer for evaluation and treatment of voice problems. The personnel at first aid placed the performer on vocal rest for one week. Following persistence of voice loss, the performer was referred for an evaluation at our practice.

This performer had a successful work history of 10 years performing in street theater within the theme park atmosphere. She had formal coaching in musical theater and her schooling included studies in musical theory, music performance, and theater training. Past medical history was unremarkable.

From the case history interview, we learned that she was unaware of the proper voicing and respiratory strategies used in performance for projecting and maintaining a "good" voice. She stated, "I have learned about 'diaphragmatic support' and placement of the head voice from my vocal coaches." Our interpretation of the patient's knowledge of voice production was that it was adequate, but not focused on the physiologic mechanisms that are necessary for developing proper breath support, that is, subglottal air pressure for her specific performance style. The performer was motivated to engage in a therapeutic process focused on remediating her current condition as well as teaching her proper mechanisms for generating vocal power and eliminating poor vocal techniques/compensations developed over the years.

Time Line

She reported a normal voice until October 2007. She experienced one incident of a vocal disturbance occurring in September 2007 where she reported screaming for approximately 10 minutes. At that point she reported "thinking" she strained her voice. Although she experienced some acute voice difficulties following this incident, she did not perceive any longstanding voice problems. She continued with her daily activities and performance following this event.

In January of 2008, she recalled a particular performance where she was not warmed up, had "no real support" during loud vocalization, and "pushed through her throat" to perform. During one of nine performances that day she stated that it "felt like a muscle was pulled in my neck." She was able to complete all nine shows but experienced a "vocal breakdown" characterized by periods of complete voice loss and excessive vocal strain.

Additionally, she was dealing with severe emotional stress from caring for a family member who was extremely ill. She stated that she had extensive periods of crying and high amounts of perceived muscle tension in her throat during these crying episodes. This situation was compounded by an unusual work schedule, which included performing 10 days without a day off.

Evaluation

Perceptual Impressions. Perceptually, her speaking voice was characterized as moderately breathy, slightly strained with frequent glottal fry ("low pitch gravel sound"). There were frequent episodes of hard glottal attacks ("punching the sounds out when talking") at the onset of voicing. Vocal loudness was perceived as excessive. Occasional voice breaks were observed during conversation that appeared to be related to the high amount of vocal strain. Extrinsic laryngeal muscle tension was determined to be moderate based on palpation of the neck muscles. She reported mild soreness with palpation of the lower neck region (hyoid and midthyroid area).

Evaluation of her singing voice revealed the highest pitch easily sung was E above middle C and the lowest was C below middle C with a 17-semitone (limited) range; pitch control during this task was fair.

Results of Laryngolaryngostroboscopy: Prior to Intervention. She was not able to tolerate the oral endoscopic exam so a topical anesthesia (Ponticaine) was sprayed in the back of the throat, enabling a complete view of the vocal folds.

- Vocal fold edge: A wide-based polyp on the left true vocal fold was identified at the junction of the anterior one-third and the posterior two-thirds of the vocal fold along with moderate vascularity. On the right true vocal fold, a moderate degree of swelling with a small soft nodular formation was observed. This formation appeared to be due to irritation from the left vocal fold pathology.

- Glottic closure: Hourglass formation
- Phase closure: Open phase predominated
- Vertical level: Vertical level was judged to be equal
- Amplitude: Vibratory amplitude was moderately decreased in both vocal folds, slightly more on the left vocal fold
- Mucosal wave: Mucosal wave was moderately decreased in both vocal folds, more on the left
- Vibratory behavior: Vibratory behavior was partially absent for the right and left, with what appeared to be greater reductions in vibration on the left side
- Phase symmetry: Phase symmetry was characterized as mostly irregular
- Hyperfunction: Hyperfunction was characterized by anteroposterior press and ventricular compression toward midline to assist with glottal closure

Intervention

A behavioral treatment approach was initiated that focused initially on modifying maladaptive behaviors associated with her performance and lifestyle. The general strategies at the onset of the behavioral program included identifying and eliminating any form of phonotrauma, initiating a modified voice rest program (no more than 2 hours of talking per day for approximately one week), and a light duty work environment, which meant her performance duties were stopped and that she worked in a job that did not require any voicing (filing). The likelihood of her going back to her performance demand and producing the same phonotraumatic behaviors was high without modifications in place and strategies to reduce phonotraumatic and strained vocal behavior in the performance.

Within the first therapy session the concept of the therapeutic voice was introduced. This was characterized by soft voice (low impact), relaxed voice production (without strain), and use of a breathy voice. The main goal of therapy was to preserve the normal mechanical properties of the vocal folds, prevent more vocal fold damage, particularly to the medial edge, as well as restore the vibratory characteristics of the damaged area.

For modifications of maladaptive behaviors and lifestyle changes some recommendations were made. These included: providing information about hydration, nutrition, sleep, and anxiety. Additionally, the external sources of stress/tension that appeared to be contributing to the voice problem were discussed with her. This included discussing performance demand, her financial reliance on her job, and her coping strategies in dealing with her ill family member, her difficulties with sleeping, and her motivation for participating in the voice therapy program. Her awareness of these factors was noted to be elevated based on her compliance with recommendations for change as well as her observed ability to learn how to monitor her phonotraumatic behaviors.

In order to relax the laryngeal musculature and reduce laryngeal height and stiffness, circumlaryngeal massage techniques were employed (Roy, Ford, & Bless, 1996). Another technique that was incorporated into this program was resonance therapy (see Chapter 7).

Results of Therapy

The performer was compliant with therapy, in that she attended all sessions. After seven weeks of voice therapy the vocal folds were re-examined with the oral endoscope and laryngolaryngostroboscopy. Review of the visual examination revealed improvement in right true vocal fold swelling including resolution of the reactive nodular formation. Slight improvements in the left vocal fold were also observed; these included a decrease in the generalized edema and vascularity with slight improvements in mucosal wave. The left true vocal fold polyp appeared to be more pronounced due to the reduction of the generalized swelling surrounding the polyp formation. The voice care team felt that the patient had exhausted behavioral management at this point in the therapeutic process. Therefore, surgical intervention was addressed with the patient. Surgery was scheduled and no complications occurred during the procedure.

Perceptual Impressions of Voice Following Surgery

Post-treatment, perceptual impressions of the performer's voice were characterized as a voice without a breathy quality, no longer any strained voice production, infrequent glottal fry, and no observed episodes of hard glottal attacks or voice breaks. The vocal loudness was adequate.

Laryngostroboscopy Following Surgery

- Vocal fold edge: Smooth bilaterally; free of laryngeal lesion and no edema present
- Glottic closure: Complete
- Phase closure: Normal
- Vertical level: Equal
- Amplitude: Normal
- Mucosal wave: Normal
- Vibratory behavior: Fully present
- Phase symmetry: Normal
- Hyperfunction: Not present

Behavioral Voice Therapy Postsurgery

Singers and actors (or any professional voice user) should be considered "vocal athletes" with the premise that working with respiratory and vocal exercise addresses the issues of strength, flexibility, and endurance as they apply to the voice. The therapy completed with this performer involved training the laryngeal muscles and avoiding misuse of the larynx. A secondary effect of this method was to train the proper mechanics of breathing in order to utilize the natural forces of the respiratory system to facilitate voice production. This provided her with the ability of producing her voice in an efficient, low-risk manner for meeting her performance and lifestyle demand. The performance schedule for this patient included a return to work on a gradual basis.

Case 3: Adolescent Singer/ Aspiring Performer

This 14-year-old performer presented to our clinic with persistent hoarseness, reported loss of vocal range, vocal loudness, pitch breaks, and long periods of complete voice loss. A typical week involved rehearsing with three different choirs and participating in her church choir weekly as a soloist. During case history interview she reported her voice was "normal and serviceable" until Wednesday or Thursday in the week, then her voice would begin to get "hoarse and breathy."

Course of Referral

This patient routinely lost her voice due to social and extracurricular school activities. Her parents, along with her school choir director, recommended a medical examination of the larynx due to chronic laryngitis. She was first seen by her primary care physician and then referred to our otolaryngology practice.

She was in overall good health. She was not taking any prescribed medications, and had no history of substance abuse. She had a history of chronic sinus infections but no known allergies. She sang with her church choir and school choral group for six years. She was involved with a vocal coach intermittently since age 11 years old and reported having an average amount of vocal training. It is relevant to comment that her family was "very active and talkative." In fact, both her mother and father have reported periods of complete loss of voice and "hoarse/breathy" voice symptoms on occasion.

Evaluation

The results of the laryngeal exam revealed a lesion (sessile polyp) along the anterior one-third of the right true vocal fold and reactive nodular formation on the left vocal fold.

Perceptual Impressions. Upon arrival to our office for a voice evaluation, the patient's vocal quality was moderately breathy with frequent voice breaks (approximately two per five-word phrase) and hard glottal attacks on back consonants (/g/, /k/).

Results of the Laryngostroboscopic Examination

- Vocal fold edge: A large polyp on the middle one-half of the right true vocal fold with reactive tissue change (possible nodular formation) on the opposite vocal fold
- Glottic closure: Hourglass, unless hyperfunctional compensatory mechanisms were employed
- Phases closure: Open phase predominated
- Vertical level: Equal
- Amplitude: Moderately limited and decreased in the right true vocal fold and judged to be slightly limited in the left true vocal fold
- Mucusal wave: Moderately limited in the right true vocal fold and judged to be slightly decreased in the left
- Vibratory behavior: Nearly absent vibratory behavior of the right vocal fold in the area of the polyp formation and slightly reduced in the left
- Phase symmetry: Always irregular
- Hyperfunction: Hyperfunction was present occasionally with the arytenoid complex moving anteriorly

Intervention

Immediately following the examination, a behavioral voice therapy program was initiated. It focused first on modifying maladaptive vocal behaviors and factors in the patient's social life, which appeared to relate to the etiology of the vocal pathology. These factors centered on her daily encounters at school. The importance of dealing with peer pressure was discussed with her as well as staying off the telephone unless urgent. We encouraged her to continue being active socially without injuring the voice and taught her strategies to use to help minimize phonotraumatic behaviors. We informed her classroom teachers about her voice use so she was not penalized for not participating orally in class discussion and projects. We believed that if these factors were not addressed the success of any further treatment would be compromised.

Treatment of the entire family unit was also essential for carryover of good vocal habits. Her parents routinely participated in our treatment sessions as did her younger siblings on occasion. The home environment was addressed with the parents in the hopes of minimizing her need to engage in phonotraumatic behaviors. The general strategies at the onset of the behavioral program included identifying and eliminating any forms of phonotrauma, initiating a modified voice rest program (no more than 1 to 2 hours of talking per day for approximately one week), use of a therapeutic voice, resonant focus, breath support/management, and laryngeal relaxation strategies as previously described in prior cases. Even though the patient was compliant with this therapeutic regimen she ultimately required surgical removal of the right true vocal fold polyp.

Surgical Procedure and Result

The patient was brought to the operating room and underwent a microlaryngoscopy with excision of the right true vocal fold polyp. The left vocal fold reactive nodular formation was left intact.

Perceptual Impressions Following Surgery. She presented back to our office for a postoperative examination and voice therapy following 4 days of complete voice rest and 3 weeks of modified voice rest (no more than two hours of talking per day) using a relaxed vocal production, good vocal hygiene, and no phonotraumatic behaviors. Her voice was still slightly breathy. This was due, in part, to the low impact voice she was using and the surgical healing process. There was no evidence of hard glottal attacks or strained-pressed voicing.

Laryngostroboscopic Results Following Surgery

- Vocal fold edge: Smooth bilaterally, free of laryngeal lesion, slight edema noted on the left true vocal fold in the area of the reactive nodular change. This edema was substantially reduced from what was observed on presurgical examinations.

- Glottic closure: Complete
- Phase closure: Normal
- Vertical level: Equal
- Amplitude: Normal
- Mucosal wave: Normal
- Vibratory behavior: Fully present
- Phase symmetry: Regular
- Hyperfunction: Not present

Behavioral Voice Therapy Following Surgery. The goals of the voice therapy program following surgery were the same as the presurgical goals. Additionally, speaking voice therapy was strongly emphasized as her singing voice was well trained given her age and vocal maturity. Therefore, more emphasis was placed on using resonance therapy teaching her how control her vocal loudness during spontaneous conversation. In addition, vocal function exercises were incorporated into her therapy regimen (Stemple, 1984). The patient was instructed on how to incorporate these strategies in a home-based therapy program throughout the week until she returned to the office for follow up therapy sessions over the next 4 to 6 weeks. A vocal "endurance/stamina" program was also implemented.

She was ultimately able to make a full return to all of her daily and extracurricular activities. She learned a great deal about vocal health and gained insight about her own vocal production. Her ability to self-monitor her own vocal production was outstanding.

Summary

Professional voice is a unique population of individuals who experience vocal difficulty. The demands of performance go beyond just vocal use and require careful assessment of many environmental variables and well as personal factors that contribute to the development and maintenance of the voice problem.

References

Aronson, A. E. (1990). *Clinical voice disorders:* An *interdisciplinary approach* (3rd ed.). New York, NY: Theime-Stratton.

Bunch, M., & Chapman, J. (2000). Taxanomy of singers used as subjects in voice research. *Journal of Voice, 14*(3), 363–369.

Carroll, L., Sataloff, R., Heuer, R., Speigel, J., Randionoff, S., & Cohn, J. (1996). Respiratory and glottal efficiency measures in normal classically trained singers. *Journal of Voice, 10*(2), 139–145.

Cohen, S. M., Jacobson, B. H., Garrett, C. G., Noordzij, J. P., Stewart, M. G., Attia, A., . . . Cleveland, T. F., (2007). Creation and validation of the Singing Voice Handicap Index. *Annals of Otolology, Rhinology, and Laryngology, 116*(6), 402–406.

Colton, R. H., & Casper, J. K. (1996). *Understanding voice problems: A physiological perspective for diagnosis and treatment.* Philadelphia, PA: Williams & Willkins.

Hirano, M., & Bless, D. (1993). *Laryngostroboscopic examination of the larynx.* San Diego, CA: Singular.

Hixon, T. J. (1987). *Respiratory function in speech and song.* Boston, MA: College-Hill Press/Little Brown and Company.

Hoffman-Ruddy, B., Lehman, J., Crandell, C., Ingram, D., & Sapienza, C. (2001). Laryngoscopic, acoustic, and environmental characteristics of high-risk vocal performers. *Journal of Voice, 15*, 543–552.

Hollien, H. (1974). On vocal registers. *Journal of Phonetics, 2*, 125–143.

Kitch, J., & Oates, J. (1994). Perceptual features of vocal fatigue as self-reported by a group of actors and singers. *Journal of Voice, 8*(3), 207–214.

Miller, R. (1986). *The structure of singing: System and art in vocal technique.* New York, NY: Schinner Books.

Moore, G. P. (1975). Ultra high speed photography in laryngeal research. *Canadian Journal of Otolaryngology, 4*, 793–799.

Raphael, B. N. (1998). Special patient history considerations relating to members of the acting profession. In R. T. Sataloff (Ed.), *Vocal health and pedagogy.* San Diego, CA: Singular.

Roy, N., Ford C. N., & Bless D. M. (1996). Muscle tension dysphonia and spasmodic dysphonia: the role of manual laryngeal tension reduction in diagnosis and management. *Annals of Otology, Rhinology and Laryngology, 105*(11), 851–856.

Sandage, M. J. & Emerich, K. (2002, July 23). Singing voice: Special considerations for evaluation and treatment. *ASHA Leader Online.*

Sataloff, R. T. (1985). Ten good ways to abuse your voice: A singers guide to a short career (part 1). *NATS Journal, 42*(1), 23–35.

Sataloff, R. T. (1987). The professional voice: Part I anatomy, function and general health. *Journal of Voice, 1*, 92–104.

Sataloff, R. T. (1988). Respiration and singing. *Journal of Voice, 2*(1), 1–2.

Sataloff, R. T. (1998). *Vocal health and pedagogy.* San Diego, CA: Singular.

Sataloff, R. T. (2006). *Vocal health and pedagogy: Advanced assessment and treatment* (2nd ed.). San Diego, CA: Plural.

Shipp, T. (1977). Vertical laryngeal position in singing. *Journal of Research in Singing, 1*(1), 16–24.

Shipp, T., & Izdebski, K. (1975). Vocal frequency and vertical larynx positioning by singers and nonsingers. *Journal of the Acoustical Society of America, 58*(5), 1104–1106.

Stemple, J. C. (1984). *Clinical voice pathology: Theory and management.* Columbus, OH: Charles E. Merrill.

Sundberg, J. (1987). *The science of singing.* Dekalb, IL: Northern Illinois University Press.

Sundberg, J., & Askenfelt, A. (1981). Larynx height and voice source. A relationship? *Speech Transmission Laboratory Quarterly Progress Status Report (KTH Stockholm), 2–3*, 23–36.

The Complete Guide to the Alexander Technique. Retrieved from http://www.alexandertechnique.com/at.htm

The Feldenkrais Method. Retrieved from http://www.feldenkrais.com/

Titze, I. R. (1994). *Principles of voice production.* Englewood Cliffs, NJ: Prentice-Hall.

VASTA. Retrieved from http://www.vasta.org/Organization/mission.html

Voice Foundation. Retrieved from http://www. voice foundation.org/

Watson, P. J., & Hixon, T. J. (1985). Respiratory kinematics in classical (opera) singers. *Journal of Speech and Hearing Research, 28*, 104–122.

Watson, P. J., & Hixon, T. J. (1991). Respiratory kinematics in classical (opera) singers. In T. J. Hixon (Ed.), *Respiratory function in speech and song.* Boston, MA: College-Hill Press.

Appendix 10–1
Glossary of Singing Terms

A cappella: Choral (one or more) singing without any instrumental accompaniment.

Alto (or also called a contralto): A low female voice.

Aria: A self-contained composition for solo voice, usually with instrumental accompaniment and occurring within the context of a larger form such as opera, oratorio.

Baritone: The male voice lying below the tenor and above the bass.

Bass: The lowest sounding male voice (lowest pitch).

Bel canto: A manner of singing that emphasizes beauty of sound, with an even tone throughout the full range of the voice; fine legato phrasing dependent on a mastery of breath control; agility in florid passage, and an apparent ease in attaining high notes.

Break: 1. In jazz, fast-moving, improvised solo, usually played without any accompaniment, that serves as an introduction to a more extended solo or that occurs between passages for the ensemble; 2. A muscle spasm causing an interruption in the normal production of sound.

Castrato: In music, a male singer who has been castrated before puberty in order to preserve the soprano or contralto range of his voice.

Coloratura (It.: "coloring"): 1. Runs, trills, and other florid decorations in vocal music. 2. A high soprano who specializes in such music.

Countertenor: A male who sings in falsetto.

Falsetto: The vocal register above its normal range; characteristically breathy and flutelike.

Fortissimo: Very loud.

Head voice: The higher register of the voice, as compared with the chest voice.

Legato: Singing smoothly with no separation between successive notes. The opposite of staccato.

Marking: When a singer chooses to sing half-voice for a rehearsal, usually because their voice is tired.

Messa di voce: A vocal exercise in which the singer initiates a note pianissimo, crescendos gradually to fortissimo, and then gradually diminuendos to pianissimo.

Mezzo forte: Moderately loud.

Ornament: Embellishments—musical flourishes that are not necessary to the overall melodic (or harmonic) line.

Parlando: Speechlike.

Patter song: A song whose text is usually humorous, sung very rapidly.

Phrasing: The realization, in performance, of the phrase structure of a work; the phrase structure itself.

Scat: Jazz singing primarily composed of syllables/vocables.

Soprano: The highest pitched general type of human voice, normally possessed only by women and boys.

Staccato: The opposite of Legato. Each note is separate from the one before and after it.

Tenor: The highest sounding range in the male singing voice.

Timbre: The characteristic quality of a sound, independent of pitch and loudness, depending on the number and relative strengths of its component frequencies, as determined by resonance.

Trill: Rapid alternation of two pitches.

Vibrato: A slight fluctuation of pitch used by performers to enrich or intensify the sound.

Vocable: A word considered as a unit of sounds or letters, without regard to meaning.

Vocalises: Vocal exercises.

Yodel: A style of singing with frequent changes between chest register and falsetto.

Chapter 11

Drug Types and Effects on Voice

This special topics chapter addresses an important area of study regarding drug treatments and their side effects. The reason this information is presented within this book is that many of the drug treatments currently prescribed to voice patients have side effects, which can affect voice treatment response. Also, many voice patients are not treated solely for their voice problem, but rather may be subject to multiple pharmaceutical therapies for treatment of coexisting conditions. Also, the terminology associated with drug administration is commonly encountered in patient medical charts and knowledge of this area is important for physician-to-clinician communication and clinician interpretation and understanding of patients' treatment response.

After reading this chapter, you will:

- Understand the definition of pharmacokinetics
- Understand the mechanisms of drug administration and drug actions
- Understand the side effects, drug interactions, nutritional considerations, and drug compliance associated with commonly prescribed medications

As advancements in research and development within pharmacology are ever changing, this special topics chapter represents the most current drug information available at the time of preparation. Additional sources are provided so that you may continue to advance your knowledge in this topic area and provide the most current information to patients with whom you work with.

Drug Interactions

Virtually all medications can cause a physiologic reaction or interaction that affects treatment response (CDER, 2001). Although some interactions are minor and not significant to patients, other interactions can exert more profound effects. Therefore, the challenge for the medical professional is to develop the most appropriate treatment plan while taking into account the numerous variables that may influence a patient's response to a drug. Some of these variables can include: mechanisms of drug interaction, disease progression, activities of daily living, and financial constraints that may alter a patient's ability to follow a regimented drug treatment plan.

Patient-Specific Factors

The patient-specific factors that may affect the outcome of pharmacological treatment include the patient's age, sex, weight, metabolic status, body response times, and use of other drugs. Therefore, within the diagnostic process it is important to gather the patient's full list of current medications, including prescribed, over-the-counter (OTC), and herbal remedies. A thorough diagnostic interview will provide other significant information including the history, disease progression, and current or past forms of treatment. With this level of understanding, voice clinicians can participate and work more efficiently in an interdisciplinary manner with the patient's physician.

Pharmacokinetics

The kidneys are primarily responsible for the processes of drug absorption, distribution, metabolism, and excretion (Pronsky, 2001). The study of these processes is referred to as *pharmacokinetics*. **Absorption** is the process by which a drug proceeds from the site of administration to systemic circulation. **Distribution** refers to the movement of the drug from one location in the body to another.

Metabolism is the process by which a drug is chemically altered by the action of enzymes, typically in the liver. How well a person responds to a particular medication is dependent on the liver's ability to process the medication. **Excretion** is the process where the drug is removed from the body.

Drug Administration

A drug can be administered by invasive or noninvasive means. Some examples of invasive administration include intramuscular (IM), where the drug is injected into the muscle and absorbed into the blood. Subcutaneous (SubQ) administration is where the drug is injected into the tissue beneath the skin. Intravenous (IV) administration is where the drug is given into a vein. This is the most expedient way to administer a drug to its desired location with the highest concentration level. With IV, the drug is directly injected into the bloodstream through the vein and has direct access to most tissues in the body. Intraventricular or intrathecal administration is where a drug is injected in the cerebrospinal fluid (Craig & Stitzel, 1986; Vogel, Carter, & Carter, 2000).

Noninvasive examples of drug administration include oral (PO) where the drug is taken by the mouth (either in tablet/capsule form or by liquid) and absorbed in the gastrointestinal (GI) tract. The drug is further broken down in the liver and then distributed to the intended tissue. Drugs administered PO includes several formulations. Controlled release tablets (SR, ER, CR) are designed to provide a long period of absorption time through the GI tract. SR: sustained release, CR: controlled release, and ER: extended release.

> Note that when a medication is delivered through means other than PO, the process of the formulation of the drug will change. The pharmaceutical companies may make a synthetic form of the drug to be delivered to the body in other forms such as through an IV.

Controlled release tablets or capsules are taken less frequently, are more convenient for patient use, and encourage higher levels of patient compliance. Multiple layer drug tablets are produced in several different compounds. A common mistake made by patients is to crush these tablets for oral intake, thereby destroying the desired drug effects. Multiple microspheres are another form of PO administration and are formulated to dissolve at different rates. Multiple microsphere capsules also should not be crushed. Clinicians working with patients who have dysphagia should caution against making recommendations for pill crushing or manipulating the oral intake without investigating the drug's delivery mechanism (Craig & Stitzel, 1986; Vogel et al., 2000).

Other noninvasive means of drug administration include topical or transdermal, where the drug is administered on the skin and then absorbed through the body. These types of drugs typically are creams, ointments, sprays, or patches and have the ability to release the drug over a controlled period of time ranging from hours to several days. Sublingual administration refers to a drug tablet being placed under the tongue. This method enables a quick absorption rate because of the increased mucosal vascularity. Buccal administration refers to the drug being placed and dissolved in the buccal (cheek) cavity and has a slower process and slower absorption rate than sublingual administration. Inhalation administration is the last noninvasive means of administration and refers to drugs that are formulated for nasal and pulmonary absorption. These include steroidal nasal sprays and bronchodilators (Craig & Stitzel, 1986; Vogel et al., 2000).

Drug Classes

Antihistamines

Many patients with voice disorders suffer from allergies, and antihistamines are one of the most common drugs used by voice patients to help with the symptoms caused by allergies.

Some antihistamines are available OTC whereas newer generation antihistamines require a prescription. The newer generation antihistamines are reported to have fewer side effects, such as drowsiness and drying of mucous membranes. Older OTC antihistamine formulations are known for their sedative effect and patients should take with caution. Antihistamines function by blocking symptoms such as runny nose, nasal congestion, watery eyes, sneezing, and prutitus (itching), (Craig & Stitzel, 1986). Since antihistamines offer only symptomatic relief, further ways to determine and control exposure to the underlying environmental allergens should be investigated.

Professional voice users should be cautioned of the potential side effects of antihistamine use, primarily the drying and/or thickening of upper respiratory tract secretions, dehydration, and sedation. Antihistamines that are combined with other drugs such as cough suppressants (codeine, or dexamethorphan) may cause further drying of secretions and sedation. However, if an antihistamine is combined with a mucolytic agent such as Guaifenesin, the drying of the mucosal secretions is minimized. And, while codeine has always been touted as the "gold-standard" in pharmacologic treatment for cough suppression, recent studies demonstrate that codeine has little to no effect on cough production (Bolser & Davenport, 2001).

Those involved in the care of professional voice users should also implement behavioral management including vocal health counseling and initiation of voice hygiene therapy to minimize the side effects from antihistamine use. If the normal balance of laryngeal mucous secretions is impaired, alterations in phonation can occur. For professional voice users, this impairment can significantly impact their livelihood (Sataloff, Hawkshaw, & Rosen, 1998).

Examples of commonly prescribed antihistamines are:

OTC (over-the-counter)

- Chlor-Trimenton (Chlorpheniramine)
- Allegra (Fexofenadine)
- Zyrtec (Certirizine)

- Claritin (Loratidine)
- Benadryl (Diphenhydramine)

Prescription Only

- Clarinex (Desloratadine)
- Xyzal (Levocetirizine)
- Atarax (Hydroxyzine)
- Astelin (Azelastine)
- Optivar (Azelastine)

Mucolytic Agents

While there is no medication that is an appropriate substitute for adequate hydration, the best mucolytic agent available is water. Mucolytics and or expectorants are helpful in counteracting the dehydration or "drying out" effects of antihistamines. Adequate respiratory and laryngeal lubrication is essential for normal vocal fold function. Respiratory secretions are directly related to the availability of water in the body. Proper hydration decreases the viscosity of mucous secretions.

Dehydration may occur as the result of athletics, environment, altitude and interference from metabolic and pharmacologic agents. The most common manufactured mucolytic agents include:

- Mucinex (guaifenesin)
- Guaifenesin

Almost all of the OTC cough suppressants are a combination of guaifenesin and dextromethorphan. For example:

- Mucinex DM
- Robitussin DM
- Tussin DM
- Dimetapp
- Vicks
- Delsym

Dextromethorphan is indicated for the temporary relief of cough caused by minor throat and bronchial irritation.

Products that contain guaifenesin such as Robitussin, Entex, and Mucinexwork to thin and enhance mucosal secretions by increasing respiratory tract fluid, and reducing the viscosity of the secretions.

Corticosteroids

Glucocorticoids are the most common class of corticosteroids used to manage acute inflammation. They are used in various dosage forms such as an oral tablet, respiratory inhaler, and injectable. Their precise mechanism of action is largely unknown, but they are thought to inhibit the inflammatory response by preventing the synthesis or action of inflammatory mediators (Burham & Short, 1997; Craig & Stitzel, 1986).

> The adrenal glands are complex endocrine glands situated near the kidney.

Oral glucocorticoids are usually administered in the form of a tapered dosing interval to avoid adrenal insufficiency. Signs of adrenal insufficiency include fatigue, anorexia, nausea, vomiting, diarrhea, and weakness (Burham & Short, 1997; Craig & Stitzel, 1986). Because of their anti-inflammatory effect, glucocorticoids are commonly used in asthmatic patients and are also effective in reducing inflammation associated with laryngitis (Sataloff, Hawkshaw, & Rosen, 1998). Corticosteroids are effective for short-term use with singers and other professional voice users who experience changes in voice quality due to vocal fold edema. Although this can be an expedited and effective treatment approach, overuse of corticosteroids must be avoided

(Sataloff et al., 1998). Corticosteroid therapy should not replace education about phono-traumatic behaviors that may bring harm to the vocal folds. Furthermore, vocal health and hygienic voice therapy programs need to be advocated by the clinician in conjunction with corticosteroid therapy to maximize voice quality improvements. Corticosteroids should be prescribed only after immune response is regulated (Burham & Short, 1997; Craig & Stitzel, 1986; Sataloff et al., 1998).

Side effects from long-term use of glucocorticoids may include gastritis, hypertension, hyperglycemia, muscle wasting, and fat redistribution (Burham & Short, 1997; Craig & Stitzel, 1986).

> Hyperglycemia is a condition in which the blood sugar is higher than normal.

Long-term inhaled steroid use may also cause patients to experience excessive laryngeal drying due to direct exposure of a variety of propellants in the steroid formulation. Other side effects include gastric irritation, fluid imbalance, electrolyte disturbances, muscle weakness, ulceration, hemorrhage, insomnia, mild mucosal drying, blurred vision, mood changes, and irritability. These effects typically do not occur after short-term use. A side effect seen in many asthmatics, which is not directly related to the use of corticosteroids, is hoarseness. Throat irritation, and coughing due to the topical release of small drug particles may lead to localized irritation (Burham & Short, 1997; Craig & Stitzel, 1986; Sataloff et al., 1998; Vogel et al., 2000).

Many asthma patients may also use bronchodilators such as Proventil, cromolyn sodium, and epinephrine, which are available as metered-dose inhalers (MDIs). Patients may also be prescribed oral forms of bronchodilators (theophylline and other xanthine derivatives). In general, each of these medications promotes the relaxation of the bronchial smooth muscle. Bronchodilators are also used to treat professional voice users. See discussion of normal pulmonary function for voice production in Chapter 1. Impairment of pulmonary function can cause serious problems for professional voice use.

Antihypertensive Agents

Antihypertensive drugs encompass a broad range of medications that are used to control hypertension. They include diuretics, ACE inhibitors, beta-blockers, calcium channel blockers, alpha-2 agonists, and angiotension receptor blockers.

Diuretics mainly work by decreasing the body's plasma volume and thereby decreasing systemic blood pressure (Burham & Short, 1997; Craig & Stitzel, 1986). Dehydration is a common side effect when using medications containing diuretics. Dehydration leads to decreased laryngeal lubrication, increased mucosal drying, and chronic laryngeal edema.

The alpha-2 agonists, like methyldopa and clonidine, work by blocking neurotransmitter release and result in less sympathetic stimulation (Burham & Short, 1997; Craig & Stitzel, 1986). Consequently, there is a decrease in heart rate and blood pressure. The side effects with these drugs include anticholinergic effects (blocking of the neurotransmitter acetylcholine). In most cases, patients may notice drying of the mucosal membranes within the upper respiratory tract.

Beta-blockers mainly block the beta-andrenergic receptors in the heart. This produces a reduction in heart rate and cardiac output and causes a reduction in blood pressure. Professional voice users take advantage of these cardiac effects to reduce performance anxiety. However, some vocalists complain of "lackluster" performances with the use of drugs like propanolol (Sataloff et al., 1998). Beta-blockers should be taken under medical supervision. Most beta-blockers must be tapered down to avoid potential problems. For example, taking a patient off beta-blockers abruptly may lead to an overstimulation of beta-receptors, which were previously blocked by the drug.

Calcium channel blockers work by blocking the calcium ion movement into the smooth muscle, causing a relaxation of vascular smooth muscle, and reducing blood pressure. Some calcium channel blockers that have been approved for use in the United States include nisoldipine (Sular), nifedipine (Adalat, Procardia), nicardipine (Cardene), bepridil (Vascor), isradipine (Dynacirc), nimodipine (Nimotop), felodipine (Plendil), amlodipine (Norvasc), diltiazem (Cardizem), and verapamil (Calan, Isoptin). These also must be tapered when discontinued, to avoid reoccurrence of symptoms (Burham & Short, 1997; Craig & Stitzel, 1986).

A very bothersome side effect of ACE inhibitors is a dry productive cough. This can lead in many cases, to a discontinuation of the drug treatment.

Examples of antihypertensive agents are:

- Diovan (Hydrochlorothiazide)
- Avapro (Irbesartan)
- Lotensin (Benazepril Hydrocholoride)
- Lopressor (Hydrocholorthiazide)
- Toprol-XL (Metoprolol)
- Hyzaar (Hydrocholorothiazide and losartan)

Antibiotics

An antibiotic is a chemical substance that has the capacity to inhibit the growth of (bacteriastatic) or to kill (bacteriacidal), other microorganisms. Antibiotics work in various ways depending on the class of antibiotic (i.e., penicillins, macrolides, and fluoroquinolones). They cause a bacteriacidal or bacteriastatic action against the bacterial organism via inhibition of basic cellular function in the infecting bacterium (Burham & Short, 1997; Craig & Stitzel, 1986). Antibiotics may be recommended in dosages large enough to achieve therapeutic blood levels rapidly. Compliance is a significant problem with patients especially with antibiotic therapy. The most important rule about antibiotics is that the patient must complete the therapy. If the course is not completed, it may have to be repeated due to an infection reoccurrence.

> Patient compliance is hard to measure and track. Improving patient compliance may include finding simple dosing schedules, refill reminders, reward systems, and frequent contact by the clinician.

Examples of antibiotics are:

- Amoxicillin (Penicillin)
- Azithromycin/Zithromax (Macrolide)
- Biaxin (Claritthromycin)
- Kefllex (Cephalexin)
- Doryx (Tetracycline)
- Avelox, levaquin, cipro (quinalone)

Antivirals

Antivirals work by preventing the release of infectious viral nucleic acid into the host cell or by inhibiting viral DNA/RNA replication (Burham & Short, 1997; Craig & Stitzel, 1986). Acyclovir is one of the most common antivirals used for cases of recurrent laryngeal nerve paresis or paralysis. Amantadine is another antiviral used primarily against influenza. It can be prescribed if a patient is going to be exposed to large group of people.

Examples of antivirals are:

- Complera (Emtricitabine)
- Truvada (Emtricitabine/Tenofovir)
- Atripla (Efavirenz)
- Combivir (Lamivudine)
- Epzicom (Abacavir/Lamivudine)

Analgesics

Analgesics are drug agents used to relieve pain. Available by prescription or OTC, analgesics include aspirin, acetaminophen, and ibuprofen. All are presumed safe for short-term use. In cases of pain relief from sore throat and laryngeal irritation with voice use, care should be taken to avoid excessive use of aspirin or ibuprofen as they may cause platelet dysfunction and predispose a patient, particularly a vocal performer, to vocal fold hemorrhage. The best alternative OTC is acetaminophen. Pain relievers available by prescription include non-steroidal anti-inflammatory drugs and the newest class of drugs referred to as the COX-2 inhibitors. Even so, great caution is still advised when taking these drugs for those at risk for bleeding, especially vocal fold hemorrhage.

Although analgesics are helpful for pain relief, care should be taken not to ignore the reason for the pain. Pain is a protective physiologic function; masking it may produce further damage that may not be reversible. Narcotic pain relief should only be prescribed in extreme cases, due to its high incidence of drug dependency and sensory impairment. The side effects could lead to an impairment of vocal performance or unconscious vocal abuse.

Examples of analgesics are:

- Aspirin (salicylate)
- Choline salicylate
- Magnesium salicylate
- Ibuprofen
- Ketoprofen (Benzoylphenyl)
- Sodium salicylate

Hormones

Hormone therapy replaces hormones no longer produced by the body or alters hormonal levels in the body. Hormones potentially have larger bodily and voice-specific effects. Androgenic hormones affect the voice significantly by producing a lowering of the fundamental frequency especially in females and a coarsening of the voice (Damste, 1967, 1968; Sataloff et al., 1998). Hormonal therapy is mainly employed to treat breast cancer, endometriosis, and post-menopausal sexual dysfunction. Birth control pills also have an androgen component that is paired up with estrogen. Ideally the balance of estrogen and progesterone is such that voice changes do not occur.

Androgen: responsible for the development of male characteristics

Estrogen: responsible for the development of female characteristics

Progesterone: responsible for regulating a women's reproductive cycle

---

In the few cases where a noticeable voice change is experienced, discontinuation of the pills will restore normal vocal function (Sataloff et al., 1998). For vocal performers that are post-menopausal it is also important for them to be placed on hormone replacement therapy to avoid the typical voice changes that follow menopause.

Thyroxine replacement is also important for restoring vocal efficiency and the "ring" or resonant voice features lost as a consequence of thyroid gland deficiency or *hypothyroidism* (Sataloff et al., 1998). Compliance is important for hormone replacement therapy to be effective. A "steady-state" in blood levels should always be maintained to optimize the drug's effectiveness. These drugs should be taken at approximately the same time each day as directed by the clinician.

Examples of hormones are:

- Prempro (conjugated estrogens and medroxyprogesterone)
- Activella (Estradiol/Norethindrone)
- Premphase (conjugated estrogens/ medroxyprogesterone)
- Estratest (esterified estrogens/ methyltestosterone)
- NuvaRing (vaginal insert ring)

Gastroenterologic Medications

There are many forms of pharmacologic therapies for gastroesophageal reflux that are available by prescription and OTC. The major groups include antacids, H2-receptor antagonists, and proton-pump inhibitors. Antacids are typically a single ingredient or a combination of aluminum hydroxide, magnesium hydroxide, and/or calcium carbonate. These products can cause diarrhea, constipation, bloating, and possibly a drying effect (Burham & Short, 1997; Craig & Stitzel, 1986). Some medications may also include simethicone, which helps with bloating discomfort. Usually, finding an antacid with the right balance of each of the ingredients will eliminate most of the bothersome side effects. If these over-the-counter medications do not offer adequate relief, the next step is to move to the H2-blockers.

The H2-blockers (histamine H2-receptor antagonist) work by being a competitive inhibitor of histamine H2-receptors. The primary component of pharmacologic activity for these types of drugs is inhibition of gastric secretion. Some of these are now available OTC. Some H2-blockers have even begun to add the antacids with the H2-blockers for a more complete relief of the GI symptoms. Stronger versions of these H2-blockers are still available by prescription. These also may cause an overall drying effect, which may be bothersome to a vocal performer.

Gastric proton-pump inhibitors (H+/ K+ATPase) do not exhibit anticholinergic or histamine H2-receptor antagonist properties, but suppress gastric acid secretion by specific inhibition of the H+/K+ ATPase enzyme system at the secretory surface of the gastric parietal cell (Burham & Short, 1997; Craig & Stitzel, 1986). These generally work extremely well; however, they are not free of side effects. Some of the side effects include diarrhea, abdominal pain, nausea, depression, and some have reported dry mouth, esophageal stenosis, esophageal ulcer, esophagitis, or constipation, but the occurrence rate is less than 1% (Burham & Short, 1997; Craig & Stitzel, 1986).

GI stimulants such as metoclopramide, stimulate motility of the upper GI tract without stimulating gastric, biliary, or pancreatic secretions (Burham & Short, 1997; Craig & Stitzel, 1986). They have some potentially serious side effects such as extrapyramidal symptoms. This side effect is seen very early in therapy, within 24 to 48 hours. The only other drug in this class is Cisapride, or Propulsid. However, it is no longer available due to its cardiac side effects. Some cases of these events have been fatal.

Other GI medications include the antispasmodics/anticholinergics, such as belladonna tincture, Dicyclomine, Clindex, Levsin, and Phenerbel-S tablets. All of these agents show a high rate of dryness on sections of the vocal tract.

Examples of gastroenterologic medications are:

- Aciphex (Raberprazole Sodium)
- Aloxi (Palonosetron)
- Axid AR (Nizatinidine)
- Canasa (Mesalamine)
- Dexilant (Dexlansoprazole)
- Dificid (Fidaxomicin)
- Nexium (Esomeprazole Magnesium)
- Prilosec (Omeprazole)

Psychoactive Medications

Antipsychotic Drugs

Antipsychotic drugs are a large group of drugs; they include antidepressants, anti-anxiolytics, anticonvulsants, mood stabilizers, and sedatives. These medications work by a variety of mechanisms and can produce many side effects. For some voice patients, antipsychotic medications may be extremely helpful. Also, with the large number of available drugs in this class, the drug therapy can be modified so it provides greater effectiveness and the least amount of side effects.

Examples of pyschoacative medications are:

- Abilify (Aripiprazole)
- Adderall (Dextroamphetamine sulfate)
- Ambien (Zolpidem)
- Geodon (Zprasidone hydrochloride)
- Haldol (Haloperidol lactate)
- Imipramine (Imipramine hydrochloride)

Antidepressants

Antidepressants are a large class of antipsychotic drugs. The older generations, which are still used, are the tricyclic antidepressants, MAO (monoamine oxidase) inhibitors. The new generation includes selective serotonin reuptake inhibitors (SSRI). Tricyclic and tetracyclic antidepressants include but are not limited to imipramine (Tofranil), amitriptyine (Elavil), doxepine (Sinequan), nortriptyline (Pamelor), and desipramine (Norpramin). Antidepressants work by inhibiting the reuptake of norepinephrine or serotinin at the presypnatic neuron (Burham & Short, 1997; Craig & Stitzel, 1986).

> Serotonin is a neurotransmitter that affects many psychological functions such as anxiety, mood, aggression, appetite, sex drive, and the sleep/wake cycle. Lack of serotonin is often associated with depression.

The side effects of these drugs include Tardive Dyskinesia, a syndrome consisting of potentially irreversible, involuntary dyskinetic movements, and anticholinergic effects such as urinary retention, constipation, dry mouth, and cardiovascular disturbances. All of these side effects may be dose related and agent specific.

MAO (monoamine oxidase) inhibitors are a class of antipsychotics that are not commonly used due to their complicated potential side effects. They are used in cases where the patient is refractory to the other classes of antidepressants.

> Refractory means the patient's symptoms are not responding to a drug treatment.

These drugs have their own side effects such as dizziness and orthostatic hypotension, but also react with many other drugs such as demoral, epinephrine, local anesthetics, and decongestants (Sataloff et al., 1998). They are also very reactive with certain foods that are rich in tyramine. These include cheese and dairy products, certain meat and fish (meat organs, meat prepared with tenderizer, and caviar), alcoholic beverages, (such as red wine, especially Chianti, beer, and ale), and certain fruits and vegetables (bananas, bean curd, avocados, and figs), (Pronsky, 2001; Sataloff et al., 1998).

These side effects can linger after discontinuation of therapy. All therapy should be tapered and new therapy with other medications should only be started after a sufficient washing out period.

The serotonin selective reuptake inhibitors (SSRIs) are the most commonly prescribed antidepressants. In most cases, they are generally prescribed as the first line of therapy. The antidepressant activity of the SSRIs is linked to their inhibition of central nervous system (CNS) neuronal uptake of serotonin. These drugs include fluoxetine (Prozac), sertraline (Zoloft), and paroxetine (Paxil). Some of their side effects include dizziness, drowsiness, dry mouth, constipation, and sexual dysfunction (Burham & Short, 1997; Craig & Stitzel, 1986; Sataloff et al., 1998).

Examples of antidepressants are:

- Lexapro (Escitalopram)
- Luvox (Fluvoxamine maleate)
- Paxil (Paraxetine hydrocholoride)
- Prozac, Prozac weekly (Fluoxetine hydrocholoride)
- Zoloft (Setraline hydrocholoride)

Anxiolytics Drugs

Anxiolytic drugs such as alprazolam (Xanax), diazepam (Valium), lorazepam (Ativan), oxazepam (Serex), clonazepam (Klonopin), chlordiazepoxide (Librium), and clorazepate (Tranxene). Their activity may involve many sites including the spinal cord causing muscle relaxation, in the brainstem having anticonvulsant properties, and limbic and cortical areas affecting emotional behavior. These activities are agent and dose specific. The side effects of these drugs include sedation, weakness, and decreased motor performance. They can be highly addictive and patients will present with withdrawal symptoms, if stopped abruptly. These drugs should not be combined with other depressants, such as alcohol, or stimulants such as cocaine and amphetamines or even OTC decongestants. These combinations can have deleterious effects.

Examples of anxiolytics drugs are:

- Antidepressants
- Antihistamines (Atarax)
- Azapirones (BuSpar)
- Benzodiazepines (Ativan, Centrax, Dalmane)
- Beta-Blockers

Anticonvulsant/Antiepileptic Drugs

Anticonvulsant drugs include a variety of agents, all possessing the ability to depress abnormal neuronal discharges in the CNS, thus inhibiting seizure activity. Some of the more common ones are phenytoin (Dilantin), carbamazepine (Tegretol), valproic acid (Depakote), and phenobarbital. All of these drugs have very serious side effects associated with them. Phenytion can cause slurred speech, mental confusion, and motor twitching. Carbamazepine side effects include adverse hematologic reactions, confusion, agitation, stomatitis, lymphadenopathy, and drowsiness. Valproic acid can also be used in the manic phase of bipolar disorder (Burham

& Short, 1997; Craig & Stitzel, 1986; Sataloff et al., 1998). Its side effects include suicidal ideation, and the more commonly seen side effects of sedation, edema of extremities, and hair loss. Phenobarbital is one of the oldest anticonvulsants on the market. It has also been used as a hypnotic. It has similar side effects as other barbiturates and sedatives. They include somnolence (sleepiness), confusion, drowsiness, and vertigo.

Mood stabilizers are used with patients that have a bipolar disorder to prevent manic and depressive recurrences. The main drug used is lithium carbonate. Its mechanism of action is to alter sodium transport in nerve and muscle cells (Burham & Short, 1997; Craig & Stitzel, 1986; Sataloff et al., 1998; Vogel et al., 2000). Lithium is available in several dosage forms, so that the dosages maybe customized to each patient's symptoms and blood levels. Some of the side effects include fine hand resting tremor, polyuria (excessive passage of urine), and mild thirst. These effects are typically transient with continued usage. Some of the more common side effects are drowsiness, fatigue, and dehydration. It is extremely important for these patients to drink large amounts of water or other adequate liquid every day while on this medication.

Examples of antiepileptic/convulsant drugs are:

- Phenytoin (Dilantin)
- Carbamazepine (Tegretol)
- Clonazepam (Klonopin)
- Pregabalin (Lyrica)

Neurologic Medications

Most drugs used for neurologic disorders have a large number of side effects; some of these side effects can be quite serious. These drugs are dosed individually, customized to each patient depending on disease progression. Any neurologic disorder is in itself debilitating and many times the drugs prescribed for the disorder can have side effects that can lead to voice and speech difficulty (Sataloff et al., 1998). Some examples of these disorders include Parkinson's disease, myasthenia gravis, multiple sclerosis, amyotrophic lateral sclerosis, cerebral palsy, Wilson's disease, Essential Tremor, Epilepsy, Tourette's syndrome, and Huntington's disease. The current form of therapy for these diseases is palliative, as there is no cure available. The goal of drug therapy is to provide maximum relief from the symptoms, slow the progression of the disease, and help the patient maintain independence and mobility.

Examples of neurologic medications are:

- Baclofen (Kemstro, Lioresal, Liofen, Gablofen)
- Fingolimod (Gilenya)
- Gabapentin (Fanatrx, Gabarone, Gralise, Horizant, Neurontin)
- Lamotrigine (Lamictal)
- Rasagiline (Monoamine Oxidase)

Parkinson's disease is a progressive disease of the brain involving the degeneration of nigral cells and the destruction of the nigrostriatal pathway resulting in loss of striatal dopamine (Marsden, 1994). Dopamine facilitates the transfer of electrical messages between nerve cells that control movement. The speech and voice characteristics associated with PD include: imprecise articulation, rapid speech rate with progressive acceleration and short rushes of speech, reduced stress of syllables, reduced loudness, and a hoarse, tremulous, and monotone voice (Darley, Aronson, & Brown, 1975; Duffy, 1995) (see Chapter 6). Drugs used to treat PD are anticholinergics such as Benzatropine (Cogentin), Biperiden (Akineton), and Trihexyphenidyl (Artane). Anticholinergics are used to alleviate tremor.

Dopaminergic replacement agents include Levodopa (L-dopa), and L-dopa in combinations with other drug agents such as Carbidopa including Sinemet and Prolopa or Amantadine (Symmetrel). Dopamine agonists are used to enhance the effects of L-dopa. Some of these drugs include apomorphine, bromocriptine (Parlodel), Pergolide (Permax) ropinerole (Requip), and pramepezole (Mirapex). Catechol-O-methyltranserase (COMT) inhibitors are used to decrease the L-dopa metabolism and in turn increase L-dopa availability. These drug agents include Tolcapone (Tasmar) and Entacapone. Monoamine oxidase-B (MAO-B) inhibitors are used for relief of symptoms and to slow the progression of PD by prolonging the availability of dopamine released into the synapse. MAO-B inhibitor drug agents include Selegiline, and Deprenyl (Eldepryl).

Anticholinergics produce a large number of side effects including blurred vision, dryness, drowsiness, confusion, memory loss, gastrointestinal disturbance, muscle cramps, skin rash, nervousness, and hallucinations. Other side effects are gastrointestinal disturbance oral dryness, orthostatic hypotension, syncope (partial or complete loss of consciousness), cardiac arrthymias, depression, confusion, dyskinesias, and psychosis (Burham & Short, 1997; Craig & Stitzel, 1986; Vogel et al., 2000). Dopamine agonist side effects include nausea, dizziness, dyskinesias, somnolence (sleepiness), and orthostatic hypotension. COMT inhibitor side effects include increased dyskineasias, nausea, and GI disturbance. MAO-B inhibitor side effects included sleep disturbance, increased dyskinesias, increased nausea when added to Sinemet, and increased liver enzymes (Burham & Short, 1997; Craig & Stitzel, 1986; Vogel et al., 2000).

As discussed in Chapter 6, myasthenia gravis is an autoimmune disease that affects the neuromuscular junction by producing antibodies that impair transmission of nerve impulses to muscle. The neurotransmitter involved in myasthenia gravis is acetylcholine (Duffy, 1995; Freed, 2000; Vogel et al., 2000). Drugs used to treat myasthenia gravis include acetlycholinestrase inhibitors (in the CNS) including pyridostigmine (Mestinon). This drug works to increase levels of acetylcholine that facilitates stimulation of movement and muscular activity. Some of the side effects of acetycholinestrase include excessive salivation, GI disturbances, and confusion. Corticosteriods are also used to treat myasthenia gravis. Side effects caused by corticosteriods were described earlier.

Multiple sclerosis (MS) is characterized as a progressive disease where there is a degeneration of myelin covering the axons (Duffy, 1995; Freed, 2000; Vogel et al., 2000). Patients with MS produce voice and speech characteristics consistent with mixed dysarthria (flaccid, spastic, and ataxic dysarthria), (see Chapter 6). Pharmacologic therapy for MS is directed at the underlying cause of the disease or directed at the symptoms from the disease progression. Corticosteroids along with other immunosuppresants such as azothioprine and cyclophosphamide are often used. Beta-interferon, is also used to slow the progression of the physical disability and prevention of exacerbations. Beta-interferon is administered by subcutaneous injection every other day so side effects include injection site reactions such as redness, swelling and irritation. Other side effects may include flulike symptoms, a worsening of symptoms, and/or depression (Burham & Short, 1997; Craig & Stitzel, 1986; Vogel et al., 2000).

Drug Compliance

As mentioned earlier, compliance refers to a patient's ability to follow through with a prescribed regimen of treatment. Compliance is a major factor of medication failures. Noncompliance is most frequently seen in the geriatric population and is due to factors such as financial limitations, multiple drug therapies, and issues associated with normal aging (i.e., confusion, memory loss, etc.). Compliance also directly relates to the patient's individual motivation. For example a patient is not feeling well so they begin pharmacologic treatment. As the patient begins to recover, a sharp decline is typically seen in compliance because the patient perceives that he no longer needs to take the prescribed medication. This choice not only affects his health status, but also is more costly because the drug therapy typically will need to be repeated. For those on a fixed income status this can bare serious consequences.

In general, patients taking multiple doses of a medication in a 24-hour period (i.e., taking a medication four times a day versus one time per day) have been shown to be less compliant. This is due to the increased frequency of dosing. Patients may either forget to take medication or try to cut back on the frequency (self directed) so that the medication will last longer and create less of a financial burden. This is frequently seen in the geriatric population as a way to contain cost. In some instances, patients may be over compliant by taking medication too frequently or overmedicating. Clinicians should counsel patients on various strategies to help minimize noncompliance. For example, pill organizers or beepers can be obtained and/or spouse or personal care providers can help monitor the drug regimen. Primary care physicians or pharmacists can help by continuing to monitor all drug therapies including prescription, OTC, and dietary supplements on a regular basis, or more frequently as health status changes.

Effects of Nutrients on Absorption of Drugs

Many foods and nutrients have the potential to interfere with pharmacotherapeutic goals. Nutrition and diet affect how a drug is absorbed, metabolized or excreted. For example, protein deficiency may lead to impaired drug metabolism. This is illustrated by an increase in sleeping time produced by barbiturates. Fat-free diets or diets that lack essential fatty acids also impair drug metabolism. The rates of drug metabolism can also be impaired by vitamin A, riboflavin, ascorbic acid (in citrus fruits, tomatoes, potatoes, and leafy green vegetables), and vitamin E deficiency states. Iron deficiency, however, has not been shown to have any effect on drug metabolism even in severe cases.

Use of alcohol affects drug therapy differently depending on the amount and type of alcohol consumed by the patient (Burham & Short, 1997; Craig & Stitzel, 1986; Pronsky, 2001). Wine can elevate the anticoagulant effect of drugs such as Coumadin. Conversely, some vegetables with high vitamin K will lower the anticoagulant effect.

The presence of certain nutrients in the GI tract affects the bioavailability and disposition of many oral medications (Pronsky, 2001). Drug-nutrient interactions can also have positive effects that result in increased drug absorption or reduced GI irritation. Knowing the significant drug-nutrient interactions can help identify which ones to avoid with certain medications, as well as the therapeutic agents that should be administered with food. For example, taking antibiotics with food may delay or prevent absorption whereas dairy products are associated with overall impaired absorption with PO drug administration (Pronsky, 2001; Sataloff et al., 1998; Vogel et al., 2000). High protein diets are also known to be associated with interfering with the absorption of L-dopa. L-dopa is an amino acid derivative and when taken with a protein meal it must compete with other amino acids from the protein meal for transport across the GI tract lining and into the blood. This in turn decreases absorption and availability to the brain (Holden, 2001; Pronsky, 2001; Vogel et al., 2000). Patients with

PD undergoing L-dopa pharmacotherapy should be advised to have their protein meal as the last meal of the day (Holden, 2001).

Food may alter the metabolism of some drugs. Modification of medication action may be experienced when combined with foods or additives. Foods or additives may produce effects similar to the desired effect of a drug, and may potentially enhance the side effects or toxicity of the specific drug. For example, high caffeine intake may increase the adverse effects of nervousness, tremor, and insomnia. Nutrients or food ingredients may produce an antagonistic effect of medication action. For example, vitamin K aids the production of clotting factors in direct opposition to the action of Coumadin (Pronsky, 2001).

The interactions continue. Caffeine is a stimulant that counteracts the antianxiety effects of tranquilizers and grapefruit juice has been shown to have adverse reactions when mixed with particular drugs (Elbe, 2001).

Drugs may also impair salivary flow causing dry mouth, increased caries, stomatitis, and glossitis. Specific drugs may also suppress natural oral bacteria resulting in oral candidiasis; for example, tetracycline, may result in oral yeast overgrowth (candidiasis). For additional and updated information recommended reading/references are listed at the end of this chapter.

Herbal Supplements/ Alternative Medicines

Alternative therapies such as herbal products are being used with increasing numbers in the United States. Approximately 25% of Americans who consult their physician about a serious health problem are employing some form of unconventional therapy, but only 70% of these patients inform their physician of such use (Eisenberg et al., 1993). Herbal remedies are prepared from a variety of plant materials including leaves, roots, bark, stems, and flowers. They can be prepared using fresh or dried ingredients and are primarily for mild or chronic ailments (Gianni & Dreitlein, 1998). The use of herbal remedies can be problematic for several reasons. Herbal products are not tested with the scientific rigor required of conventional drugs, and they are not subject to the approval process of the U.S. Food and Drug Administration (FDA). Herbal products therefore cannot be marketed for the diagnosis, treatment, cure, or prevention of disease. Nonetheless, the Dietary Supplement Health and Education Act of 1994 allows these products to be labeled with statements explaining their effect (i.e., alleviation of fatigue) or their role in promoting general well-being (i.e., enhancement of mood or mentation) (Public Law No. 103-417, 1994). Analysis of some of the effects of herbal products shows that they sometimes closely resemble claims of clinical efficacy for various diseases or conditions. Unlike conventional drugs, herbal products are not regulated for purity and potency (Public Law No. 103-417, 1994). Thus, some of the adverse effects and drug interactions reported for herbal products could be caused by impurities (e.g., allergens, pollen, and spores) or batch-to-batch variability. In addition, the potency of an herbal product may increase the possibility of adverse effects (Cupp, 1999).

Many consumers of herbal remedies incorrectly believe that as it is a "natural" remedy it must be better for your body. Patients who use herbal therapies are recommended to consult their physician. Yet, although this is true, patients often find that their medical professionals do not have enough information available to them regarding herbal supplements. As a result, physicians are often unable to predict any interactions that herbal remedies may have when mixed with traditional medications. This can leads to misdiagnosing and/or mistreatment of a patient's medical condition. Patients who are considering or currently taking herbal supplements should be properly advised of the impact it can have on the existing medical condition. In short, a physician or other licensed medical professional specializing in alternative therapy should be advising and overseeing alternative/herbal treatment. Kush et al. (2007) and Surrow (2000) have listed common herbal qualities and actions of herbs and vitamins, some of which are included in this discussion.

Because dietary supplements are becoming increasingly popular, clinicians need to ask questions about patient use and stay up to date on trends in dietary supplement use, with the realization that for most supplements the adverse effects and potential for drug interactions are not well characterized (Cupp, 1999).

Some questions to ask patients who may be taking herbal products include:

- Are you taking an herbal product, herbal supplement, or other "natural remedy?" If so, are you taking any prescription or nonprescription medications for the same purpose as the herbal product?
- Have you used this herbal product before?
- Are you allergic to any plant products? Are you pregnant or breast-feeding? (Cupp, 1999)

Anti-inflammatories

Nickjeh (1999) and Surrow (2000) have listed common herbal qualities and actions of herbs and vitamins, some of which are included in this discussion. For further information, consult a licensed medical professional specializing in alternative therapy. Anti-inflammatories include herbs that soothe inflammation or decrease the inflammatory response of the tissue directly. Some anti-inflammatories include Echinacea, which is extracted from a purple coneflower. It works by increasing the num-

ber of immune cells and decreases inflammation, coughs, colds, sore throats, tonsillitis, and external wounds. Its use is advocated within the first 24 hours of the onset of cold symptoms. Echinacea should not be taken for more than eight weeks, as long-term effects are unknown. A patient should avoid using Echinacea if allergic to pollen or if their immune system is compromised. Goldenseal is another popular anti-inflammatory used to stimulate the immune system. This should not be taken for more than 2 weeks at a time as it may kill good bacteria in the digestive tract. Goldenseal is to be avoided if a patient has high blood pressure or is pregnant. Chamomile is an anti-inflammatory used as a soothing and relaxing effect. It relaxes the lining of the digestive tract and promotes healing of nausea, indigestion, gastritis, and colitis, and it relieves allergies and hay fever much like an antihistamine. It is also used for insomnia and drug withdrawal. Chamomile may cause an allergic reaction in those allergic to pollen. Slippery Elm is used to soothe irritated mucous membranes of the larynx and ulcers.

Antimicrobials

Antimicrobials help the body destroy disease-causing microorganisms, and help the body strengthen its own resistance to infection. Some antimicrobials include Echinacea, Goldenseal, vitamin C (no more than 1,000 mg every 2 hours), rose hips, licorice (avoid taking with high blood pressure), and garlic (limit use if taking blood-thinning medications).

Antispasmodics

Herbals are also sold as antispasmodics. Antispasmodics serve to ease cramps in smooth and skeletal muscles. Some antispasmodics include chamomile and valerian. Valerian is a natural tranquilizer and is used to relieve pain and muscle spasms. Valerian contains natural compounds that depress the nervous system and relieve anxiety. This should not be taken with alcohol or any medication that causes drowsiness. Long-term use is linked with headache, insomnia, and stomach upsets.

Astringents

Astringent reduces irritation and inflammation and creates a barrier against infection. Astringents are helpful in to heal wounds and burns. Some common astringents include red sage, yarrow, raspberry leaves, white oak bark, saltwater, and cayenne pepper.

Bitters

Bitters work by triggering a sensory response in the central nervous system leading to a range of responses including stimulating appetite, aiding in liver's detoxification, increase bile flow, toning, and stimulating effect on mucosal lining. Wormwood is a bitter currently used.

Demulcents

Demulcent works to soothe and protect irritated or inflamed tissue. Some common demulcents include zinc, slippery elm, vitamin A, and vitamin E. These work to decreased gastric acids, decrease diarrhea, and decrease muscle spasms.

Special Populations

Drug Dosing for the Pediatric and Geriatric Populations

Age is a factor when dosing not only for the pediatric population but also for the geriatric population. These two groups show very different rates of drug metabolism than the average adult. However, drug dosing is tested on the average male adult's metabolism.

When dosing for the pediatric population one should not assume that the very young are just "little adults." With children it is not always appropriate to dose a child based on a fractional adult recommended dose. From a physiologic perspective, early childhood drug-metabolizing enzyme activity is very low. These rates of biotransformation do increase dramatically to adult levels at or about the age of puberty, but prior to that the activity levels are low. In the geriatric populations multiple drug usage is common, and this polypharmacy may cause interactions, which lead to increased side effects, subtherapeutic levels or drug toxicity. With age, drug absorption is less complete or slower due to altered gastrointestinal motility, reduced blood flow due to decreased cardiac output, and reduction in absorptive surfaces. The distribution of the drugs are also effected in the elderly due to hypoalbuminemia (low amounts of albumin, a plentiful protein in the blood), changes in the drug binding sites, reduced muscle mass, increase in the proportion of body fat, and a decrease in total body water. Drug metabolism and excretion are also affected by age. As blood flow is decreased in the kidneys and the liver, a higher incidence of drug toxicity is encountered.

Drug Treatment for Spasmodic Dysphonia

Spasmodic dysphonia (SD) is described Chapter 6. One of the drug treatments of SD is botulinum toxin type A (Botox™). Botox™ is a complex protein produced by clostridium botulinum, which is an anaerobic bacteria. The mechanism of its action is to block neuromuscular conduction by binding to the receptor site on the motor nerve terminal, inhibiting the release of acetylcholine thereby producing muscle paralysis (Craig & Stitzel, 1986). Botox™ should be used with caution in patients with already existing neuromuscular disease to avoid a compounding effect. Patients with a history of anticoagulation will tend to bruise easily and may have a bleeding problem from the actual insertion of the needle. This side effect is not just specific to Botox™ treatment but holds true with any injectable drug.

Drugs That Can Cause Dysphagia

There are only a few reports indicating drugs that may cause symptoms of dysphagia (difficulty swallowing). These drugs include anti-infective drugs including demeclocycline (Declomycin), doxycycline (Vibramycin), minocycline (Dynacin), oxytetracycline (Terramycin), tetracyclinc (Achromycin), and an autonomic nervous system drug, pilocarpine hydrochloride, that increases salivary gland secretion of the salivary glands. Only a few drugs are advocated in treating dysphagia symptoms. These include Buspirone (an anti-anxiety drug) (Hanna, Feibusch, & Albright, 1997), nifedipine (cardiovascular system drug), and Cisapride (Propulsid), which has been found beneficial in PD and other degenerative diseases. It works by stimulating serotonin receptors, which enhances the release of acetycholine and increases GI motility (Perez, Smithard, Davies, & Kalra, 1998; Vogel et al., 2000).

Summary

Due to the development of new medications, the following recommended readings include books, peer-reviewed articles, and Web sites that can be used for updating information reviewed in this chapter.

Recommended Readings

Brown, C. (2001). Overview of drug interactions, *U.S. Pharmacist.* Retrieved August 31, 2008 from http://www.uspharmacist.com
This Web site is maintained by U.S. Pharmacist, *which is a monthly journal providing pharmacists, students, and other health care professionals with up-to-date, peer-reviewed clinical articles relevant to contemporary pharmacy practice.*

Drugs.com http://www.drugs.com/drug_interactions.html. This site explains the mechanisms of each drug interaction and the interactions between drugs and food.

Harris, S. *Herbal drug interaction handbook.* Retrieved August 31, 2008 from http://www.foodmedinteractions.com

Holden, K. (2000). *Eat well, stay well with Parkinson's disease.* Fort Collins, CO: Therapy Five Star Living Inc.

Physicians desk reference for nutritional supplements. (2007). Montvale, NJ: Medical Economics Company Inc.

The medicine corner. Retrieved March 8, 2012 from www.themedicinecorner.com

Mobile Device Downloads

Epocrates—Medical App Developer. Clinical reference tool for the mobile device. http://www.epocrates.com/mobile .

References

Bolser, D. C., & Davenport, P. W. (2007). Codeine and cough: An ineffective gold standard. *Currents Opinions in Allergy and Clinical Immunology, 7*(1), 32–36.

Burham, T. H., & Short, R. M. (1997). *Drug facts and comparisons.* St. Louis, MO: Wolters Kluwer.

Center for Drug Evaluation and Research (CDER). (2001). Retrieved from http://www.fda.gov/cder/index.html

Craig, C. R., & Stitzel, R. E. (1986). *Modern pharmacology* (2nd ed.). Boston, MA: Brown and Co.

Cupp, H. J. (1999). Herbal remedies: Adverse effects and drug interactions. In *American Academy of Family Physicians.* Retrieved from, http://www.aafp.org

Damste, P. H. (1967). Voice changes in adult women caused by virilizing agents. *Journal of Speech and Hearing Disorders, 32*, 126–132.

Damste, P. H. (1968). Virilization of the voice due to anabolic steroids. *Folia Phoniatrica, 16*, 10–18.

Darley, F. L., Aronson, A. E., & Brown, J. R. (1975). *Motor speech disorders*. Philadephia, PA: W. B. Saunders.

Dietary Supplement Health and Education Act of 1994. Public Law No. 103–417, 1994.

Duffy, J. R. (1995). *Motor speech disorders: Substrates, differential diagnosis and management*. St. Louis, MO: Mosby-Year Book.

Eisenberg, D. M., Kessler, R. C., Foster, C., Norlock, F. E., Calkins, D. R., & Delbanco, T. L. (1993). Unconventional medicine in the United States: Prevalence, costs, and patterns of use. *New England Journal of Medicine, 328*, 246–252.

Elbe, D. (2001). *Grapefruit juice drug interactions*. Retrieved from http://www.powernetdesign.com/grapefruit/

Food and Drug Administration (FDA). Retrieved from http://www.fda.gov/

Freed, D. (2000). *Motor speech disorders: Diagnosis and treatment*. San Diego, CA: Singular.

Gianni, L. M., & Dreitlein, W. B. (1998). Some popular OTC herbals can interact with anticoagulant therapy. *U.S. Pharmacist, 23*(80), 83–86.

Hanna, G. L., Feibusch, E. L., & Albright, K. J. (1997). Buspirone treatment of anxiety associated with pharyngeal dysphagia in a four-year-old. *Journal of Child and Adolescent Psychopharmacology, 7*, 137–143.

Holden, K. (2001). *Parkinson's disease: Guidelines for medical nutrition*. Fort Collins, CO: Therapy Five Star Living.

Kush, R. D., Bleicher, P., Raymond, S., Kubich, W., Marks, R., & Tardif, B. (2007). *PDR for herbal medicines* (4th ed.). Montvale, NJ: Thomson Healthcare.

Marsden, C. D. (1994). Parkinson's disease. *Journal of Neurology, Neurosurgery, and Psychiatry, 57*, 672–681.

Perez, I., Smithard, D. G., Davies, H., & Kalra, L. (1998). Pharmacological treatment of dysphagia in stroke. *Dysphagia, 13*, 12–16.

Pronsky, Z. Food medication interaction. (2001). Retrieved from http://www.foodmedinteractions.com

Sataloff, R. T., Hawkshaw, M., & Rosen, D. (1998). Medications: Effects and side effects in professional voice users. In R. T. Sataloff (Ed.), *Vocal health and pedagogy*. San Diego, CA: Singular.

Surrow, J. (2000). *Rationale use of herbal medicines for singers*. Presentation at the XIII Annual Pacific Voice Conference, San Diego, CA.

Vogel, D., Carter, J., & Carter, P. (2000). *The effects of drugs on communication disorders* (2nd ed.). San Diego, CA: Singular.

Appendix 11–1
Chapter 11 Glossary

ACE inhibitors: Decreases angiotesion II chemicals from contracting muscles that surround the blood vessels and causes them to increase pressure by narrowing the vessel.

Advanced: Further along in development.

Agonist: Combines with a receptor on the cell to produce a reaction.

Alpha-2 agonist: Decreases blood vessels in the heart, kidneys, and periphery in order to decrease the blood pressure.

Alveoli: Tiny saclike air spaces in the lung where carbon dioxide and oxygen are exchanged.

Anticholinergic: Inhibits nerve impulses from acetylcholine neurotransmitters.

Anticoagulant: Prevents the formation of blood clots.

Antispasmodics/anticholinergics: Decreases cramping in the stomach, by slowing down the stomach activity.

Anxiolytic: Relieves anxiety.

Beta-blockers: Blocks epinephrine (adrenaline) and causes the heart to beat slower and thereby reduces blood pressure.

Bioflavonoid: Protects blood vessels using water-soluble plant pigments.

Bronchodilator: Widens the lung's air passage.

Calcium channel blockers: Block calcium from entering the cells of the heart and thereby slowing the heart rate.

Cox-2 inhibitors: Block enzymes that cause pain and swelling from inflammation of the joints.

Electrolyte: Regulates the flow of various ions across the cell membrane.

Extrapyramidal: Regulates muscle reflexes.

Gastritis: Reduces inflammation of the stomach.

Gingival hyperplasia: Reduces overgrowth of gum tissue.

H2-receptor antagonist: Decreases stomach acid, by binding to cell and limiting acid production.

Hepatic: To do with the liver.

Hyoid: U-shaped bone at the base of the tongue that is suspended in the neck. Site for multiple muscular attachments that support the larynx.

Hyperglycemia: High levels of glucose in the blood.

Metabolite: Changes stored energy into used energy.

Mucolytic: Enzymes that break down mucus.

Metoclopramide: Increases muscle contractions in the upper digestive tract and increases the rate at which the stomach empties into the intestines.

Orthostatic hypotension: Lowers blood pressure when standing up, causes dizziness.

Nigral cells: Produces the chemical dopamine and are located in the substantia nigra.

Palliative: Relieves the symptoms of the disease without curing.

Plasma: Fluid portion of the blood, with no cells.

Platelet: Small pieces of bone marrow cells in the blood.

Proton-pump inhibitor: Blocks the enzyme on the wall of the stomach that produces the acid.

Somnolence: Drowsiness.

Stomatitis: Inflammation of the mucous tissue in the mouth.

Subglottis: The area below the vocal folds.

Viral nucleic acid: Attachment of a virus to a living cell (with macromolecules composed of nucleotide chains), incorporating their own genetic materials.

Reference

Webster's New World Medical Dictionary. Retrieved from http://www.mayoclinic.com

Glossary

Abdomen: Portion of the body lying between the thorax and the pelvis.

Abduction: Open; away from midline.

Abductor SD (Ab-SD): Spasms in muscles that open vocal folds and interrupt speech, causing breathy or voice breaks. A form of dystonia, thought to be of neurological orgin.

Abilify: Is an antipsychotic medicine used to treat the symptoms of schizophrenia and bipolar disorder.

Acid and Enzymes: Chemical substances, within the stomach, that help break up (digest) food. An increased level of acid (measured by low pH) can lead to stomach ulcers, heartburn, and esophagitis.

Actin: One of two protein filaments of the myofilament. Myosin is the other protein filament.

Aciphex: Aciphex (rabeprazole) is used to treat gastroesophageal reflux disease (GERD) and other conditions involving excessive stomach acid.

Action Potential: Occurring at the surface of the nerve or muscle tissue at the moment of excitation. An electrical potential change that is of short-duration, period of negativity called the spike potential and secondary changes in potential called after-potentials.

Activella: Increases the risk of developing endometrial hyperplasia, a condition that may lead to cancer of the lining of the uterus.

Acute: Of short duration, new.

Adam's Apple: Layman's term for the anterior projection of the thyroid cartilage, especially in men. Formed by the joining to the two thyroid lamina.

Adderall: Is a central nervous system stimulant. It affects chemicals in the brain and nerves that contribute to hyperactivity and impulse control.

Adduction: Closed; toward midline.

Adenoid: The enlarged or hypertrophied pharyngeal tonsil.

Adenoidectomy: Excision of adenoids.

Adenosine triphosphate (ATP): A molecule in the cell through which energy is produced, released, and regenerated.

Adenosine triphosphate-creatine phosphate (ATP-CP): A high-energy molecule that combines with adenosine diphosphate (ADP) to generate adenosine triphosphate (ATP).

Advanced Laryngeal Cancer: T3 = complete non-movement of one vocal fold; T4 = invades thyroid cartilage or structures outside of the voice box.

Airway Symptoms: Breathing complaints.

Allegra: A brand name antihistamine drug used in the treatment of hay fever and similar allergy symptoms.

Aloxi: Blocks the actions of chemicals in the body that can trigger nausea and vomiting.

Alveoli: Tiny air sacs in the lungs which are surrounded by many blood vessels, facilitating the exchange of oxygen and carbon dioxide gases.

Ambien: A sedative and is used for the short-term treatment of insomnia by helping you fall asleep.

Amoxicillin: Amoxicillin is a penicillin antibiotic. It fights bacteria in your body. Amoxicillin is used to treat many different types of infections caused by bacteria.

Amplification: Increasing the amplitude of a signal to increase the "gain" (measurable or detectable changes in time-variation for purposes of recording playback data.

Amplitude: The degree to which there is lateral excursion of the vocal folds.

Amplitude/Intensity: Perceptual correlate is volume or loudness; also called energy; measured by the amplitude or magnitude of the sound wave generated in decibels (dB).

Analog-to digital (A/D) processing: Conversion of an analog signal to digital form using a computer hardware devices (A/D board or converter). An analog signal is time- and amplitude-varying and continuous. Digital processing, or digitization, divides the signal into discrete bits of information that are encoded numerically.

Androgen: A steroid hormone, such as testosterone or androsterone that controls the development and maintenance of masculine characteristics.

Anterior: Front.

Anterior Commissure: Anterior juncture of the true vocal folds.

Anticholinergic: An agent that is antagonistic to the action of parasympathetic or other cholinergic nerve fibers.

Antihistamines: Antihistamines are used to relieve or prevent the symptoms of your medical problem.

Antihypertensive Agents: A drug aimed at reducing high blood pressure (hypertension).

Aphonia: Complete voice loss.

Aphonic breaks: A break or interruption in vocal fold vibration/phonation.

Articulation: (1) a joint or juncture of bones; (2) movement and placement of the articulators during speech production.

Articulators: Those structures responsible for modifying the acoustic properties of the vocal tract; i.e., tongue, lips, soft and hard palate, teeth.

Artificial Ventilation: Machine-assisted breathing.

Arytenoid Cartilages: Pair of pyramid-shaped cartilages that serve as posterior attachment of the vocal folds. Movement is responsible for adduction and abduction of the vocal folds.

Arytenoid Fixation: Restricted joint motion of the arytenoid joint that can lead to abnormal-sounding voice and incomplete closure of the vocal folds.

Aspiration: Choking or coughing when swallowing food, drink, or saliva. Foreign materials enter the airway instead of the esophagus.

Aspirin: Aspirin is in a group of drugs called salicylates. It works by reducing substances in the body that cause pain, fever, and inflammation.

Astelin: An antihistamine. It blocks the effects of the chemical histamine in your body.

Ataxia: Incoordination of muscle movement.

Atripla: Prevents the human immunodeficiency virus (HIV) from reproducing in your body.

Avapro: Avapro (irbesartan) is in a group of drugs called angiotensin II receptor antagonists. Irbesartan keeps blood vessels from narrowing, which lowers blood pressure and improves blood flow.

Axial Rotation: Abnormal tilt of the vocal folds during high pitch sound production.

Axid AR: Nizatidine works by decreasing the amount of acid the stomach produces. Nizatidine is used to treat ulcers in the stomach and intestines.

Azothioprine: Azothioprine is a drug that suppresses the immune system.

Baclofen: Baclofen is used to treat muscle symptoms caused by multiple sclerosis, including spasm, pain, and stiffness.

Bacteriacidal: Destroying bacteria.

Bacteriastatic: Inhibiting growth or multiplication of bacteria; an agent that so acts.

Ballistics: (1) the study of the motion of projectiles; (2) movements resulting from sudden muscle contractions, which are continued by the forces of inertia.

Ballistic Stretching: Active, forceful stretching of the muscle, returning immediately to resting length.

Barium Swallow Esophagram: X-ray imaging of the esophagus during swallowing.

Barrett's Esophagus: Abnormal surface appearance of the esophagus due to replacement of the normal surface cells; often seen as an ulcer and can be precancerous.

Basal Ganglia: Part of the brain that is likely involved in spasmodic dysphonia (SD); located deep in the cerebral hemispheres and the upper brainstem.

Basement Membrane: Layer of extracellular material upon which surface cells rest.

Bernoulli's Principle: Pressure is perpendicular to the direction of fluid flow. Thus, if volume fluid flow is constant, velocity will increase at an area of constriction with a corresponding decrease in pressure at the constriction.

Beta-Andrenergic Receptors: Any of various cell membrane receptors that can bind with epinephrine and related substances that activate or block the actions of cells containing such receptors.

Beta-Blockers: Prevent stimulation of the beta adrenergic receptors at the nerve endings of the sympathetic nervous system and therefore decrease the activity of the heart.

Benzodiazepines: A benzodiazepine receptor antagonist.

Biaxin: Biaxin (clarithromycin) is a macrolide antibiotic. Clarithromycin fights bacteria in your body.

Bilateral: Both sides.

Biliary: Of or relating to bile or the bile duct.

Biopsy: Removal of a small piece of possibly abnormal tissue to examine under a microscope to determine presence or absence of malignancy.

Botulinum Toxin, Type A (Botox): A short-lasting medical mixture, injected into the vocal fold to temporarily limit mobility.

Boyle's Law: At any given temperature the volume of gas varies in inverse proportion to the pressure exerted upon it.

Breathy: Audible escape of air; a weak vocal tone; glottal insufficiency.

Bronchoscopy: Examination of the airway above the lungs using an instrument (scope) that also allows for biopsy and culture.

Broyle's Ligament: Anterior commissure tendon.

Canasa: Treating various forms of mild to moderate inflammation of the colon.

Capillaries: Blood vessels that connect larger vessels and together form a network within the body.

Carbamazepine: Used to treat epileptic seizures and nerve pain such as trigeminal neuralgia.

Chorditis: Inflammation of the vocal folds.

Chronic: Long-term, long-lasting.

Chronic Cough: Cough that has lasted an abnormally long time.

Chronic Intermittent: Goes away, then returns again—even several months to years later.

Claritin: An antihistamine that reduces the effects of natural chemical histamine in the body. Histamine can produce symptoms of sneezing, itching, watery eyes, and runny nose.

Clavicular Breathing: Use of upper check and shoulder muscles with excessive movement during inspiration.

Clonazepam: Clonazepam is used to treat seizure disorders or panic disorder.

Combivir: Lamivudine and zidovudine are antiviral medications. They are in a group of human immunodeficiency virus (HIV) medicines called reverse transcriptase inhibitors. This medication helps keep the HIV virus from reproducing in the body.

Complera: Complera contains a combination of emtricitabine, rilpivirine, and tenofovir. Emtricitabine, rilpivirine, and tenofovir are antiviral drugs that prevent preventing HIV (human immunodeficiency virus) cells from multiplying in the body.

Compliance: The action or fact of complying with a wish or command.

Compounding Conditions: Condition that can complicate an existing abnormality or make it worse.

Computed Tomography (CT): Specialized radiologic imaging technique that allows visualization of soft tissue and bone with greater detail than a simple x-ray.

Condyloma: Papilloma; a wartlike growth.

Contact Ulcer: Benign bilateral ulceration of the vocal folds that occurs over the vocal process of the arytenoids cartilages; usually the result of vocal abuse, and may result in hoarseness and laryngeal pain; more common in men than women, and only rarely observed in children.

Contralateral: On the opposite side of the body.

Corticosteroids: It reduces swelling; used for many conditions, among them: allergic reactions, skin diseases, blood disorders, and eye problems.

Coup Deglotte: Forceful starts to phonation.

Cricoarytenoid Joint: A synovial joint formed between the cricoid and arytenoid cartilages.

Cricothyroid muscle: Intrinsic laryngeal muscle primarily increasing vocal fold length and the elevation of vocal pitch.

CT Scan: Computed tomography scan.

Cyclophosphamide: A synthetic cytotoxic drug used in treating leukemia and lymphoma and as an immunosuppressive agent.

Damping: To cause a decrease in amplitude of successive waves or oscillations.

Dead Air: Air in the respiratory tract that does not enter into gas exchange, that is, air in the mouth, nasal cavities, pharynx, larynx, and trachea.

Decibel (dB): A quantitative unit of relative sound intensity or sound pressure, based on the logarithmic relationship of amplitudes or pressures of two wounds, one of which serves as the reference.

Deglutition: Swallowing.

Delayed Emptying: An abnormally slow movement of stomach contents into the small intestine (could be a sign of stomach muscle malfunction).

Delayed Esophageal Clearance: When esophageal muscle contraction is weak or uncoordinated, moving the food into the stomach is delayed.

Dexilant: Dexlansoprazole decreases the amount of acid produced in the stomach.

Diagnosis: The determination of the cause of a disease.

Diaphragm: Major muscle of inspiration.

Diaphragmatic Breathing: Use of the diaphragm to produce an outward movement of the abdomen in inhalation.

Differential pressure: Difference between two pressures, where pressure 1 serves as the reference pressure, typically atmospheric pressure.

Dificid: Is an macrolide antibiotic that works by killing sensitive bacteria.

Diovan: Is a thiazide diuretic (water pill) that helps prevent your body from absorbing too much salt, which can cause fluid retention.

Diplophonia: Two frequencies produced simultaneously, resulting in rough sounding quality.

Direct Laryngoscopy: Direct visualization of the larynx by speculum/mirror or laryngoscope.

Distribution: The extent of a ramifying structure such as an artery or nerve and its branches.

Diuretics: Diuretics are medicines that help reduce the amount of water in the body.

Doryx: Doxycycline is a tetracycline antibiotic. It fights bacteria in the body.

Double-Probe pH Monitor: Test that uses a small tube placed through the nose into the esophagus with two sensors that measure acid levels.

Driving Pressure: Flow of a gas from higher to lower regions of pressure concentrations.

Dysarthria: Difficulty forming words; presenting with imprecise consonants, hard-to-understand speech.

Dysfluent Speech: Abnormal speech pattern of stuttering characterized by stops and repetitions of sound segments.

Dyskinesia: Impaired control of voluntary movement.

Dyspepsia: Heartburn or discomfort after eating.

Dysphagia: Difficulty swallowing.

Dysphonia: Voice impairment and /or change in pitch, loudness, or quality.

Dysphonia Plica Ventricularis: Condition in which sound is made using the false vocal fold.

Dysplasia: Disorderly pattern of cell maturation.

Dyspnea: Perceived difficulty breathing.

Dystonia: Central nervous system disorder causing a disorder of movement.

Edema: Swelling.

Effusion: Fluid escape from its natural vessels into a body cavity.

Electroglottograph: Instrument that measure the relative conductance or impedance between two small electrodes placed on either side of the larynx; indicates vocal fold contact for each vibratory cycle.

Electrolarynx: A handheld device that enables speech after a laryngectomy by producing an external vibration that mimics the vibration of the vocal folds.

Electromyography: Device for recording electric currents from an active muscle to produce an electromyogram.

Emphysema: Chronic, irreversible disease of the lungs characterized by abnormal enlargement of air spaces in the lungs accompanied by destruction of the tissue lining the walls of the air spaces.

Empiric Therapy: Treatment trial that often helps determine diagnosis.

Endometriosis: A condition in which bits of the tissue similar to the lining of the uterus (endometrium) grow in other parts of the body.

Endomysium: Connective tissue surrounding the entire muscle.

Endoscopy: Visual examination of the interior of a hollow body organ by use of an endoscope.

Endotracheal Tubes: Breathing tubes.

Enzymes: Organic catalysts that speed up specific chemical reactions during metabolism.

Epimysium: Connective tissue surrounding the entire muscle.

Epithelium: Layer of surface cells covering the larynx.

Epzicom: It is in a group of human immunodeficiency virus (HIV) medicines called reverse transcriptase inhibitors.

Erosive Esophagitis: Inflammation and irritation of the esophagus.

Erythema: Redness.

Esophageal Stenosis: Narrowing of the esophagus.

Esophageal Strictures: Abnormal narrowing along the food pipe.

Esophagitis: Inflammation of the esophagus.

Esophagus: Muscular passage connecting the mouth or pharynx with the stomach.

Essential Tremor: Tremor of unknown cause (usually of the hands and head) that develops in older people; often mistaken for Parkinsonism but is not life-threatening and can usually be kept under control.

Estratest: Esterified estrogens are female sex hormones necessary for many processes in the body.

Estrogen: Any of a group of steroid hormones that promote the development and maintenance of female characteristics of the body.

Exacerbations: Aggravation: action that makes a problem or a disease worse.

Excisional Biopsy: Removal of part or all of the abnormal tissue for microscopic examination.

Excretion: The act or process of discharging waste matter from the blood, tissues, or organs.

Exercise-Induced Asthma: Airway limitation and airway distress co-occurring with exercise or high ventilatory task demands.

Exercise Physiology: Scientific study of human muscles and muscle movement, especially as they relate to physical exercise and athletic development.

Exhale: To expel air from the lungs by breathing.

Expectorate: To cough up and spit out material from the lungs, bronchi, and trachea.

Expiratory Reserve Volume: Maximum volume that can be expired beyond tidal volume expiration (1500–2000 cc).

External Intercostal Muscles: Muscles of the rib cage that facilitate inspiration. They are positioned between the ribs in such a way that, when these muscles contract, the ribs are lifted and tilted.

Extralaryngeal Speech Techniques: Alternative methods for voice for patients who have experienced a laryngectomy.

False vocal folds: Ventricular folds.

Falsetto: Unnatural or artificially high-pitched voice or register especially for a male.

Fatigue: Temporary loss of strength.

Fauces: Passage from the mouth to the pharynx, surrounded by soft palate, palatine arches, and the base of the tongue.

FEES: Flexible endoscopic examination of swallowing.

Fibroblasts: Cell that gives rise to connective tissue.

Filters: Method of including (passing) and excluding (filtering) specified levels of energy in the signal, usually in the course of signal processing. A "low-pass" filter excludes energy at high frequencies; a "high-pass" filter excludes energy at low frequencies; and a "band-pass" filter excludes energies higher or lower than a specified band of frequencies.

Fingolimod: It works by keeping immune cells trapped in your lymph nodes so they can't reach the central nervous system (brain and spinal cord).

Flow: Movement of a quantity of gas through an area.

Flow Glottogram: Signal obtained from inverse filtering the oral airflow collected with a pneumotachograph mask.

Flow Rate (volume velocity): Speed (and direction) of flow per unit time.

Flow Volume: Quantity of flow.

Focal: Concentrated within a small area.

Focal Dystonia: Neurological movement disorder affecting muscle within one part of the body.

Forced Expiratory Volume: The maximum volume of air expired from the lungs in a specific time interval when starting from maximum inspiration.

Forced Vital Capacity: Vital capacity measured with subject exhaling as rapidly as possible.

Formant: One of the regions of concentration of energy, prominent on a sound spectrogram that collectively constitute the frequency spectrum of a speech sound.

FRC: Functional residual capacity.

Frequencies: Speed at which the vocal folds vibrate.

Functional Voice Disorder: Disorder arising from nonorganic and nonneurological causes.

Fundamental Frequency: Lowest periodic waveform of vocal fold vibration. Fundamental frequency is the reciprocal of the pitch period ($f_0 = 1/T$) and is measured in hertz (Hz).

Gabapentin: Used to treat some types of seizures and for postherpetic neuralgia.

Gag Reflex: Pharyngeal reflex.

Gastric Dysmotility: Abnormal contraction of stomach muscles.

Gastroesophageal Reflux Disease (GERD): Backflow of stomach fluids into the esophagus; perceived as "heartburn."

Gender: Assignment of masculinity or femininity; how people perceive their role in society.

Geodon: Geodon is used to treat schizophrenia and the manic symptoms of bipolar disorder (manic depression) in adults and children who are at least 10 years old.

Glissando: Series of ascending or descending notes on the musical scale.

Globus Pharyngeus: Feeling of a lump in the throat.

Glottal Attack: Hyperadduction of the vocal folds at phonation onset.

Glottal Chink: Space between the vocal folds when they are adducted, commonly in the posterior, cartilaginous region of the vocal folds in women and young children.

Glottal Cycle: Vibratory cycle.

Glottal Fry: Lowest vocal register, characterized by a very low fundamental frequency.

Glottal Incompetence: Incomplete vocal fold closure.

Glottal Resistance: Pressure across the glottis divided by the flow through the glottis.

Glottal Stop: Approximation of plosive sound made by stopping and releasing the breath stream at the level of the glottis.

Glottic: Referring to the vocal fold area.

Glottic Closure: The degree that the vocal folds approximate during the closed phase of vibration.

Glottis or Rima Glottides: Opening between the two vocal fold margins.

Glottograph: Instrument used to measure the relative amount of light that shines through the glottis; indicates that extent of the glottal opening but not the shape.

Glucocorticoids: Any of a group of anti-inflammatory steroid-like compounds, such as hydrocortisone, that are produced by the adrenal cortex, are involved in carbohydrate, protein, and fat metabolism, and are used as anti-inflammatory agents.

Granuloma: An inflammatory tumor or growth composed of granulation tissue.

Graft Migration: Shifting of an implant.

Granulation Tissue: Tissue that is formed as part of the tissue healing and repair process after injury or surgery.

Haldol: Haloperidol is used to treat schizophrenia. It is also used to control motor and speech tics in people with Tourette's syndrome.

Harmonic: A frequency that is an integral multiple of the same basic frequency.

Harmonic-to-Noise Ratio: Alternative term for signal-to-noise ratio; a measure of the "normalcy" of vocal fold vibration.

Harsh: Irregular vocal fold vibrations resulting in a combination of hoarse and breathy voice quality.

Hashimoto's: Chronic inflammation of the thyroid characterized by goiter or thyroid fibrosis.

Heartburn: Burning sensation in the stomach, typically extending toward the esophagus.

Hemoptysis: Coughing up blood.

Hemorrhage: Bleeding within the body.

Hiatal Hernia: Abnormal junction (or connection) between the stomach and the food pipe (esophagus).

Hiatus: Opening, as in the case of an opening between two muscles.

Hoarseness: Sound production characterized by aperiodic vocal fold vibrations.

Humibid: Temporarily relieving cough due to the common cold, upper respiratory tract infections, sinus inflammation, sore throat, or bronchitis.

Human Papilloma Virus (HPV): Virus that causes recurrent respiratory papillolmatosis; HPV also causes genital warts.

Hyaluronic Acid: Mucopolysaccharide serving as a viscous medium in the tissues of the body and as a lubricant in joints.

Hydration: Process of providing an adequate amount of liquid to bodily tissues.

Hyoid Bone: U-shaped bone at the root of the tongue, only bone in the laryngeal framework which serves as an attachment to many extrinsic laryngeal muscles.

Hyperfunction: Increased supraglottic tension or the presence of false fold adduction.

Hyperfunctional: Reduced function; low muscular effort.

Hyperglycemia: The presence of an abnormally high concentration of glucose in the blood.

Hyperkinesia: Increase in movement resulting in spasticity or tremor.

Hypernasal: Excessive, undesirable amount of perceived nasal cavity resonance during phonation.

Hyperthyroidism: Abnormal functioning of the thyroid, in which too much thyroid hormone is released.

Hypokinesia: Reduction of movement resulting in rigidity.

Hyponasal: Lack of resonance for the three phonemes /m/, /n/, and /nj/ resulting form a partial or complete obstruction in the nasal tract.

Hypophonia: Form of dysphonia characterized by a soft or whispered voice.

Hypothyroidism: Abnormal functioning of the thyroid, in which too little thyroid hormone is released.

Hypoxia: Deficiency of oxygen in inspired air.

Hytuss: Immediate-release capsules are used for: relieving symptoms of an unproductive cough and mucus in the chest due to colds, flu, or hay fever.

Hyzaar: Hyzaar (hydrochlorothiazide and losartan) is used to treat high blood pressure and to reduce the risk of stroke in people with hypertension.

Hyzine: Hyzine is used for: treating anxiety. It is also used to cause sedation before and after general anesthesia.

Ibuprofen: Ibuprofen is a nonsteroidal anti-inflammatory drug (NSAID). Ibuprofen works by reducing hormones that cause inflammation and pain in the body.

Imipramine: Imipramine affects chemicals in the brain that may become unbalanced. Imipramine is used to treat symptoms of depression.

Impaired Esophageal Clearance: Abnormal emptying or clearance of esophagus.

Implant Extrusion: Implant is "rejected" and pushed outward.

Inferior: From below.

Inferior Laryngeal Artery: Laryngeal artery supplying the back part of the larynx.

Inflammation: Response to injury that results in swelling, redness, and/or pain.

Inflammatory Reaction: The injury healing response.

Inflammatory Tissue: The cells and substances found in the areas where there is response to injury, such as inflammation.

Inhalant: Medication, anesthetic, or other compound in vapor or aerosol form, taken by inhalation.

Insomnia: Insomnia is the inability to obtain an adequate amount or quality of sleep. The difficulty can be in falling asleep, remaining asleep, or both.

Inspiration: The inhalation of air into the lungs.

Inspiratory Reserve Volume: The volume of air that can be inspired after normal tidal inspiration (1500–2500 cc).

Inspiratory Stridor: Audible inspiration typically due to increased airway resistance produced by airway narrowing.

Intensity: (1) Correlate of physical energy and the degree of loudness of a speech sound; (2) sound energy present in a signal, represented by waveform amplitude.

Interval Scale: Measurement scale that quantifies differences between values.

Intonation: (1) pattern or melody of pitch changes in connected speech; (2) the rise and fall of pitch in an individual's voice during speech.

Intracordal cyst: An abnormal membranous sac found just below the epithelium of the vocal fold.

Intrafold Injection: Injection of substance within the vocal fold.

Intramuscular: Within the muscular substance.

Intraoral Pressure: The amount of pressure measured in the mouth during a stop plosive. Can serve as an estimate of subglottal pressure.

Intrathecal: Within a sheath; through the theca of the spinal cord into the subarachnoid space.

Intravenous: Within or administered into a vein.

Intraventricular: Pertaining to the space within a ventricle or to the conduction system within the walls of a ventricle.

Intubation: Insertion of a tube into the glottal space.

Inverse Filtering: Method used to estimate the source of voice speech.

Ipsilateral: On the same side of the body.

Irritable Larynx Syndrome: Myriad symptoms related to upper airway irritation; can result in laryngeal spasm.

Jackson's Syndrome: Unilateral paralysis of the soft palate, larynx, sternocleidomastoid and trapezius muscles, and hemiatrophy of the tongue; results from lesions of the vagus, spinal accessory, and hypoglossal nerves.

Jitter: Measure of cycle-to-cycle variability in fundamental frequency. Can be expressed in absolute measures or as a percentage referenced to the fundamental frequency.

Joint: The articulation of two or more bones.

Keflex: Keflex (cephalexin) is used to treat infections caused by bacteria, including respiratory infections and ear infections.

Keratosis: Any skin disease characterized by a warty growth.

Ketoprofen: Ketoprofen is in a group of drugs called nonsteroidal anti-inflammatory drugs (NSAIDs). Ketoprofen works by reducing hormones that cause inflammation and pain in the body.

Kilohertz (kHz): One thousand cycles per second.

Kinematics: Study of motion or movement.

Kinesiology: Study of human muscle movement.

Kinesthesia, kinesthesis: (1) an awareness of the movement or position of the speech muscles and structures; (2) sense of movement originating from sensory end organs in muscles, tendons, joints, and sometimes the canals of the ear.

Kinesthetic Cue: Use of the awareness of the position of the articulators or their correct pattern of movements as an aid in teaching the correct production of a speech sound.

Kinetic: Relating to movement of motion.

Kymograph: Instrument that graphically records the different articulatory movements.

Lamina Propria: Nonmuscle part of the vocal fold, directly underneath the epithelium of the vocal fold.

Lamotrigine: An anti-epileptic medication, also called an anticonvulsant. Lamotrigine is used either alone or in combination with other medications to treat epileptic seizures in adults and children.

Laparoscopically: Surgery or visualization performed without cutting open the body; instead, special "tools" and cameras are inserted through small holes in the body.

Laryngeal Anomaly: Pathologic condition of the vocal folds and related structures; vocal folds and related structures.

Laryngeal Electromyography (LEMG): Test that measures electrical signals to nerve inputs to muscles.

Laryngeal Examination: Examination of the larynx.

Laryngeal Framework Surgery: Surgical modification of the laryngeal cartilage framework so the vocal folds can close better or have more tension, allowing improved sound production.

Laryngeal Injection Augmentation: Injection of a variety of synthetic or natural materials into the vocal fold to optimize vocal fold closure in order to enhance vocal fold vibration, thus improving voice. Also called vocal fold injection or vocal fold augmentation.

Laryngeal Reinnervation: Re-establishing nerve inputs to the laryngeal muscles.

Laryngeal Stroboscopy: Using a synchronized flashing light that allows visualization of vocal fold vibration in slow motion.

Laryngeal Web: Membranous tissue that extends across the glottis from one vocal fold to the other; usually located in the anterior part of the larynx and varying in size from a small membrane filling the anterior commissure to a structure extending to the vocal processes of the arytenoid cartilages, thereby occluding most of the airway; webs may be congenital or the result of an injury, and may connect the ventricular folds or span the larynx subglottally.

Laryngectomy: Surgery to remove the larynx.

Laryngitis: Inflammation of the vocal folds.

Laryngocele: Irregular air sac that connects with the cavity of the larynx and produces a tumorlike lesion that may be visible on the outside of the neck.

Laryngofissure: Surgical procedure in which the larynx is directly exposed by dividing the thyroid cartilage in the midline; permits adequate exposure for the surgical handling of lesions that cannot be attacked satisfactorily via the oral route, yet are not sufficiently extensive to require total laryngectomy.

Laryngologist: An ear, nose, and throat doctor who specializes in voice care.

Laryngology: Science of the anatomy, physiology, and diseases of the larynx.

Laryngomalacia: Presence of soft laryngeal cartilage; in extreme cases, severe breathing problems may be present.

Laryngopathy: Disease of the larynx.

Laryngopharyngeal Reflux (LPR): Backflow of stomach fluids to the laryngopharynx.

Larngopharynx: Refers to the area of the larynx and lower back part of the throat (hypopharynx).

Laryngoscope: (1) Specialized scope to view the larynx; (2) Any of several types of endoscopes used in examining or operating upon the interior of the larynx.

Laryngoscopy: An endoscopic examination of the larynx.

Laryngospasm: Sudden inability to breathe due to closing off of the airway.

Laryngostenosis: Contraction or stricture of the larynx.

Larynx: Voice box; composed of vocal folds, muscles, and framework cartilage; highly specialized structure atop the windpipe responsible for sound production, air passage during breathing and protecting the airway during swallowing.

Larynx Preservation: Term used when a treatment choice for cancer is designed to maximally retain the laryngeal structures without compromising the chances of cure.

Lateral Cricoarytenoid Muscle: An intrinsic laryngeal muscle that serves to adduct the vocal folds.

Lateral Fixation: Immobility of the vocal fold to move to the side.

Lateralization Thyroplasty: Manipulation of the larynx so the vocal folds lie farther apart.

Laterally: Away from midline.

Lee Silverman Voice Treatment: A programmatic treatment for the rehabilitation of voice disorders associated with Parkinson's disease.

Lesion: Any localized, abnormal structural change in the body.

Leukoplakia: Benign growth of thick whitish patches which may be found on the vocal folds; considered to be a precursor of cancer.

Lexapro: Is an antidepressant in a group of drugs called selective serotonin reuptake inhibitors.

Loft Register: Falsetto voice.

Lombard Effect: An adjustment in vocal loudness when in the presence of environmental noise.

Long-Term Average Spectrum: Analysis that allows the generation of a fast Fourier transform generated spectrum.

Lopressor: A thiazide diuretic (water pill) that helps prevent your body from absorbing too much salt, which can cause fluid retention.

Lotensin: Is used to treat high blood pressure (hypertension).

Loudness: Perceptual correlate of intensity.

Low Esophageal Pressure: Decreased pressure within the esophagus or at its sphincters that results in the backflow of stomach fluids into the esophagus and/or larynx.

Low Pitch: Perceptual correlate of a low fundamental frequency.

Lower Esophageal Sphincter: The "gate" where the esophagus connects to the stomach.

Lupus: Any of several inflammatory diseases characterized by skin lesions.

Luvox: An antidepressant in a group of drugs called selective serotonin reuptake inhibitors.

Lymph Nodes: The connection and repository sites of the lymphatic system, the system of tissue drainage within the body; it is often the method of cancer spread.

Lymphadenopathy: A disease affecting the lymph nodes.

Magnesium Salicylate: Magnesium salicylate is a nonsteroidal anti-inflammatory drug in a group of drugs called salicylates. This medicine works by reducing substances in the body that cause pain, fever, and inflammation.

Maligant: Cancerous; having abnormal cells that cause cancer.

Malinger: To feign illness or disability, especially to avoid work, obtain compensation, or arouse sympathy.

Malocclusion: Any deviation from normal occlusion.

MAO (Monoamine Oxidase.): Medicines that relieve certain types of mental depression.

Mastication: The act of chewing food in preparation for swallowing and digestion.

Maximum Flow Declination Rate: A measure made from the inverse filtered airflow waveform that relates to the speed of vocal fold adduction.

Maximum Phonation Duration: Greatest amount of time a sound can be sustained after inhaling as much air as possible.

Medialization Laryngoplasty: Surgery that brings the vocal fold together to improve vocal fold vibration during sound production.

Medialization Thyroplasty: A surgical procedure used to medlialize the vocal folds.

Medially: Toward midline.

Metabolism: The sum of the physical and chemical processes in an organism by which its material substance is produced, maintained, and destroyed, and by which energy is made available.

Metastasis: The transfer of disease to another part of the body.

Metastasize: The spreading of cancer beyond its original location.

Metoclopramide: Metoclopramide (INN) is an antiemetic and gastroprokinetic agent. Thus, it is primarily used to treat nausea and vomiting.

Microlaryngoscopy: Examination of the larynx with a scope with special magnification capability.

Microspheres: A microscopic globule of radio-labeled material.

Mitochondria: Subcellular structures found in cells that contain aerobic metabolism.

Modal Register: Most common vocal pitch.

Monotone: Constant fundamental frequency, an unvaried tone.

Motor Signals: Nerve signals that trigger muscle movement.

MPT: Abbreviation for maximum phonation time.

MRI: Abbreviation for magnetic resonance imagine.

Mucolytic Agent: Substance that helps to dissolve mucus in the airway.

Mucolytics: Capable of dissolving, digesting, or liquifying mucus.

Mucosal: Lining, such as that which covers the larynx.

Mucomyst: Acetylcysteine is a mucolytic drug that breaks down mucus, the substance that lubricates many parts of the body such as the mouth, throat, and lungs.

Mucosal Wave: Movement of the vocal fold cover in lateral, longitudinal, and vertical waveform motion.

Multifactorial Etiology: Multiple causes of a disorder.

Multifactorial Voice Disorders: Voice disorders resulting from more than one cause.

Muscle Tension Dysphonia: Abnormal-sounding voice due to loss of normal muscle coordination or inappropriate muscle contraction.

Myasthenia Gravis: Disease of impaired transmission of motor nerve impulses, characterized by episodic muscle weakness and easy fatigability, esp. of the face, tongue, neck, and respiratory muscles: caused by autoimmune destruction of acetylcholine receptors.

Myoelastic Aerodynamic Theory of Voice Production: Theory that the vocal folds are subject to well established aerodynamic principles and are set into vibration by the subglottal pressure and that the frequency of vibration is dependent upon their length in relation to their tension and mass. These factors are primarily regulated by the interplay of the intrinsic laryngeal muscles.

Nasal Coupling: Condition in which the velum is lowered to allow air to pass directly through the nose.

Nasopharynx: Space joining the throat and nasal cavity.

Nerve Transposition: Taking nerve and muscle from another part of the body and grafting the new nerve into the paralyzed muscle.

Neurolaryngologist: Laryngologist who specializes in the neurologic cause of voice disorders, including nonlarynx disease.

Neurological Voice Disorders: Voice problems caused by abnormal control, coordination, or strength of voice box muscles due to an underlying neurological disease such as stroke, Parkinson's disease, multiple sclerosis, myasthenia gravis, Lou Gehrig's disease, or ALS.

Neurologist: A physician who specializes in conditions of the brain.

Neutralize: In the case of acids, it means to balance and reduce.

Nexium: Nexium decreases the amount of acid produced in the stomach. Nexium is used to treat symptoms of gastroesophageal reflux disease.

Nissen Fundoplicaion: This surgery tightens the lower food pipe sphincter so that it can perform better as a barrier to stomach fluid backflow.

Nodule: A small, rounded mass or lump.

Noise: Aperiodic or random distribution of acoustical energy.

Noy: Unit for a subjective measusre of perceived noisiness indicated in terms of how loud a sound appears to a listener.

NuvaRing: NuvaRing contains ethinyl estradiol and etonogestrel, a combination of female hormones that prevent ovulation (the release of an egg from an ovary).

Objective: Impartial, unbiased, measureable.

Oblique Arytenoid Muscles: Intrinsic laryngeal muscle that adducts the vocal folds when contracted.

Oblique Line: Line that, meeting or tending to meet another, makes oblique angles with it.

Occlusion: Closure or blockage of a blood vessel.

Omohyoid Muscles: Extrinsic laryngeal muscle, depresses the larynx when contracted.

Oral Cavity: The part of the mouth behind the teeth and gums that is bounded above by the hard and soft palates and below by the tongue and the mucous membrane connecting it with the inner part of the mandible.

Oral Pressure: Pressure measured within the mouth.

Oral Resonance: Vibration of the tissues within the oropharynx.

Ordinal Scale: Measurement scale where there is no fixed difference between the values.

Organic: Relating to an organ or structure.

Oropharynx: The part of the pharynx between the soft palate and the upper edge of the epiglottis; the pharynx as distinguished from the nasopharynx and laryngeal pharynx.

Oscillation: Repeated and regularly fluctuating movement above and below some mean value.

Oscillogram: Graph traced by an oscillograph.

Ossification: Act or process of becoming a bony formation.

Odynophagia: Pain on swallowing.

Odynophonia: Pain on speaking.

Otalgia: Pain originating elsewhere that is felt in the ear.

Otolaryngologist: An ear, nose, and throat physician specialist.

Otology: Study of disorders of the ear and related structures.

Oxidative Phosphorylation: Process in the respiratory chain that synthesizes ATP during the transfer of electrons to molecular oxygen.

Pachyderma: Thickening of the tissue in between the vocal folds at the back of the larynx.

Palliative: Relieving pain or alleviating a problem without dealing with the underlying cause.

Palpation: Method of examination in which the examiner feels the size or shape or firmness or location of something.

Pancreatic: Of or involving the pancreas; "pancreatic cancer."

Papilloma: Wartlike growth caused by the human pailloma virus (HPV).

Paradoxical Vocal Cord Disorder (VCD): Inappropriate and uncontrollable movement of the vocal folds; vocal folds adduct (instead of abduct) on inspiration; vocal fold abduct (instead of adduct) on phonation.

Paralysis: Complete loss of nerve input to a muscle, resulting in complete loss of muscle function.

Paramedian: Slightly lateral of midline; slightly abducted position.

Paresis: Partial paralysis; partial loss of nerve input to a muscle, resulting in muscle weakness.

Partial Glossectomy: Surgical resection of a portion of the tongue.

Partial Laryngectomy: Surgery to remove part of the larynx while attempting to keep voice production.

Pathologist: Physician who examines tissue and cells (e.g., from biopsies), often using a microscope, to determine complete diagnosis.

Pathology Analysis: Examination of tissue and cells to determine full diagnosis, often completed using a microscope.

Paxil: An antidepressant belonging to a group of drugs called selective serotonin reuptake inhibitors.

Pedunculated: Wartlike tumor with a slim stalk.

Perception: What is perceived or conceptualized.

Periactin: An antihistamine (trade name Peiactin) used to treat some allergic reactions.

Perichondrium: Fibrous connective tissue membrane of cartilage.

Periodicity: (1) regularity of the timing of successive cycles; (2) quality of recurring at regular intervals.

Peristalsis: Esophageal muscle contractions that move food into the gastrointestinal tract.

Perturbation: (1) Disturbance in the regularity of the waveform that often times correlates to perceived roughness or harshness; (2) measures of variability or instability in a quasi-periodic waveform.

Pesin: Stomach enzyme.

pH Levels: Acid levels.

Pharmacokinetics: The process by which a drug is absorbed, distributed, metabolized, and eliminated by the body.

Pharyngeal Constrictor Myotomy: Surgical incision to divide or release muscular fibers of the pharyngeal complex.

Pharyngoesophageal Tract: Throat (pharynx) + food pipe (esophagus).

Phase Closure: Ratio of open-to-close phase of the glottis during one full vibratory cycle. Rated from videostroboscopy.

Phase Symmetry: Rating completed during videostroboscopy of whether the right and left vocal folds are moving symmetrically during phonation.

Phenytion: Phenytoin is an anti-epileptic drug, also called an anticonvulsant. It works by slowing down impulses in the brain that cause seizures.

Phonation: Sound production/voice production.

Phonation Threshold Pressure: (1) Minimal amount of subglottal pressure needed to initiate vocal fold vibration; (2) minimal pressure needed to set the vocal folds into oscillation, considering variables of tissue damping, mucosal wave, vocal fold thickness, prephonatory glottal width, and transglottal pressure.

Phonetogram: Graphical representation of frequency and intensity contours.

Phonomicrosurgery: Highly specialized surgery to improve voice (phonosurgery) using microsurgical techniques and highly magnified views (microsurgery) to provide microscopic detail.

Phonosurgery: Surgery to improve or maintain voice.

Phonotrauma: Trauma to the larynx caused by (sometimes abusive) vocal usage.

Physiology: Science and study of the function of living beings.

Pitch: Perceived frequency of sound production (high or low).

Pitch Breaks: An interruption in the frequency of vibration.

Pitch Detection Algorithm (PDA): Mathematical equation designed to detect the fundamental frequency of a speech waveform. Several methods are used commonly: zero-crossing, peak-picking, and waveform matching with autocorrelation.

Pitch Period: Length of time it takes for one cycle of vocal fold vibration. The pitch period is the reciprocal of fundamental frequency ($T = 1/F$).

Placebo: Substance having no pharmacological effect but given merely to satisfy a patient who supposes it to be a medicine. Not the active preparation.

Platelet: A small colorless disk-shaped cell fragment without a nucleus, found in large numbers in blood and involved in clotting.

Pneumotachograph: Differential pressure-sensing device that measures the drop in pressure when airflow passes across a known mechanical resistance (e.g., wire-mesh screen).

Polycondritis: Degenerative disease characterized by recurrent inflammation of the cartilage in the body.

Polyp: Projecting growth from a mucous surface.

Polypoid Corditis: Another term for Reinke's edema.

Positron Emission Tomography: Test that can help assess internal organ function by measuring electric changes.

Postcricoid Space: The space behind the cricoid cartilage.

Posterior: From the back.

Posterior Cricoaytenoid Muscle: An intrinsic laryngeal muscle that when contracted abducts the vocal folds.

Posterior Laryngitis: Inflammation of the back of the larynx.

Postnasal Drip: Feeling of a drip in the back of the throat.

Pre-epiglottic Space: Space in front of the epiglottis.

Pregabalin: Pregabalin is an anti-epileptic drug, also called an anticonvulsant. It works by slowing down impulses in the brain that cause seizures.

Premphase: Treatment of moderate to severe vasomotor symptoms due to menopause treatment of moderate to severe vulvar and vaginal atrophy due to menopause.

Prempro: Prempro (conjugated estrogens and medroxyprogesterone) is used to treat the symptoms of menopause such as hot flashes and vaginal dryness.

Presbylarynx: Age-related changes to laryngeal structure and function.

Presbyphonia : Age related dysphonia.

Pressure: Force per unit area.

Prilosec: Prilosec is used to treat symptoms of gastroesophageal reflux disease (GERD) and other conditions caused by excess stomach acid.

Primary Tumor: First tumor in development; the original site of a spreading cancer.

Professional Voice: Use and need of the voice for a paid occupation.

Progesterone: A steroid hormone released by the corpus luteum that stimulates the uterus to prepare for pregnancy.

Progressive Relaxation: Technique for teaching an awareness of the state of tension in muscle groups throughout the body and an ability to bring about decreased tension when under stress sometimes used in stuttering and voice therapy.

Prosody: Variation in stress, pitch, and rhythm of speech.

Proton-Pump Inhibitors: Stomach acid reducers.

Proximal: Toward the center of the body.

Prozac: Used to treat major depressive disorder, bulimia, obsessive-compulsive disorder, and panic disorder.

Prutitus: Itching.

Pseudobulbar Palsy: Motor neuron disease, includes difficulty with speech, voice, and swallowing.

Pseudocysts: Appearance of a true cyst.

Psychogenic Dysphonia: An impairment of voice cause by an emotional origin.

Puberphonia: Abnormally high pitch, adolescent sounding voice that is present after puberty.

Pulse Register: Sound generation characterized by very low fundamental frequency.

Pushing Technique: Voice therapy technique used to help medialize the vocal folds during phonation**.**

Quality: Texture of a tone, dependent on its overtone content that distinguishes it from others of the same pitch and loudness.

Quantization: Division of amplitude in an analog signal into discrete numeric values. The greater

the quantization levels, the more adequately the amplitude waveform is represented.

Radiation: Process in which energy is emitted as particles or waves.

Radiofrequency Ablation: Type of radio wave surgery.

Radiographic Imaging: Tests that allow flims (pictures) of the inside of the body (e.g., x-ray, CT scan, MRI, etc.).

Rasagiline: Works by increasing the levels of certain chemicals in the brain. Rasagiline is used to treat the symptoms of Parkinson's disease.

Recurrent Laryngeal Nerve (RLN): Branch of vagus nerve to that innervates the intrinsic laryngeal muscles.

Recurrent Respiratory Papillmoatosis (RRP): Wartlike growths in the airway passages caused by the human papilloma virus.

Reflux: Backflow of stomach fluids which contain acid and enzymes.

Reflux Laryngitis: Voice disorder caused by backflow of stomach fluids to the throat and larynx; a type of supraesophageal GERD.

Reflux Precautions: Lifestyle changes that a patient follows to minimize backflow of stomach fluids (reflux) such as (but not limited to) sleeping with the head elevated, refraining from lying down after a meal, refraining from food that increase acidity in stomach fluids or refraining from foods associated with relaxation of the esophageal sphincter.

Refluxers/Upright Refluxers/Daytime Refluxers: Patients with reflux laryngitis in whom the backflow of stomach fluids occurs in the upright (sitting/standing) position; often not associated with heartburn.

Refractory: A substance that is resistant to heat.

Reinke's Edema: "Swelling in Reinke's space"; voice disorder from accumulation of gelatinous substance in Reinke's space.

Reinke's Space (Superficial Lamina Propria): Vocal fold layer right underneath the vocal fold epithelium; really not an empty space — a layer in the vocal fold composed of cells, special fibers, and substance (extracellular matrix); has key role in vocal fold vibration.

Resection: Surgical removal of a structure.

Residual Volume: Volume of gas/air remaining in the lungs after maximum expiration; the residual lung volume that cannot be expelled (1000–1500 cc).

Resistance: Loss of drug effect.

Resonance: Intensification of vocal tones; increased amplitude of vibration in the vocal tract, natural vibrating frequency of tissue.

Respiration: Act of breathing.

Respiratory Papillmatosis: Viral infection of the vocal folds that can be a precursor to cancer.

Resting Tremor: Common symptom of Parkinson's disease, involuntary movement when body part is at rest, typically the hands.

Rigid Laryngoscopy: Examination of the larynx in which a rigid telescope is used; this examination provides the clearest magnified detail of the laryngeal structures, but the patient is unable to articulate during the examination.

Rigidity: Physical property of being stiff and resisting bending; the quality of being rigid and rigorously severe.

Rotameter (flow meter): Measures airflow within a closed tube. Measurement device that relies on gravity and the physical properties of the tube to make its measurement.

S/Z Ratio: Indicator of glottal closure, and by extension an indicator of laryngeal pathology, computed by dividing the maximum phonation time for the phoneme /s/ by the maximum phonation tome for the phoneme /z/.

Sarcoidosis: Disease of unknown cause, characterized by granulomatous tubercles of the skin, lymph nodes, lungs, eyes, and other structures.

Scarring: Development of fibrotic tissue. A sign of tissue damage.

Screamer's Nodes: Term used to describe vocal fold nodules.

Sampling Rate: Number of samples per second of a digital signal. The greater the sampling rate, the more information obtained for signal processing.

Selective Laryngeal Abbuctor Denervation-Reinnervation: Operation in which nerves to two nonworking muscles that close (adduct) the vocal folds are cut (denervated) and replaced (re-innervated) with functioning nerves.

Semitone: Unit devised for comparison of frequencies (e.g., 200 hertz to 400 hertz represents a 12-semitone range). The semitone scale includes all of the notes (sharps and flats included) on the musical scale and is logarithmic. Reflects the perceptual attributes of the human ear.

Sensory Nerves: Nerves that carry signals of sensation.

Serotonin Reuptake Inhibitors: Any substance that interferes with a chemical reaction, growth, or other biologic activity.

Sessile: Wartlike tumor with no stalk.

Shimmer: Measure of the cycle-to-cycle variability in waveform amplitude.

Signal (or harmonic)-To-Noise Ratio: Mathematical ratio of periodic energy (signal) to random or aperiodic energy (noise) in a given signal.

Sjogren's Syndrome: Chronic inflammatory autoimmune disease that results in dryness of mucous membranes (especially eyes and mouth).

Smoker's Laryngitis: Another term for Reinke's edema; often associated with a history of smoking.

Sodium Salicylate: A nonsteroidal anti-inflammatory agent that is less effective than equal doses of aspirin in relieving pain and reducing fever.

Somnolence: Sleepiness: a very sleepy state.

Spasmodic Dysophonia: Neurogenic voice disorder caused by irregular and uncontrollable spasms within muscles controlling the opening and closing the vocal folds.

Spectrogram: Visual display of a speech signal across time (horizontal axis), giving information about frequency (vertical axis) and intensity (gray or color variation) in the display.

Spectrum: Plot of signal energy (intensity) by frequency at a single point in time.

Speech Disorder: Malfunction of the tongue and/or lip muscles resulting in misarticulation.

Spirometer: Flow volume measurement device (wet and dry varieties); records the total amount of air blown across a sensing device (dry) or volume of water displaced (wet) during exhalation.

Stephens-Johnson Syndrome: Severe autoimmune disorder causing erythema and inflammation of mucous membranes.

Stiffness/nonvibrating portion/adynamic segment: Commonly expressed as a percentage of the full length of the membranous portion of the vocal fold.

Stomatitis: Inflammation of the mucous membrane of the mouth.

Strained-Strangled: Perceived strain or pushed vocal quality during phonation.

Stridor: Noisy breathing, usually cause by obstruction or narrowing of the airway; stridor is a sign of difficulty passing air—any breathing difficulty needs immediate medical attention.

Stripping: A "radical" surgical procedure that removes ("strips") the top layers of vocal folds resulting in severe vocal fold scarring and abnormal voice; due to the resultant damage, this procedure is currently rarely used.

Stroboscopy: Examination in which a strobe light is combined with a rigid or flexible laryngoscopy to produce a slow-motionlike view of vocal fold vibration.

Stroke: Condition in the brain cause by too little or too much blood supply, resulting in poor function of the parts of the body controlled by the affected areas of the brain.

Squamous Cell Cercinoma: Cancer composed of a certain type of cell called squamous cells, usually found in lining cells.

Subcutaneous: Located, found, or placed just beneath the skin; hypodermic.

Subglottal Pressure: Lung pressures below the glottis, when the vocal folds are adducted. Subglottic pressure: estimated clinically using intraoral pressure peaks produced during an unvoiced plosive consonant; a measure of the tracheal (respiratory) driving pressure used during phonation.

Subglottic Larynx: Below the glottis.

Subglottic Stenosis: Narrowing below the vocal folds.

Subglottic Tumor: Tumor below the glottis.

Subglottis: Below the glottis (area of the vocal folds).

Subharmonic: Oscillation that has a frequency that is an integral submultiple of the frequency of a related oscillation.

Sulcus: Long, narrow, shallow furrow or groove, as on the surface of the brain bordering the gyri or in the oral cavity.

Superficial Lamina Propria: Top layer of the lamina propria that plays a key role in vocal fold vibration; loosely structured; located just underneath the cell lining (epithelium) covering the vocal folds.

Superior Laryngeal Artery: Provides blood supply to the larynx and mucous membranes of the larynx.

Superior Laryngeal Nerve (SLN): Branch of vagus nerve to cricothyroid muscle involved in control of pitch.

Supraglottic Larynx: Above the glottis.

Supraglottic Tumor: Tumor in the larynx above the glottis.

Supraglottis: Above the glottis (area of the vocal folds).

Surgical Excision/Surgical Resection: Removal through a surgical procedure.

Symmetry: Extent to which the left and right vocal folds appear to move as mirror images.

Syncope: Temporary loss of consciousness caused by a fall in blood pressure.

Talbolt's Law: Persistence of vision on the retina; the human retina cannot perceive more than five separate images per second (each image "rests" 0.2 seconds on the retina) and, when presented in succession, are fused into one apparent continuous image. Thus, a series of still images presented at this rate (or faster) will be perceived visually as a connected, moving image.

Teflon: (1) Ineffective polymer used as an injectable for vocal fold medialization procedures; (2) polymer used as an injectable for vocal fold medialization procedures; seldom used.

Thyroarytenoid: Relating to the thyroid and arytenoid cartilages.

Thyroarytenoid (TA) Muscle: Muscle within the vocal fold.

Thyroid Cartilage: Largest cartilage in the larynx. Fused thyroid plates form thyroid notch (Adam's apple).

Thryoid Gland: Major hormone regulator of the body located in the neck area.

Thyroplasty: Surgical procedure in which a silicone wedge is placed in the thyroid cartilage to "push" the vocal fold into midline.

Tidal Volume: Pulmonary term which measures air volume per breath; also know as resting volume, usually measured as 500 cc.

Timbre: Hoarseness, harsh voice, abnormal voice quality due to abnormal vocal fold vibration.

TNM Staging: T, tumor type; N, lymph nodes involved; M, metastasis or spread to other body parts.

Tobacco: Leaves of the tobacco plant smoked or ingested.

Topical Anesthesia: Substance applied to the surface to decrease sensation, such as sensation to pain.

Toprol-XL: Metoprolol is in a group of drugs called beta-blockers. Beta-blockers affect the heart and circulation (blood flow through arteries and veins).

Total Glossectomy: Complete surgical resection of the tongue.

Trachea: Windpipe; connects lungs to larynx.

Tracheomalacia: Collapse of the walls of the trachea caused by soft or weakened cartilage.

Tracheostomy: Breathing tube placed directly into the trachea, below the area of the larynx.

Transcutaneous Approach: Entering through the skin; can refer to drug administered.

Transducer: Device that converts energy from on form to another, for example, flow or pressure into an electric signal.

Transoral Laryngoscopy: Viewing of the larynx through the mouth using a specialized instrument called a laryngoscope.

Trauma: Body wound or shock produced by sudden physical injury.

Treatment: An act or manner of rehabilitation.

Tremor: Involuntary movement of the body or limbs, as from disease, fear, weakness, or excitement.

Trill: To sing or play with a vibratory effect.

Trismus: Spasm of the muscles associated with mastication.

Truvada: Emtricitabine and tenofovir are antiviral drugs that work by preventing HIV (human immunodeficiency virus) cells from multiplying in the body.

Tumor: An abnormal, circumscribed growth of cells in any animal or plant tissue.

Tyramine: A colorless crystalline amine found in mistletoe, putrefied animal tissue, certain cheeses, and ergot, or produced synthetically.

UES: Acronym for upper esophageal sphincter, the muscular "gate" within the esophagus located below there the throat (pharynx) separates into respiratory and digestive pathways.

Ulcer: A lesion of the skin or mucous membrane such as stomach lining that is accompanied by formation of pus and necrosis of surrounding tissue, usually from inflammation or ischemia.

Ulceration: Development of an ulcer.

Ultrahigh speed photography: Technique used for visualing vocal fold movement in real time. Frame speed is up to 4000 frames/sec.

Ultrasound: Sound with a frequency greater than 20,000 Hz, approximately the upper limit of human hearing; the application of ultrasonic waves to therapy or diagnostics, as in deep-heat treatment of a joint or imaging of internal structures.

Unilateral: Exists on one side.

Upper Respiratory Infection: An infection of the breathing tract above the lungs (e.g., the common cold and cough).

Upstanding: Classification of a cancer to a higher level (more serious) based on pathology analysis of removed tumor.

U-tube manometer: Pressure measurement device; a bent glass tube with external measurement index, filled with liquid (usually water of mercury).

Vagus Nerve: Cranial nerve X, projecting from the medulla of the brainstem; branches serve to innervate innervation to the larynx.

Valsalva Manuver: Forceful expiration against a closed glottis.

Varix: Permanent abnormal dilation and lengthening of a vein.

Vascularity: The state of blood vessel development and functioning in an organ or tissue.

Ventricle: Space; a cavity.

Ventricular Fold: Tissue that lies above and lateral to the true vocal folds; also called false vocal folds.

Ventricularis: Space, or "ventrical," between the true vocal folds and false vocal folds.

Verrucous Carcinoma: Cancer associated with verrucous vulgaris.

Verrucous Vulgaris: Warty, lobulated lesion caused by HPV, can be a precursor to cancer.

Vibration Cycle: Rapid opening and closing of the vocal fold occurring approximately 100 to 400 times per second depending on age and sex of the individual producing the sound production.

Vidal Capacity: The total volume of air that can expired after maximal inhalation (3500–5000 cc for normal healthy males); VC is affected by height, weight, and age.

Videoendoscopy: Unternal view of the body aided by video recording.

Videokymography: Technique designed for direct observation of vocal fold movement allowing high-speed scanning up to 8000 frames/sec.

Visi-Pitch: Clinical instrumentation tool allowing visualization of fundamental frequency and relative intensity in real time on a computer display.

Visual Analog Scale: Testing technique for measuring subjective or behavioral phenomena in which a subject selects from a gradient of arranged in linear fashion.

Vocal Abuse: Normal vocal behaviors used in excess, leading to vocal fold injury (e.g., excessive loudness or cough).

Vocal Cords: Anatomically less-precise term, laymen's term, for vocal folds.

Vocal Fatigue: Voice tiring; reported complaint of "tired talking," the need to use increased effort to talk, especially after a period of prolonged voice use.

Vocal Fold Atypia: Noncancerous, but irregular cells in vocal fold epithelium; often leads to cancer; often recurs after removal.

Vocal Fold Cyst: Firm mass of material contained within the sac, usually on only one vocal fold.

Vocal Fold Early Cancer: Cancer of vocal fold epithelium that is confined to the vocal folds and has not spread.

Vocal Fold Edema: Swelling of the vocal folds.

Vocal Fold Epithelium: Top cell layer of the vocal fold; surface lining of vocal folds composed of squamous cells.

Vocal Fold Granuloma: Pale, sometimes red, mass on vocal folds resulting from irritation; contains inflammatory cells ad new blood vessels; usually found over arytenoids cartilages at the site of contact during coal fold closure.

Vocal Fold Immobility: Absence of vocal fold movement.

Vocal Fold Lesions: Refers to vocal nodules, vocal polyps, and vocal cysts.

Vocal Fold Paralysis: No movement of the vocal fold.

Vocal Fold Paresis: Abnormally limited movement of the vocal fold.

Vocal Fold Phonomicrosurgery: Special skilled surgery of the vocal folds using endoscopic tools called microlaryngeal instruments, and techniques to enable maximum preservation of the vocal fold structure.

Vocal Fold Polyp: Lesion usually seen on only one vocal fold; characteristically red due to increased blood vessel supply or blood within lump.

Vocal Folds: Either of two pairs of folds of muscularized mucous membrane projecting into the larynx and used for sound production.

Vocal Fold Trauma: Injury to the vocal fold.

Vocal Hygiene: Program of vocal health, usually introduced in voice therapy, that uses strategies to preserve vocal fold tissue and normal vibratory characteristics of the vocal folds.

Vocal Hyperfunction: Results from an overuse of the vocal fold muscles, causing excessive adductory force.

Vocal Ligament: Band that extends on either side from the thyroid cartilage to the vocal process of the arytenoids' cartilage.

Vocal Misuse: Abnormal vocal behaviors that cause stress or injury to the vocal folds (e.g., excess tension while speaking).

Vocal Overuse: Normal voice behavior that "takes is toll" with time (e.g., singer after many years of performing).

Vocal Pedagogy: Training or teaching voice mechanisms.

Vocal Range: Spectrum of "voice pitch" and vocal loudness from low pitch to high pitch and low loudness to high loudness.

Vocal Tract: Cavity above the vocal folds including the pharyngeal, oral, and nasal cavities that cha shape the sound source vibration into distinctive speech sounds by modifying the movement and placement of the articulators.

Vocal Tract Articulators: Tongue, lips, and palate and other oral and laryngeal structures that help make voice sound precise and controllable.

Vocalis Muscle: Belly of the thyroarytenoid muscle, comprises the vibrating edge of the vocal fold.

Vocalization: To produce with the voice.

Voice Handicap Index: Tool that is used to help voice patients identify the amount of disability a voice disorder creates for them. Divided into physical, social, and emotional categories.

Voice Onset Time: Time from when a consonant is released and voicing begins.

Voice Pathophysiology: Impact and cause of voice disorders on voice function.

Voice Range Profile: See Phontetogram.

Voice Surgeon: Laryngologist specializing in laryngeal surgery.

Volume: Term used for describing the loudness of the voice, also used a measurement for defining the space taken up by an object.

VRQOL: Voice-Related Quality of Life. An index used to define the impact of a voice disorder on the quality of life.

Warm-Wire Anemometer: Flow measurement device; as airflow passes over (and cools) the warm metal wire, its electrical resistance changes, and flow magnitude can be predicted from the change in resistance of the wire.

Webbing: The formulation of scar tissue between the vocal folds.

Whisper: Complete breathiness; increased airflow through slightly abducted vocal folds.

Wilson's Disease: Disease caused by abnormal metabolism of copper, causing increased blood levels of copper and copper metabolites.

Wound: An injury, usually involving division of tissue or rupture of the mucous membrane, due to external violence or some mechanical agent rather than disease.

Xerostomia: medical term for "dry mouth."

Yawn-Sigh: Voice therapy technique; the patient is instructed to simulate a real yawn and is the process is completed with a sigh.

Zithromax: Zithromax (azithromycin) treats infections caused by bacteria, such as respiratory infections, skin infections, and ear infections.

Zoloft: An antidepressant in a group of drugs called selective serotonin reuptake inhibitors (SSRIs). Zoloft affects chemicals in the brain that may become unbalanced and cause depression, panic, anxiety, or obsessive-compulsive symptoms.

References

Dictionary.com. (2008). Retrieved from Dictionary.com Web site: http://dictionary.reference.com/

Keith , S. G., & Carole, S. M. (1995). *Vocal exercise physiology*. San Diego, CA: Singular.

Nicolosi, L., Harryman, E., & Krescheck, J. (1989). *Terminology of communication disorders in speech-language-hearing* (3rd ed.). Baltimore, MD: Williams & Wilkins.

Schwartz, S. K. (2004). *The source for voice disorders: Adolescent and adult.* East Moline, IL: LinguiSystems.

Stemple, J. C., Glaze, L. E., & Klaben, B. G. (2000). *Clinical voice pathology: Theory and management* (3rd ed.). San Diego, CA: Singular.

Voiceproblem.org. (2008). Retrieved from The Voice Problem Web site: http://www.voice-problem.org

Zemlin, W. R. (1998). *Speech and hearing science: Anatomy and physiology.* (4th ed.). Needham Heights, MA: Allyn and Bacon.

Index

Page numbers in **bold** indicate references to figures.